OBSTETRICS BY TEN TEACHERS

OBSTETRICS BY TEN TEACHERS
17th edition

Edited by

Stuart Campbell DSc (Lond), FRCP (Ed), FRCOG, FACOG
Professor of Obstetrics & Gynaecology
St George's Hospital Medical School, London, UK

Christoph Lees BSc, MRCOG
Consultant in Obstetrics & Maternofetal Medicine
Rosie Maternity Hospital, Addenbrooke's NHS Trust, Cambridge, UK

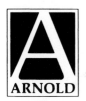

A member of the Hodder Headline Group
LONDON
Co-published in the USA by Oxford University Press Inc., New York

First published in Great Britain 1917 as *Midwifery*
Eleventh edition published 1966 as *Obstetrics*
Seventeenth edition published in 2000 by
Arnold, a member of the Hodder Headline Group,
338 Euston Road, London NW1 3BH
http://www.arnoldpublishers.com

Co-published in the United States of America by Oxford University Press Inc.,
198 Madison Avenue, New York, NY10016
Oxford is a registered trademark of Oxford University Press

Whilst the advice and information in this book are believed to be true and accurate at the
date of going to press, neither the authors nor the publisher can accept any legal responsibility or liability for any errors or omissions that may be made. In particular (but without limiting the generality of the preceding disclaimer) every effort has been made to
check drug dosages; however it is still possible that errors have been missed. Furthermore,
dosage schedules are constantly being revised and new side effects recognized. For these
reasons the reader is strongly urged to consult the drug companies' printed instructions
before administering any of the drugs recommended in this book.

British Library Cataloguing in Publication Data
A catalogue record for this book is available from the British Library

Library of Congress Cataloging-in-Publication Data
A catalog record for this book is available from the Library of Congress

ISBN 0 340 71986 9 (pb)
ISBN 0 340 74082 5 (pb, International Students' Edition)

2 3 4 5 6 7 8 9 10

Commissioning Editor: Fiona Goodgame, Aileen Parlane
Project Editor: Catherine Barnes
Production Editor: James Rabson
Production Controller: Iain McWilliams
Copy-editor & page layout: Jane Tozer
Illustrators: Sue Tyler and Kate Nardoni
Cover design: Terry Griffiths

Typeset in 9.5 pt Minion
Printed and bound in India by Ajanta Offset and Packaging Ltd, New Delhi

What do you think about this book? Or any other Arnold title?
Please send your comments to feedback.arnold@hodder.co.uk

Contents

List of contributors

Stuart Campbell DSc (Lond) FRCP (Ed) FRCOG, FACOG (Hon)
Professor of Obstetrics & Gynaecology
St George's Hospital Medical School
London

James Drife MD FRCP (ed) FRCSEd FRCOG
Professor of Obstetrics & Gynaecology
Academic Unit of Paediatrics & Obstetrics & Gynaecology
University of Leeds

William Dunlop PhD HBCRB FRCSEd FRCOG
Head of School of Surgical & Reproductive Sciences
University of Newcastle

Dr Jason Gardosi MD MBBS FRCSE MRCOG
Director of West Midlands Perinatal Institute
Birmingham

Donald Gibb MD MRCP FRCOG
Independent Consultant
Hospital of St John and St Elizabeth
London

JG Grudzinskas BSc MD FRACOG FRCOG
Professor of Obstetrics and Gynaecology
Department of Obstetrics and Gynaecology
St Bartholomew's and The Royal London School of Medicine & Dentistry
London

Kevin Harrington MD MRCP1 DCH MRCOG
Consultant & Senior Lecturer
Academic Dept. of Obstetrics and Gynaecology
St Bartholomew's and The Royal London School of
   Medicine & Dentistry
The Homerton Hospital
London

Phillip Hay MBBS FRCP
Senior Lecturer in Genitourinary Medicine, St George's
Hospital Medical School
London

Des Holden PhD MRCOG
Consultant Obstetrician & Gynaecologist
Royal Sussex County Hospital
Brighton, Sussex

Richard Johanson MA BSc MD MRCOG
Consultant Obstetrician and Gynaecologist
Senior Lecturer in Perinatology
North Staffordshire Hospital and Keele University

Christoph Lees BSc MRCOG
Consultant in Obstetrics & Maternofetal Medicine
Rosie Maternity Hospital, Addenbrooke's NHS Trust,
Cambridge

Kypros Nicolaides BSc MRCOG
Professor of Obstetrics & Gynaecology
and Director, Harris Birthright Unit,
King's College Hospital, London

Margaret R Oates DPM FRCPsych
Senior Lecturer in Psychiatry
University of Nottingham
Hon Consultant Nottingham Health Care Trust
Nottingham

Janet M Rennie MA MD FRCP FRCPCH DCH
Consultant in Neonatal Medicine
King's College Hospital
London

Michael Robson FRCS MRCOG
Consultant Gynaecologist & Obstetrician
South Buckinghamshire NHS Trust
Wycombe Hospital
Buckinghamshire

Neil Sebire MBBS MD
Research Fellow
Harris Birthright Unit
King's College Hospital
London

Abdul H Sultan MD MRCOG
Consultant Obstetrician & Gynaecologist
Mayday University Hospital
Surrey

E Malcolm Symonds MB.BS(Adel) MD FRCOG FFPHM
FACOG(Hon) FRANZCOG(Hon)
Professor Emeritus
Faculty of Medicine and Health Sciences
University of Nottingham

Basky Thilaganathan MD MRCOG
Director, Fetal Medicine Unit
St George's Hospital Medical School
London

J Guy Thorpe-Beeston MA MD MRCOG
Consultant Obstetrician
Chelsea & Westminster Hospital
London

Preface

Obstetrics by Ten Teachers is the oldest and most respected English language textbook on this subject and it is an awesome responsibility to ensure its continuing success. The fundamental changes occurring in obstetrics are such that we felt that only a complete rewrite by a new team of contributors would suffice. Not only that, but we have broken with some of the traditions as well. For example, although we have kept the title, you will see that we have now many more than ten teachers contributing to this volume, which reflects the increasing subspecialization within our subject. So what are these fundamental changes? Before discussing these, it would be useful to outline the development of obstetrics from its origins to where we are today.

Originally our subject was called midwifery and almost all ancient historical records show that babies were delivered only by women. This was because it was deemed immodest for a female patient's genitalia to be seen by a man. In the 17th century, the male midwife started to appear, as they were frequently required to deal with obstructed labour. A key development was the invention of the obstetric forceps by the Chamberlens, a Huguenot family practising in England. The Chamberlens kept their secret for more than a century, although it is almost certain that Peter Chamberlen the Elder was the pioneer in their development. The greatest eminence in obstetrics in the 17th century was undoubtedly Francois Mauriceau, Chief of Service at the Hotel Dieu in Paris, who educated a whole generation of physicians and midwives in France and also in England through his book 'Traite des malaidies de femmes grosses…'. Interestingly, his book was translated into English by Hugh Chamberlen, son of Peter, who had unsuccessfully tried to persuade Mauriceau to adopt obstetric forceps. Chamberlen's visit to Paris turned into disaster when Mauriceau mischievously challenged him to deliver a woman in obstructed labour due to a small rachitic pelvis. Chamberlen failed dismally, but the money he earned from the translation of Mauriceau's book was some consolation.

Perhaps the most important figure in the development of obstetrics as a science was William Smellie, a Scottish doctor practising in the poorer parts of London, who described the modern concept of the mechanism of labour in his 'Treatise on the Theory and Practice of Midwifery', published in 1752 and through his knowledge of this mechanism and the diameters of the pelvis and fetal head, described the safer delivery of the baby in obstructed labour. Smellie was a great teacher of both midwives and physicians and over a ten-year period personally trained 900 students in the management of over 1000 labours. Part of the secret of his popularity was that he donated part of the student fee to the mother. Through his influence, the male midwife or obstetrician

was central to the development of obstetric care up to the present day. One of Smellie's pupils was William Hunter, a fellow Scot, who opened the first anatomy school in London and pioneered many advances in obstetric anatomy, including the proof that the uterine and fetal circulations in the placenta were separate. Hunter became the first society obstetrician and delivered 12 of Queen Charlotte's 16 children. He will, however, be remembered as a scientist and as an influential obstetrician who fought against the interventionist practices of the time in obstetrics, such as the routine manual removal of the placenta and the ill-considered use of the obstetric forceps.

During the late 18th and early 19th centuries, great strides were made in the prevention of maternal infection, especially puerperal fever. Ignac Semmelweis of Vienna was the first to prove the contagious nature of puerperal fever and to demonstrate how it could be prevented. Semmelweis identified a three-fold increase in maternal mortality in women delivered by doctors and medical students compared to those delivered by midwives. In carefully documented research he made the important connection that students, who worked in the postmortem room and went straight from there to the labour ward, transferred the 'putrid particles' that caused puerperal fever to the mothers. In 1847 Semmelweis instructed his students to wash their hands after scrubbing them with a solution of chloride of lime, which resulted in a dramatic fall in maternal mortality in his ward from 11.4 to 1.2 per cent within two years. Semmelweis is a particularly tragic figure, whose impressive research was rejected by senior obstetricians in the first clinic in Vienna and his subsequent dismissal and insanity have become the stuff of legend. Semmelweis to some extent contributed to his fate by his inarticulacy, his impenetrable prose and his paranoia. Nevertheless, through his influence, the adoption of aseptic and antiseptic techniques led to a dramatic fall in maternal deaths from infection throughout the remainder of the 19th century.

Another 19th century preoccupation was the relief of pain in labour, which in those days was frequently protracted over days and could end in an excruciatingly painful instrumental delivery or Caesarean Section. James Young Simpson, Professor of Midwifery at Edinburgh University, was the first to use ether anaesthesia in labour, and shortly afterwards in 1848, introduced chloroform, which was simpler to administer. Simpson was a brilliant and innovative obstetrician and his discovery of chloroform was through self-experimentation during evening sessions at his home when he and his junior assistants would inhale various substances to find the ideal anaesthetic. Simpson had to overcome much criticism from those who believed pain to be a purifying experience and it was not until Queen

Victoria had chloroform administered for the birth of her eighth child, Prince Leopold, in 1853, that Simpson's work was fully vindicated.

Chloroform also featured in the revolutionary method of treating eclampsia, introduced in 1900 by Vasili Stroganoff, a Russian obstetrician. Next to infection, eclampsia was the leading cause of maternal mortality in the 19th century and on average 25 per cent of women died from the condition, usually from cerebral haemorrhage and asphyxia. Stroganoff realized that the key to successful treatment of this condition lay in preventing repeated convulsions until labour supervened or was induced. In addition to a cocktail of chloroform, chloral hydrate and morphine, the patient was nursed in a quiet darkened room, and any procedures were reduced to a minimum and performed under chloroform narcosis. The Stroganoff technique was quickly adopted throughout the world with an immediate five-fold reduction in maternal mortality from eclampsia.

With the dramatic reduction in maternal mortality during the twentieth century, especially following the introduction of antibiotics and blood transfusion, attention progressively moved towards the second patient, i.e. the fetus, and means of reducing perinatal mortality and infant handicap. At the turn of the twentieth century, Adolphe Pinard in Paris and John Ballantine in Edinburgh pioneered programmes of antenatal care to improve the outcome for the fetus. Ballantine's work in particular, described in his book 'Antenatal Pathology and Hygiene: The Embryo and Foetus', presaged the development of perinatal medicine. The late 1950s and early 1960s saw the rapid introduction of techniques to evaluate fetal wellbeing with the aim of reducing perinatal mortality. The monitoring of fetal wellbeing in labour was improved by the development of the electronic fetal heart monitor by Edward Hon of Yale University, while Erich Saling of Berlin was the first to sample fetal blood directly during labour to assess fetal acid base status. The concept of treating the fetus in utero was pioneered by Albert Lily of Auckland, New Zealand, who was the first to treat fetal anaemia as a result of rhesus disease by means of antenatal fetal blood transfusion. Above all the development of ultrasound as a diagnostic technique and its application in the assessment of the fetus by Ian Donald in Glasgow in 1958 totally revolutionized our ability to evaluate fetal wellbeing prenatally. Of all the advances in modern obstetrics, Donald's stands supreme. Nowadays it would be impossible to practice safe and modern obstetrics without the ultrasound scanner, which is used to diagnose fetal abnormalities, monitor fetal growth, assess placental function and guide biopsy needles for prenatal diagnosis and therapy.

The twentieth century witnessed an increasing medicalization of obstetric care and by 1990 virtually all births were in hospital. The arguments in favour of this trend were simple and persuasive; the falling maternal and perinatal mortality rates were due to the increased surveillance and access to emergency care that only hospitals could provide. Opposition to this practice began in the 1930s with Grantley Dick-Reed, an English general practitioner, whose classic book 'Natural Childbirth' began a movement which, although rejected in England, was taken up by Fernand Lamaze in France. Dick-Reed and Lamaze believed that pregnancy and labour were physiological processes and that excessive medicalization and the hospital environment could in themselves cause complications through fear and tension. In the UK there is now a strong move to devolve antenatal care for uncomplicated pregnancies to general practitioners and Midwives in the community and to encourage home births in such cases. This formed the basic thrust of the 'Changing Childbirth' report by the expert maternity group in the early 1990s. This document also advanced the concept of the midwife as an independent practitioner taking the lead in 'normal' pregnancy whilst complicated pregnancy is dealt with by obstetricians. So the wheel has come full circle, although it is important that the gains made in reducing maternal and perinatal mortality must not be lost. The future must lie in a close collaboration between obstetrician, general practitioner and midwife to provide prospective parents with an informed choice of safe options for the delivery of their baby.

We have tried in this book to describe not only the most up-to-date evidence-based obstetric practice, but also to reflect these modern attitudes to the delivery of care to the pregnant woman and her partner, their fetus and the newborn. Also, for the first time, we have addressed some of the ethical and medicolegal dilemmas confronting obstetricians and midwives and we have tried to provide an approach to dealing with such problems. We also discuss the quality and outcomes of the service we provide which has become of pre-eminent importance. The two confidential enquiries: into maternal deaths, and stillbirths and deaths in infancy have assumed a central position in our efforts to make pregnancy and childbirth safer for mothers and babies. It is often overlooked that obstetrics was the first speciality to institute a systematic, nationwide audit of mortality through the confidential enquiry into maternal deaths first published half a century ago.

Obstetrics is perhaps the most exciting of all medical specialities; dealing with the problems of early human development and demanding knowledge of genetics, general medicine, surgery and emergency care. We hope this book will convey our continuing love for this exciting speciality and that it will enthuse a new generation of obstetricians to make pregnancy and childbirth an even safer and more fulfilling experience for parents in this new century.

STUART CAMPBELL
CHRISTOPH LEES

Acknowledgements

The editors would like to thank the following people for their contributions to this book.

Sammy Lee PhD, FIBMS, DipFertCouns(Lond)
Senior Embryologist, Portland Hospital, London

Gonzalo Moscoso MD, PhD
Senior Lecturer in Early Human Development,
St George's Hospital Medical School, London

Nicola Flack MRCOG
Fetal Medicine Specialist, Harris Birthright Unit, King's
College, London

Tim Coltart MD FRCOG FRCS
Consultant Obstetrician and Gynaecologist,
Queen Charlotte's Hospital, London

Bernard Benoir MD
Consultant Obstetrician
Ashet Hospital, Nice, France and
Princess Grace Hospital, Monaco
For the image on the front cover

Commonly-used abbreviations

AC	abdominal circumference	IVF	in vitro fertilization
ACTH	adrenocorticotrophic hormone	IVH	intraventricular haemorrhage
AF	amniotic fluid	LFTs	liver function tests
AFI	amniotic fluid index	LH	luteinizing hormone
AFP	alpha-fetoprotein	LIF	leukaemia inhibitory factor
APCR	activated protein C resistance	LMP	last menstrual period
APH	antepartum haemorrhage	LSCS	lower segment Caesarean Section
APTT	activated partial thromboplastin time	MC&S	microscopy, culture and sensitivities
ARM	artificial rupture of membranes	MCV	mean corpuscular volume
BPD	biparietal diameter	MRI	magnetic resonance imaging
CDH	congenital diaphragmatic hernia	MROP	manual removal of placenta
CMV	cytomegalovirus	MSU	midstream specimen of urine
CPD	cephalo-pelvic disproportion	NAD	nothing abnormal detected
CRH	corticotrophin-releasing hormone	NEC	necrotizing enterocolitis
CRL	crown–rump length	NIDDM	non-insulin-dependent diabetes mellitus
CSF	cerebrospinal fluid	NND	neonatal death
CT	computerized tomography	NNU	neonatal unit
CTG	cardiotocograph	NTD	neural tube defect
CVA	cerebrovascular accident	OA	occipito-anterior
CVS	chorion villus sampling	OFD	occipito-frontal diameter
DIC	disseminated intravascular coagulation	OP	occipito-posterior
DVT	deep vein thrombosis	OT	occipito-transverse
ECG	electrocardiograph	P	para
ECV	external cephalic version	PCA	patient-controlled anaesthesia
EDD	estimated date of delivery	PCR	polymerase chain reaction
EEG	electroencephalogram	PE	pulmonary embolus
EFW	estimated fetal weight	PET	pre-eclamptic toxaemia
ERPC	evacuation of retained products of conception	PI	pulsatility index
ESR	erythrocyte sedimentation rate	PIH	pregnancy-induced hypertension
ET	embryo transfer	PMR	perinatal mortality rate
FBS	fetal blood sampling	PPH	postpartum haemorrhage
FEV_1	forced expiratory volume in one second	PPIH	proteinuric pregnancy-induced hypertension (pre-eclampsia)
FL	femur length		
FM	fetal movements	PPROM	preterm prelabour rupture of membranes
FSE	fetal scalp electrode	Rh	Rhesus
FTA	fluorescent treponemal antibody test	RI	resistance index
G	gravida	SCBU	special care baby unit
GnRH	gonadotrophin-releasing hormone	SFH	symphysis–fundal height
GP	general practitioner	SGA	small for gestational age
GTN	glyceryl trinitrate	SLE	systemic lupus erythematosus
Hb	haemoglobin	SOL	stimulation of labour
HC	head circumference	SROM	spontaneous rupture of membranes
hCG	human chorionic gonadotrophin	STOP	suction termination of pregnancy
hGH	human growth hormone	SVD	spontaneous vaginal delivery
HIE	hypoxic ischaemic encephalopathy	TCD	trans-cerebellar diameter
HIV	human immunodeficiency virus	TOP	termination of pregnancy
hPL	human placental lactogen	TOS	trial of scar
HPV	human papillomavirus	TPHA	Treponema pallidum haemagglutination assay
HSV	herpes simplex virus	TRH	thyrotrophin-releasing hormone
HVS	high vaginal swab	TTTS	twin-to-twin transfusion syndrome
IDDM	insulin-dependent diabetes mellitus	USS	ultrasound scan
IOL	induction of labour	VDRL	venereal diseases research laboratory test
IUD	intrauterine death	VE	vaginal examination
IUGR	intrauterine growth restriction	WR	Wasserman reaction

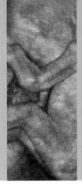

Chapter 1

Obstetric history taking and examination

OVERVIEW

Taking an obstetric history and performing an examination are quite different from the typical medical or surgical equivalents. By reading this chapter you will become conversant with the theory of history taking and examination before examining a pregnant woman on your own. Remember that the whole area of reproductive medicine is complex, with psychological, pathological and physiological components to it. This means that sometimes questions in the history must be asked particularly discretely and the obstetric examination must always be performed with sensitivity.

HISTORY TAKING AND EXAMINATION IN OBSTETRICS

A detailed and careful obstetric history is essential not only for the assessment of the mother and fetus, but to provide clues as to how to manage a woman's antenatal care and what level of risk to assign to it. During a pregnant woman's first visit to hospital, the booking history is taken by a midwife and may be entered directly into a computer. A further visit to an obstetrician should be arranged if there are aspects in the history that are considered to be high risk. A physical examination is usually performed by an obstetrician if there are known medical or obstetric disorders. The 'booking' history and examination is dealt with in more detail in the antenatal care chapter (Chapter 8). Here, we will deal with the more general aspects of history taking and examination. A template for a sample obstetric history and examination is provided later on (page 5).

The background to a history

The obstetric history should include a synopsis of a woman's background level of risk. By this, we mean various general factors that the obstetrician will need to consider when tailoring the management plan of a particular woman. Simple things, such as enquiry about maternal age (one of the oldest screening tests in the history of antenatal care), are particularly important because of the increased risk of chromosomal disorders with increasing maternal age, and the greater likelihood of gynaecological and medical disorders with increased age. Added to this, though not always relevant to it, are whether there was a prolonged period of infertility or if assisted conception techniques were required, whether the pregnancy was planned or unplanned ('accidental'), and the attitudes of the mother and father to the pregnancy.

Just consider, for instance, the impact that age and reproductive record might have in planning management in the following scenarios of two women in preterm labour at around 24 weeks.

1. A woman aged 42, in her first pregnancy, trying for 8 years and finally conceiving after three cycles of IVF. Partner is a professional who is very supportive over this pregnancy.
2. A woman aged 26, with three live, well babies. Lives at home with children; has split up with the father of this pregnancy.

The woman in scenario 1, for whom this is quite possibly the last chance for a pregnancy, would quite likely request that every possible obstetric and neonatal effort be made in optimizing the chances of survival for her baby. However, the management plan might be very different for the woman in scenario 2, for whom a healthy baby might be far more important, and who would perhaps be more concerned about the risks of having a handicapped child. The management plan for delivery (whether caesarean or vaginal), resuscitation and neonatal care would be quite different in these two cases. This is why it is so important to be aware of the background to a pregnancy, as well as the facts about the pregnancy itself.

Dating a pregnancy

Conventionally, we date a pregnancy from the first day of the last menstrual period (for this purpose only we shall refer to this day as LMP), not from the date of actual conception or implantation. This means that from the LMP, the estimated date of delivery will be exactly 280 days (40 weeks). For this relationship to hold true, ovulation (and hence conception), should occur 14 days after the LMP. This cannot be held to be true in the circumstances outlined in the box below, in which case the dates and assessment of estimated date of delivery (EDD) must be calculated according to dating ultrasound. It is important to note that the EDD is taken as 40 weeks from the LMP, although term is defined as 37–42 weeks of gestation, and it is within this gestation range that most women deliver.

A relatively simple way to calculate the EDD from the LMP is to subtract 3 from the month (this is the same as adding 9), and add 7 to the days. For example, an LMP of 14th October gives an EDD of (14+7) = 21st of (10–3 = 7) July of the following year.

A discrepancy in dates between those calculated from LMP and those determined by ultrasound, usually means that the date of conception is not exactly two weeks from the last menstrual period, i.e. ovulation occurred later or earlier than expected. A difference of more than ten days between menstrual dates and ultrasound crown–rump length (CRL) between 6 and 14 weeks, or of biparietal diameter (BPD) between 14 and 24 weeks, usually means ultrasound dates should be used. However, in the late second and third trimesters, ultrasound dating can be many weeks out and must be applied carefully. Otherwise, a problem with fetal growth may be overlooked and put down to 'wrong dates', which may have disastrous consequences.

Specific dating issues are discussed in Chapter 8, Antenatal care.

Key Points

Factors making menstrual dates unreliable in dating

- Irregular periods (anything other than a 28-day cycle)
- Breastfeeding within two months of becoming pregnant
- Contraceptive pill usage within three months of becoming pregnant
- Pregnancy occurring whilst using hormonal treatment (HRT, LHRH agonists)
- Assisted conception techniques (IUI, IVF, ovulation induction)

Subfertility in the history

It is important to determine whether a pregnancy is 'spontaneously' conceived, or the result of assisted conception. Assisted conception puts a pregnancy at a higher risk level. This is partly because there are genuine obstetric risks associated with certain assisted conception techniques. For instance, placental problems, specifically placenta accreta and postpartum haemorrhage, are associated with IVF; pre-eclampsia with donated eggs. Maternal age, a strong obstetric risk factor on its own, is often higher for women undergoing assisted conception. Further-

Pre-existing medical diseases

Major pre-existing medical diseases that may impact on pregnancy (risks are shown in parentheses)

- diabetes mellitus (hypo/hyperglycaemia; fetal congenital abnormalities, macrosomia, stillbirth)
- hypertension (pre-eclampsia more common)
- renal disease (hypertension, pre-eclampsia, urinary infections, immunosuppression)
- thrombophilia or previous history of deep venous thrombosis/pulmonary embolism (thrombosis; potential risks of anticoagulants)
- connective tissue disease such as systemic lupus erythematosus, antiphospholipid syndrome (SGA babies, pre-eclampsia)
- sickle cell disease (sickle crisis)
- epilepsy (fetal abnormalities; increased risk of fits due to too low dose medication)
- thyroid disease (fetal thyroid problems)

Pre-existing conditions

Previous pregnancy

- obese or very slim (>100kg or <45kg)
- assisted conception
- deep vein thrombosis/pulmonary embolism
- psychiatric condition
- smoker or excess alcohol consumption
- pre-eclampsia
- SGA infant
- major medical condition
- multiple pregnancy
- preterm delivery
- age (<20 or >35)
- heavy vaginal bleeding
- Caesarean section
- any pelvic mass or tumour
- Major antepartum or postpartum haemorrhage
- stillbirth or neonatal loss

more, for many couples undergoing assisted conception, this pregnancy may represent their only chance of having a baby and obstetric risks that would be considered acceptable to a young pregnant woman with no complications (such as allowing a pregnancy to proceed to 42 weeks before intervening) would certainly not be appropriate for them.

A pregnancy is dated in a different way if it is the result of IVF. With current practice, a woman becoming pregnant following IVF will not have a proper LMP. It is therefore assumed that the day of embryo transfer (ET) will equate roughly to 14 days after the LMP. In 'spontaneous' pregnancies the median day of conception is about day 14 so this is not an unreasonable assumption. Thus to calculate an EDD, count 14 days back from the day of ET; this will give the LMP from which the EDD can be calculated.

Obstetric risk factors

As already explained, certain conditions (psychological and social) can impact in a major way on a pregnancy and the subsequent management and outcome of that pregnancy. Also important are medical and obstetric conditions that are either pre-existing, or occurred in a previous pregnancy. For example, certain conditions, such as pre-eclampsia may be more likely to occur in a first pregnancy (approximately 8 per cent incidence), but if it did occur in a first pregnancy, the chances of it occurring in a second are slightly higher (around 12 per cent). However, if the first pregnancy was not affected by pre-eclampsia, a second pregnancy (providing the father is the same as with the first) is highly unlikely to be affected (<1 per cent incidence). This makes pre-eclampsia a very obvious and important risk factor for a future pregnancy. Other conditions which might recur include preterm labour and delivery of a small for gestational age (SGA) fetus. There are also potential complications such as antepartum and postpartum haemorrhage that not only are liable to recur, but become more common at the extreme of high parity. The presence of large pelvic masses such as fibroids, large ovarian cysts, or previous pelvic surgery could all affect the pregnancy adversely by forcing surgical intervention antenatally, or affecting the mode and timing of delivery.

Parity: gravida and para

Many risks of pregnancy and delivery are related to the number of previous pregnancies and the woman's reproductive record. Therefore, the parity and gravidity of the mother is important.

- 'Gravida' records the total number of pregnancies,

irrespective of outcome. This term can only be used if the woman is currently pregnant.
- 'Para' records the number of livebirths irrespective of gestation, or of stillbirths that have reached 24 weeks.

Using this scheme, the outcome of pregnancies that didn't reach viability is unknown. It is therefore important to carefully determine the number of ectopic pregnancies, terminations of pregnancy and miscarriages that have occurred. Sometimes these details are very personal and your patient may not wish her partner/mother/friend to know about them. Be very careful not to disclose or tactlessly ask questions in front of companions unless your patient says she is happy for them to stay throughout the history taking.

These details may be added as a '+ x' superscript to the 'para' as shown below, for example:
- Currently pregnant, having had one first trimester termination of pregnancy and one normal delivery at term: G3 P1^{+1}

- A woman in her first pregnancy: G1 P0
- A woman, not currently pregnant, having had three miscarriages, an ectopic pregnancy and a stillbirth at 28 weeks: Para 1^{+4}

There is a move away from this verbal shorthand towards a more simple and open categorization, which is equally acceptable:
- This lady is in her second ongoing pregnancy, having had one normal delivery and one early termination of pregnancy.
- …is in her first ongoing pregnancy.
- …has no living children, having had four first trimester losses and one stillbirth.

The obstetric past history

This records details of every pregnancy, in chronological order.
- Date of delivery and delivery gestation.

CASE HISTORY

Mrs A is a 23-year-old secretary in her first ongoing pregnancy, who has presented this morning to the labour ward with fresh vaginal bleeding at 26 weeks' gestation.

Her LMP was 23rd March giving her an EDD of 30th December; these dates agree with a first trimester scan. Her gestation today is 26 weeks and 2 days. She has had no serious problems in her pregnancy to date, until she awoke early this morning with some dull lower abdominal pain and her underwear was soaked with fresh blood. The baby was moving well and she had no contractions, nor did any liquor leak. She called immediately for an ambulance and arrived on labour ward approximately half an hour later.

She tells me that the doctor who saw her on admission did not feel that her symptoms warranted immediate delivery. Blood tests were sent, and she was given an injection of what she was told was steroid and commenced on the cardiotocograph (CTG), which was normal. She was told that an internal speculum examination showed that the cervix was closed and there was some old blood in the vagina.

Her last ultrasound was the anomaly scan at 21 weeks, at which time the baby's growth was normal and the placenta wasn't low lying. She had a normal cervical smear 6 months ago, and has not had intercourse for several weeks.

There is nothing of note in her gynaecological history. Her periods are normally regular, not heavy, lasting for three days out of every 28–30 days. Mrs A had not been using any contraception for six months prior to becoming pregnant. She has had one first trimester termination of pregnancy 2 years ago. She has never had a gynaecological operation, nor genital infection. She is otherwise fit and well, though does suffer from mild asthma, which has never required hospitalisation. She occasionally uses an inhaler for this. She has never had a major operation. She is taking iron and folic acid tablets; and started taking folic acid two months before becoming pregnant. She is allergic to penicillin.

Mrs A smokes 5/day, doesn't drink alcohol except on rare occasions, and lives with her husband and his two children from a previous marriage. She lives in a house which she and her husband co-own. There is no family history of serious illnesses; both her mother and father are still alive though her father has hypertension and late onset diabetes.

In summary, Mrs A awoke this morning with symptoms suggestive of an antepartum haemorrhage at 26 weeks' gestation. Her condition has stabilized since then, with no further bleeding and an active baby. She has been given intramuscular steroids. The clinical picture is suggestive of a small placental abruption, though I would perform a further ultrasound to exclude placenta praevia.

- Antenatal problems.
- Length of labour, and whether spontaneous or induced.
- Type of delivery and complications (whether Caesarean Section, spontaneous vaginal or assisted).
- Weight of baby(ies) (kg).
- Age of baby/child now and any salient conditions (e.g. learning difficulties, cerebral palsy, etc.).
- Name of baby (optional).

Template history

It is vital to have a simple template in your mind for history taking. This should form the basis of an antenatal clerking. Here is a list, in approximate order of presentation, of things you should ask.

Demographic details
- Name
- Age
- Occupation
- Reason for being in hospital/outpatient/in antenatal clinic

This pregnancy
- Gestation
- LMP
- EDD by LMP, any discrepancy with ultrasound dates
- Singleton/multiple (chorionicity)
- Planned/accidental

Presenting problems in this pregnancy
- Details of the presenting complaint
- Gestation at onset
- Symptoms
- Signs
- Action that has been taken
- Her concerns
- Likely obstetric outcome
- What she has been told about this

Ultrasound scans (this may be integral to the section above)
- How many scans, when were they performed and why? What was the result of these scans?

Specific problems earlier in pregnancy
- Backache, hyperemesis, per vaginal bleeding, constipation, anaemia, urinary problems

Always ask:
- Is (are) the baby(ies) moving (after 20 weeks)?
- Do you have any contractions?
- Have you lost any fluid or blood from your vagina?

Past reproductive record
- Number of previous ongoing pregnancies: gestation at delivery, type of delivery, sex and weight of baby. Any complications in previous pregnancies
- Stillbirths, neonatal deaths, terminations of pregnancy, miscarriages and ectopics

Useful extras
- Blood group
- Rubella status
- Sickle/thalassaemia status
- Hepatitis B/HIV status
- Folic acid supplements

Gynaecological history
- Periods: regular or irregular
- Cycle length & days of bleeding
- Contraceptive history; date when contraceptives stopped
- Sexually transmitted diseases (ask about pelvic inflammatory disease, chlamydia, gonorrhea, hepatitis B, HIV)
- Cervical smear (when was your last smear test and was it normal?)
- If not, ask why, what was done (colposcopy, LLETZ biopsy) and when is the recall?
- Any previous gynaecological operations/conditions (e.g. fibroids, previous myomectomy, endometriosis, TOPs)?

Past medical and surgical history
- Relevant medical conditions and treatment
- All operations, and whether under general or local anaesthetic

Drugs
- Include iron tablets, folic acid, vitamins
- Ask specific detail about antihypertensive, diabetic, anti-epileptic and thyroid medications

Allergies
- Ask specifically about antibiotics and anaesthetics

Family history
- Diseases such as diabetes and hypertension, also ovarian and breast carcinoma

Social history
- Marital status
- Working or not
- Partner's occupation
- Help at home
- Housing
- Smoking? How many cigarettes/day?
- Alcohol? How many units/wk?
- Illicit drugs? Which and how often? Self injection?

Summary
- Name, age, gestation, single/multiple gestation, current problem/situation; action taken (investigations, plan etc.).

Special situations in history taking

Remember the following special situations in history taking:

IVF pregnancies:
- Always ask the underlying reason for infertility (e.g. blocked Fallopian tubes, polycystic ovaries, male factor).
- Are the oocytes or sperm from donors? (This may be confidential information.)
- How many attempts (cycles) of IVF were there before successful pregnancy?
- Remember to calculate the EDD by assuming the LMP is 14 days prior to the ET date

Antepartum haemorrhage (APH)
- Can happen after 24 weeks only.
- The most important thing is to differentiate a serious APH (abruption, placenta praevia) from local causes of bleeding.
- The only cause of fetal bleeding is the rare but potentially disastrous condition of vasa praevia.

Always ask:
- Was there pain with the bleeding (abruption), or painless (dull ache at worst) (praevia)?

- Did the baby stop moving with the bleeding (abruption)?
- Did your womb go hard as if you were having a contraction? (abruption)
- Where was the placenta on scan? Were you told it was low lying? (praevia)
- Do you feel generally unwell? (abruption)
- Have you had intercourse in the last 12 hours? (praevia; local causes)
- Have you had a recent smear test (you must not miss rare but important cervical pathology)? *Remember that an abruption is more dangerous to the fetus, and praevia more dangerous to the mother.*

Mid-pregnancy loss
(Note: cervical weakness is a better term to use than incompetence.) Ask:
- How many terminations/miscarriages and at exactly what gestation?
- Was there a leak of amniotic fluid first, followed by miscarriage (more suggestive of infection), or was there very little pain or signs of anything amiss until you were about to miscarry (cervical weakness)?
- Has a transvaginal ultrasound or laparoscopy been performed when not pregnant? (There may be an anatomical abnormality, such as bicornuate uterus.)

EXAMINING THE OBSTETRIC PATIENT

An obstetric examination is unique in medicine; there are several specific techniques that you must be conversant with that are not required in other specialties. See Figure 1.1 for a quick guide.

An obstetric examination should start generally, and end specifically. This means that the initial assessment as you walk across the examination room must include just stopping for a second or two, and looking at your patient from across the room to determine agitation, anxiety, mood, etc. Smile at your patient, introduce yourself by name and ask her name. Shake her hand.

(Note: If you are very pressed for time, for example in an examination situation, then say, 'I am going to ask you lots of questions, and have only got a few minutes to obtain all the answers so don't think I'm rude if I answer your questions at the end. Thank you'.)

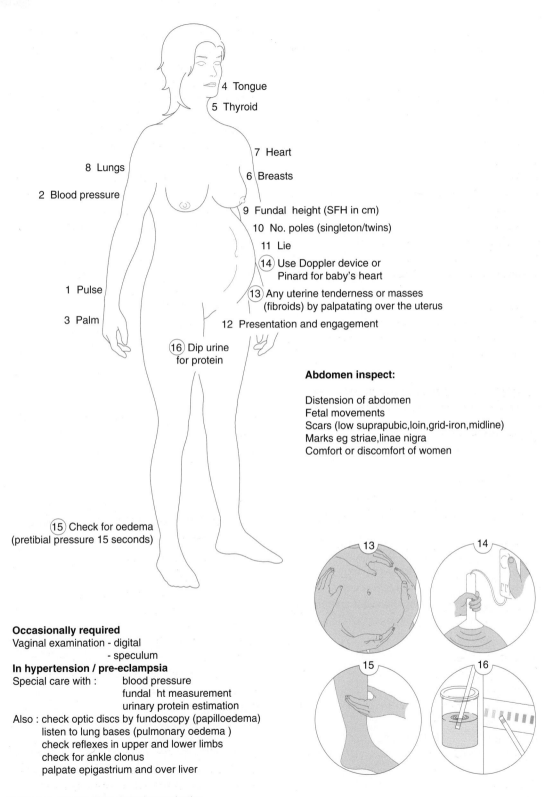

4 Tongue

5 Thyroid

7 Heart

8 Lungs

6 Breasts

2 Blood pressure

9 Fundal height (SFH in cm)

10 No. poles (singleton/twins)

11 Lie

(14) Use Doppler device or
Pinard for baby's heart

1 Pulse

(13) Any uterine tenderness or masses
(fibroids) by palpatating over the uterus

3 Palm

12 Presentation and engagement

(16) Dip urine
for protein

Abdomen inspect:

Distension of abdomen
Fetal movements
Scars (low suprapubic,loin,grid-iron,midline)
Marks eg striae,linae nigra
Comfort or discomfort of women

(15) Check for oedema
(pretibial pressure 15 seconds)

Occasionally required
Vaginal examination - digital
- speculum
In hypertension / pre-eclampsia
Special care with :   blood pressure
fundal ht measurement
urinary protein estimation
Also : check optic discs by fundoscopy (papilloedema)
listen to lung bases (pulmonary oedema)
check reflexes in upper and lower limbs
check for ankle clonus
palpate epigastrium and over liver

Figure 1.1 The complete obstetric examination.

A booking examination should include a woman's height and weight. From this, the body mass index (BMI) can be calculated:

$$BMI = \frac{weight\ (kg)}{(height\ (m))^2}$$

For example, a woman weighing 80 kg who is 2 m tall has a BMI of 80/2x2; i.e. 20. The habit of slavishly recording maternal weight gain is not effective in predicting those likely to give birth to SGA infants but, there is an increased risk of perinatal complications in association with a booking maternal weight of <45 kg (associated with SGA) or >100 kg (associated with abnormal glucose tolerance). In the assessment of risk of cephalo-pelvic disproportion and the likelihood of an operative delivery, the maternal height and even shoe size are of significance. The shorter a woman is, and/or smaller her shoe size, the possible greater likelihood of cephalo-pelvic disproportion in labour.

A full obstetric examination will include checking the woman's pulse rate, looking at her hands (nails for anaemia, palms for the redness associated with pregnancy). At a booking examination it is good practice (though largely discontinued now) to listen to the heart and lungs.

Measure blood pressure in the 'semi recumbent' (45°) position (Fig. 1.2). In the UK, the diastolic blood pressure is taken at Korotkoff IV (muffling) not V (disappearance) of the sound, but there are differences from country to country. Taking Korotkoff V, a very small minority of women will have a diastolic blood pressure of zero! Remember that you must use a large blood pressure cuff for overweight women, or else you will obtain a falsely high reading.

An examination of the thyroid gland and breasts is an important part of a first assessment. Although rarely found, a goitre could have potential implications for both mother and fetus in pregnancy if associated with thyroid gland dysfunction. The real value of a breast examination is to pick up any suspicious masses. Breast cancer is rare but not unknown in pregnancy (approximately 1:10,000 pregnancies in the UK) and it is thought to be a more rapidly evolving carcinoma because of later detection due to an increase in breast mass, and hormonal influences. The five-year survival of breast cancer detected in pregnancy is 50 per cent of that in age-matched non-pregnant women. Examination of the nipples to detect retraction or inversion, which can affect breastfeeding is unlikely to be of practical value as no helpful or successful antenatal preventive or curative measure has been found.

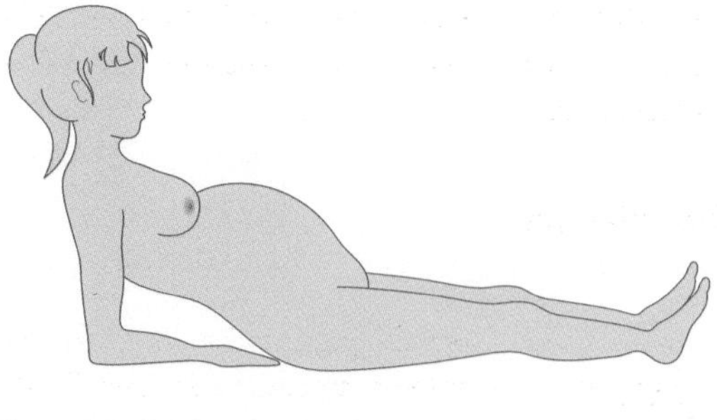

The abdominal examination

Always make sure that the patient looks comfortable, is lying semi recumbent and has a sheet covering her waist and legs, which may be bare. You must examine from the woman's right side.

Remember this order for examining the abdomen: inspection, palpation and auscultation.

Inspection

- Assess shape and size of the uterus, and any obvious asymmetry of the abdomen; fetal movements.
- Look for surgical scars (always check the loins) (kidney transplant); suprapubically (Caesarean Section, ectopic pregnancy); grid-iron (appendix); umbilicus (laparoscopy); midline (bowel or ovarian operations).
- Striae gravidarum (stretch marks) and linea nigra (pigmented vertical line running from umbilicus to symphisis pubis) are always commented on though their relevance is questionable.

Palpation

Firstly, measure the fundal height by placing the ulnar border of the left hand gently at the fundus of the uterus, and measuring with a tape in centimetres to the pubic symphysis (Fig. 1.3a). The measurement in cm should give an estimation of gestational age in weeks, i.e. +/- 2 cm from 20–38 weeks (Fig. 1.4).

Figure 1.2 Abdominal palpation.

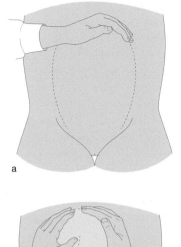 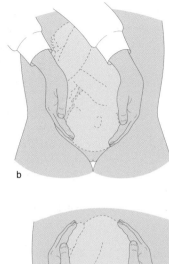

a b

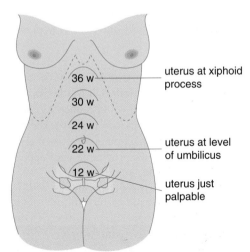

c d

Figure 1.3 a–d Engagement of the fetal head in the maternal pelvic brim assessed. (a) Palpating the uterine fundus. (b) Assessing engagement of the fetal head. (c) and (d) Palpating fetal poles.

36 w — uterus at xiphoid process

30 w

24 w

22 w — uterus at level of umbilicus

12 w — uterus just palpable

Measuring symphysis — fundal height

1 palpate for pubic symphysis
2 apply tape measure
3 stretch tape to fundus
4 turn tape measure over to read cms

Figure 1.4 Measuring symphysis–fundal height.

Then palpate fetal poles to determine presentation and lie (Fig. 1.3b, c and d). When establishing head engagement in the third trimester, it is better to gently palpate with two hands facing down over the abdomen as pictured, than to prod around with Paulik's grip (Fig. 1.5), which in non-experienced hands is painful.

To establish the lie of the fetus, palpate gently using both hands as shown in Figures 1.3c and d and 1.6.

It is important to make eye contact with the woman you are examining every few seconds; you may be hurting her by palpating too firmly.

After you have palpated the uterus, gently palpate for kidney tenderness (note that kidneys are displaced upwards by a pregnancy) and liver and spleen enlargement.

Auscultation

For a fetus with a cephalic presentation, it is relatively easy to palpate the anterior shoulder and listen for the fetal heart at this point. If you cannot hear the fetal heartbeat using a Pinard stethoscope, you must use a

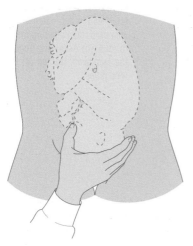

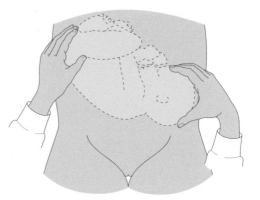

Figure 1.6 Abdominal palpation of fetus lying transversely.

Figure 1.5 Palpation of the lower pole of the uterus by Paulik's method.

hand-held Doppler apparatus ('sonicaid'), or failing this, perform an ultrasound scan. You will obviously have to modify the position for auscultation if the fetus is in the transverse or breech positions.

Internal examination

A pelvic (vaginal) examination is not routinely performed unless specifically indicated. Occasionally it is necessary to obtain a cervical smear for cytology when one is due. In normal circumstances, it is advisable for the smear to be performed postpartum, as both the sampling of the cervix and interpretation of smears during pregnancy is difficult. It is reasonable to perform a smear test if it had never been obtained before, or where a smear has not been performed for some time.

To perform a digital examination, commonly called vaginal examination (VE), or a speculum examination, ask your patient to lie comfortably on her back, usually with a slight tilt (for example a pillow wedged under the right side of her back), and the knees drawn up with the ankles together. You should have asked her to remove her underwear, and a sheet may be placed covering her abdomen and genitalia. The procedure should be performed in the presence of a female third party (for example a nurse or midwife). Both hands should be gloved.

For a digital examination, the labia are gently parted with the left hand, and index and forefinger of the right hand gently introduced into the vagina. They may be advanced until the cervix is palpated. In later pregnancy, this will provide information on the length and consistency of the cervix (Bishop score), and this allows an assessment of favourability for induction of labour (Table 1.1).

A digital vaginal examination should not be performed in the following circumstances:

- with suspected placenta praevia (risk of precipitating haemorrhage);
- when there is prelabour rupture of membranes (risk of introducing infection);
- when consent is withheld (this goes without saying).

A speculum examination (Fig. 1.7) must be taught practically rather than described. A gentle speculum examination is less likely to introduce ascending infection, and may be used to visualize the cervix in prelabour rupture of membranes, or even if a placenta praevia is suspected. The same steps apply as above, with the following adjustments:

- select an appropriately sized speculum;

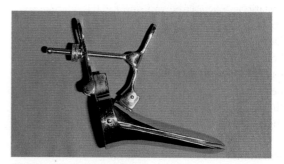

Figure 1.7 A Cusco speculum.

Table 1.1 – Bishop score

Score	0	1	2	3
Dilatation of cervix (cm)	0	1 or 2	3 or 4	5 or more
Consistency of cervix	Firm	Medium	Soft	-
Length of cervical canal (cm)	>2	2–1	1–0.5	<0.5
Position	Posterior	Central	Anterior	-
Station of presenting part (cm above ischial spines)	3	2	1 or 0	Below

- the speculum should be pre-warmed to avoid the discomfort of cold metal;
- lubricating gel or water should be applied to the mouth of the speculum;
- the labia are parted with the left hand, and speculum held with the right;
- the speculum is inserted through the introitus with the jaws in the vertical plane; it is gently rotated while being advanced into the horizontal plane;
- the speculum's jaws are slowly opened once the speculum is advanced fully into the vagina;
- at this point, the ratchet nut can be tightened;
- a light source should be at hand to enable easy visualisation of the cervix and vaginal walls;
- on removing the speculum, close the jaws gently and slowly to avoid catching vaginal epithelium in them.

Special situations in the obstetric examination

Twins

As for singleton, except: Comment on SFH, with the caveat that the measurement is unreliable in multiple gestation. When asked to listen for the fetal hearts, you should ask for both a Pinard stethoscope and a Doppler sonicaid so that you can hear both heart-beats separately and simultaneously. Or alternatively, use one Doppler sonicaid to hear two separate heart-beats at different rates in distinctly different parts of the abdomen. If unable to do this, suggest perform-ing a twin CTG for satisfactory monitoring.

Don't worry if you can't determine the lie and pre-sentations of both twins. Usually, however, you should be able to feel the presenting part of the first twin. In practice this is the most important observa-tion on which decision making as to the mode of delivery is based; you can therefore say: 'Twin 1 is longitudinal, with a cephalic presentation, however I am unable to define the lie of the second twin.'

Remember that women with twins are more likely to exhibit signs of anaemia, varicose veins and oedema.

Don't be pressured to make up any findings or confabulate; not only is it a bad habit, but you are also likely to get found out!

Hypertension/pre-eclampsia

Take special note of blood pressure, and check a specimen of urine for protein. Check for pretibial and sacral oedema. To check for oedema you must press gently but firmly with thumb or forefinger for at least 20 seconds.

If BP is very raised, check upper and lower limb reflexes, and examine for clonus.

Remember to look with an ophthalmoscope at the fundi for hypertensive changes: silver wiring, arteriovenous nipping and papilloedema.

Listen to the lung bases for pulmonary oedema, which can occur in severe pre-eclampsia.

The SFH may be reduced compared to gestation so you must measure and record this carefully.

Fibroids

Large fibroids can cause major problems throughout pregnancy, especially at and just after, delivery. It is therefore relevant and important to determine the size, position and number of fibroids antenatally. This will in turn allow decisions to be made regard-ing the mode and timing of delivery.

Remember that the SFH may be much larger than the gestational age equivalent measurement.

Palpate fibroids for tenderness: tenderness, pain and nausea indicate possible red degeneration of a fibroid (not uncommon in pregnancy).

Determine fetal presentation carefully: large fibroids may cause malpresentation (transverse or breech is common).

Twins and fibroids may co-exist: both are more common in certain ethnic groups (central Africans).

Present your examination

Finally, remember that every doctor or midwife presents a history and examination in a slightly different way, and it is human to have foibles and pet hates! It is therefore mandatory for you to adapt these generic templates to the individual situation, be it for examination purposes or for a Consultant labour ward round!

Key Points

- Introduce yourself
- Be courteous to the patient
- Check that menstrual and ultrasound dates match
- Start your history of the patient with a one or two line introduction including name, age, parity, gestational age and reason for referral
- Make your patient comfortable and ask her to lie semi-recumbent
- Examine gently, preferably with a chaperone regardless of your gender
- End your history and examination with a short one or two line summary which includes a likely diagnosis and proposed investigations/treatment

CASE HISTORY

Mrs Akbar is 1.7 metres tall and weighs 55 kg. Her blood pressure is 130/80, pulse regular and there is mild pitting oedema of the ankles.

Thyroid examination was normal and there were no lumps, adenopathy or tenderness of the breasts.

The abdomen is symmetrically distended consistent with pregnancy. There is a linea nigra present, and some striae gravidarum (stretchmarks) are visible. A lower transverse suprapubic scar is evident, as is a right-sided grid-iron scar.

The symphysis–fundal height is 32 cm. The pregnancy is singleton, with longitudinal lie and cephalic presentation. The head is five-fifths palpable, hence not engaged. I could see and feel fetal movements and on auscultation using a Doppler sonicaid, the fetal heart was heard at a rate of approximately 130 beats per minute.

Urinalysis revealed a trace of protein only.

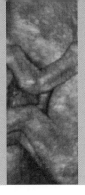

Chapter 2

Modern maternity care and changing childbirth

OVERVIEW

Much has changed since the start of the twentieth century. Maternal and perinatal mortality is now far lower and there is not the same potential for reducing these rates much further. The emphasis of maternity care must still enshrine as its core the health and safety of the mother and her baby, but it should now also concentrate on providing a welcoming and supportive environment for pregnancy and delivery.

Up until the Second World War, antenatal care was a rather haphazard process usually undertaken by General Practitioners. Only women with potentially serious problems, or those with enough money, found themselves referred to obstetricians. Most (more than 90 per cent) of deliveries were at home, attended by the local midwife and, if necessary, by a GP. In the the days from the turn of the century to the 1920s, maternal mortality was a major problem; 1 in 250 women died in childbirth. The modern pharmacological treatments for both postpartum haemorrhage (PPH) and sepsis, which killed most women, were unavailable (Fig.2.1).

The National Birthday Trust Fund was founded in 1928 to reduce maternal death in childbirth; the situation was indeed dire in the UK at that time (Fig. 2.2).

The development of a pattern of structured antenatal care: the 1940s and 1950s

The integration of healthcare services and hospitals in the UK within the National Health Service (NHS) in 1948 allowed the development of a structured, unified system for antenatal care. Pregnant women were booked at the local hospital, under the auspices of a Consultant Obstetrician, who was directly responsible for their care.

The major problems at the time stemmed from the diseases and disorders then prevalent:

- iron deficiency anaemia: due to poor diet and too many pregnancies too closely spaced;
- malnutrition: predisposed to by poverty and poor education;

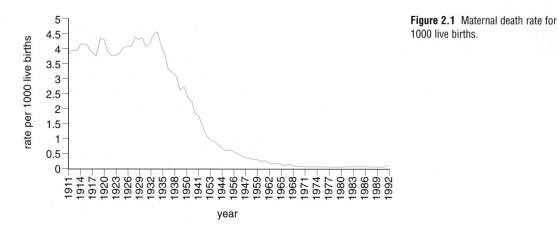

Figure 2.1 Maternal death rate for 1000 live births.

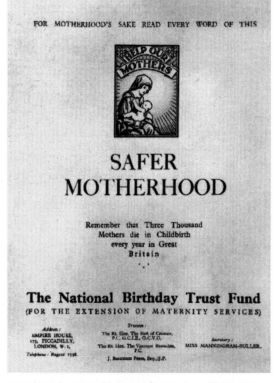

Figure 2.2 'For Motherhood's Sake Read Every Word of This' – a leaflet produced by the National Birthday Trust Fund in the early 1930s. (Reproduced courtesy of the Wellcome Institute Library, London.)

- cardiac diseases: aortic and mitral valvular disease, due to rheumatic fever;
- chronic respiratory illness due to tuberculosis and chronic bacterial lung infections.

This lead to a system of care, in widespread use until relatively recently, of 'medical booking' at the start of pregnancy to exclude by examination cardiovascular and respiratory diseases, and regular antenatal visits to record blood pressure, urinalysis, weight, fetal condition and maternal haemoglobin level. Fixed patterns of antenatal care, largely unchanged from the early decades of this century, were slavishly followed until they began to be questioned in the 1980s.

Increased hospital births: the 1960s and 1970s

The advent of the NHS, incorporation of new medical technologies to antenatal care and delivery, and decrease in both maternal and perinatal mortality, lead to the 'hospital revolution'. The prevailing wisdom strongly implied that the safest, and nicest, place to give birth was a hospital. Here a mother could be looked after by highly trained health professionals (doctors and midwives) and her delivery conducted in the quickest and most efficient way. During this time, from 1960 to 1979, the hospital delivery rate increased from 25 per cent to 99 per cent, and anyone requesting a home delivery was regarded as really quite unusual. It should not be overlooked, however, that in 1960 the perinatal mortality rate (stillbirths plus first week deaths) in the UK was 30 per 1000; this is now around 8 per 1000. It is not easy to tease out of these figures the relative contributions of improved nutrition, sanitation, midwifery and medical care, or indeed, hospital care.

The introduction of technology: cardiotography and ultrasound

The move towards hospital delivery was no doubt fuelled by a belief in the infallibility of modern technologies. During the 1960s, the cardiotocograph (CTG) became a frequent fixture on the labour ward. This is an automated method of detecting and printing out a record of the fetal heart rate, initially made by microphone and later by Doppler ultrasound or by fetal electrocardiogram (ECG). Tremendous faith was placed in its ability to discern abnormal patterns of heart rate and hence detect fetal asphyxia. By the late 1960s and early 1970s, there was a strong prevailing feeling within the obstetric establishment that CTG recording in labour would drastically reduce the number of babies suffering from birth asphyxia. This in turn lead to a media and public demand for the use of this technology.

Ultrasound scanning, first adapted for obstetric use in the late 1950s by Professor Ian Donald in Glasgow, became available in most hospitals throughout the late 1970s and 1980s. By the end of the 1980s, most women were being subjected to at least one ultrasound scan during their pregnancy. Although the ability of ultrasound to assess fetal growth and wellbeing and amniotic fluid volume, and detect placental site, multiple gestation and congenital defects was not in doubt, its value as a generally applied screening tool was controversial.

The consumer backlash: the 1990s

It is not easy to pinpoint precisely why a backlash against medicalization and hospitals occurred in the early 1990s, except to say with the benefit of retrospect, that it was bound to happen. Several factors contributed to this, although none on its own was dominant, and the unease led to a Government Select Committee Report on maternity services in 1993. Significantly, the Select Committee concluded, in sharp distinction to the Maternity Services Advisory Committee's 1984 report, that '...the conclusion that the policy of encouraging all women to give birth in hospitals cannot be justified on grounds of safety'.

Other factors contributed to the rethinking of maternity services; these included:

- The emergence of strong and well organized lay organizations, such as the National Childbirth Trust, to lobby for the rights of pregnant women.
- The increasing prominence of female pregnancy experts; often authors who viewed pregnancy from a predominantly subjective angle. Some sought to politicize the situation as a battle against the traditional 'male obstetrician' role model. This made good newsprint and galvanized the debate.
- A general realization within the obstetric profession that some technologies were being inappropriately applied, leading to an excess of intervention and not improving outcome for mothers or their babies.
- Funding problems within the NHS that by the early 1990s were making NHS maternity units look generally unkempt and certainly unwelcoming.
- The appearance of antenatal clinics as overcrowded 'conveyor belts', with a long waiting time and poor communication between professionals and a lack of continuity in care.
- A persistence, or perceived persistence, of old-fashioned and unnecessary medical and midwifery interventions such as routine enemas and episiotomy. In reality, there were few hospitals where this was the case.
- The development of the concept of midwives as competent independent practitioners in their own right.
- Cost: hospitals are expensive to run!

Changing Childbirth: the report of the Expert Maternity Group

This report, first published in 1993, attracted a great deal of publicity within both the lay and medical arenas. Its authors articulated the concerns that had been building up over a number of years regarding the over-medicalization of pregnancy and childbirth. The Expert Maternity Group comprised lay members and representatives from the worlds of politics, midwifery, journalism and management consultancy. Significantly, the group contained only one obstetrician. It should also be stressed that the document was not based on any factual or audited data or any systematic survey of the views of pregnant women; it was more a 'snapshot' view of perceived public opinion regarding the definition of the roles of midwives and doctors.

It identified a number of principles of good maternity care:

- The woman must be the focus of care. She should be able to feel that she is in control of what is happening to her and able to make decisions about her care, based on her needs, having discussed matters fully with the professionals involved.
- Maternity services must be readily and easily accessible to all. They should be sensitive to the needs of the local population and based primarily in the community.
- Women should be involved in the monitoring and planning of maternity services to ensure that they are responsive to the needs of a changing society. In addition, care should be effective and resources used efficiently.

In addition, various key points were reiterated throughout this report:

- a named midwife as the lead professional;
- the right to deliver at home;
- good access to community/GP based care;
- identification of high- and low-risk women;
- empowerment of mothers over their choice over method of delivery, and who they want to accompany them in labour.

One goal of the Changing Childbirth report was to redefine the role of the obstetrician as a specialist in complicated pregnancy, rather than as a doctor involved in normal, low-risk pregnancy. This is not a concept that should frighten obstetricians, as it should allow for much more efficient targeting of high-risk pregnancies for close care and supervision, while low-risk pregnancies can be dealt with in the community by midwives and GPs.

The role of the obstetrician was outlined as:

- the lead professional for women with complicated pregnancies;
- an adviser on actual and suspected abnormalities;
- the person responsible for the care of women who have obstetric emergencies;
- a provider of technical skills beyond the expertise of midwives/GPs;
- the practitioner of fetal medicine;
- a teacher of junior medical staff and medical students;
- increasingly, involved as an administrator and manager, and a researcher.

Have these ideas been implemented? At the time of publication of Changing Childbirth (1993), ten indicators of progress were identified as achievable within five years:

1. All women should carry their own notes.
2. Every woman should know one 'named midwife', responsible for continuity of care.
3. At least 30 per cent of women should have a midwife as the lead professional.
4. Every woman should know their lead professional.
5. At least 75 per cent of women should know the person who cares for them during their delivery.
6. Midwives should have direct access to some beds in all maternity units.
7. At least 30 per cent of women delivered in a maternity unit should be admitted under a midwife.
8. The number of antenatal visits for women with uncomplicated pregnancies should have been reviewed.
9. All front line ambulances should have a paramedic able to support the midwife who needs to transfer a woman to hospital in an emergency.
10. All women should have access to information about services available in their locality.

The five-year timescale has now passed, and many of the indicators of progress are no nearer to being implemented than they were at the time of their inception. The reasons for this include a gross shortage of midwives within the NHS, insufficient funds to remedy this problem and the inability of the Emergency Services to respond to the demands placed on them. At present, fewer than 2 per cent of women have home births, which suggests that the hospital birth is here to stay and that this is where we should concentrate on improving the environment.

New developments

The development of antenatal care in the millennium: ideas for the future

Antenatal care for the coming decades must enshrine the following aims:

- the life and health of the mother;
- the life and health of the baby(ies);
- the emotional satisfaction of those involved.

It is this last point that has often been overlooked, and which must now be developed in the UK, Europe and North America as we begin the new millennium. The challenge is to accommodate the emotional satisfaction of potential parents whilst, at the same time, not compromising the impressive reduction in maternal and perinatal mortality that has been achieved over the post-war decades. This will be no mean feat, and essentially means a radical overhaul of the way we teach obstetrics, train obstetricians and deliver care antenatally, in labour and the postnatal period.

Key Points

- Maternal mortality has reduced forty-fold in the UK since the beginning of the century: but there is still scope for improvement, for instance by reducing venous thrombo-embolic deaths
- In areas of the world where maternal mortality remains high, initiatives such as ensuring access to contraception, improving the safety of transfused blood and providing temperature-stable oxytocic agents to prevent postpartum haemorrhage, are far more relevant than attempting to reduce risks from thromboembolism
- Modern maternity care should direct technology to those that need it, whilst reducing unnecessary medicalization of completely normal pregnancy

References for further reading

Changing Childbirth. Part 1: Report of the Expert Maternity Group. London: HMSO, 1993.

Williams SA. (ed.) *Women and childbirth in the twentieth century.* Stroud, Gloucestershire, UK: Sutton Publishing Ltd., 1997.

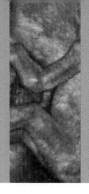

Chapter 3

Maternal and perinatal mortality: the confidential enquiries

OVERVIEW

The death of a woman in childbirth is now a rare event in the UK. Yet maternal death was once commonplace here and still is, sadly, in many countries of the world. A nation's maternal mortality rate is a basic indicator not just of the quality of its health care but of its attitude towards women. Although the safety of the mother is now taken for granted in this country, people are well aware that pregnancy carries risks for the baby's life. It is standard practice for each hospital to monitor the numbers of its stillbirths and neonatal deaths, and any change in the perinatal mortality rate is of local concern. Perinatal mortality is now also being examined on a nationwide basis in England, Wales and Northern Ireland, and new lessons are being learned about why babies die.

Maternal and perinatal deaths in the UK are subject to confidential enquiry, conducted mainly by doctors and midwives. Why 'confidential'? Surely a public enquiry is better than investigation behind closed doors? Public enquiries, however, inevitably become confrontational and lead to defensiveness among the staff involved. A confidential enquiry gives people the chance to be frank in discussing what went wrong, and to suggest how care can be improved. The findings of the national confidential enquiries are made public in regular reports.

Audit in obstetrics

For many years obstetricians have prided themselves on taking the lead in clinical audit. Monitoring mortality rates is one of the most basic ways of checking the effectiveness of a clinical service. Other specialties, such as general surgery, are only now beginning to introduce this form of public audit. Mortality rates are fundamental to the audit process: death is undeniably important, the diagnosis is unarguable and the figures are readily available from the Registrar General. There is of course much more to obstetric care than simply ensuring that mother and baby survive pregnancy and childbirth.

Nowadays we audit rates of intervention, non-fatal adverse outcome, satisfaction among women and long-term health outcomes. Nevertheless safety is paramount. In developing countries maternal and perinatal mortality rates are the main indicators of the quality of maternity services, and they demand constant vigilance even in developed countries.

MATERNAL MORTALITY

In order to make accurate historical or international comparisons, clear definitions are needed; deaths can be maternal, direct, indirect, late or fortuitous.

Definitions

Maternal death
Death of a woman while pregnant, or within 42 days of termination of pregnancy, from any cause related to, or aggravated by, the pregnancy or its management, but not from accidental or incidental causes.

Direct
Deaths resulting from obstetric complications of the pregnant state (pregnancy, labour and puerperium), from interventions, omissions, incorrect treatment or from a chain of events resulting from any of the above.

Indirect
Deaths resulting from previous existing disease, or disease that developed during pregnancy and which was not due to direct obstetric causes, but which was aggravated by the physiologic effects of pregnancy.

Late
Deaths occurring between 42 days and one year after abortion, miscarriage or delivery that are due to direct or indirect causes.

Fortuitous
Deaths from unrelated causes that happen to occur in pregnancy or the puerperium.

Maternal mortality rate
This is generally defined as the number of deaths from obstetric causes per 100,000 maternities. 'Maternities' are the number of mothers delivered of registerable live births at any gestation, or stillbirths of 24 weeks or later.

The global picture

The WHO estimates that there are over half a million maternal deaths every year in the world: 4000 of these occur in developing countries. Rates are highest in Africa, as shown in Table 3.1. The lifetime risk of pregnancy is also shown in Figure 3.1.

In Table 3.1, maternal mortality rates shown are higher in Europe than in North America because of relatively high rates in Eastern Europe. Rates in Western Europe are similar to those in North America, as are those in Australia and New Zealand.

In some rural parts of Africa maternal mortality rates are higher than 1000 per 100,000 live births. The combined problems of high fertility and high maternal mortality in some of the world's poorest countries mean that a woman's lifetime risk of dying of pregnancy-related causes is as high as 1 in 7. In addition, for every mother who dies, as many as 15–20 will suffer serious long-term complications.

Table 3.1 – World Health Organization estimates of maternal mortality (around 1988)

Region	Live births (millions) per year	Maternal deaths (thousands)	Maternal mortality /100,000	Total fertility	Lifetime risk of death from pregnancy
Africa	26.7	169	630	6.1	1 in 23
Asia	81.2	310	380	3.4	1 in 71
Latin America	12.2	25	200	3.4	1 in 131
USSR	5.2	2	45	2.3	1 in 863
Europe	6.4	1	23	1.7	1 in 2288
North America	4.0	1	12	1.8	1 in 4006
World	137.6	509	370	3.4	1 in 73

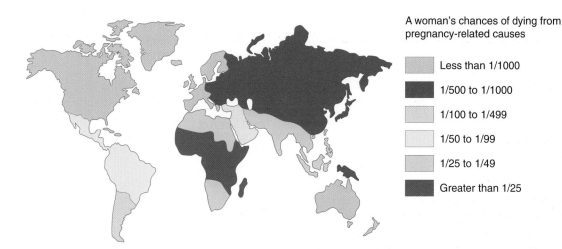

A woman's chances of dying from pregnancy-related causes

Less than 1/1000

1/500 to 1/1000

1/100 to 1/499

1/50 to 1/99

1/25 to 1/49

Greater than 1/25

Figure 3.1 World map showing risk of pregnancy-related death.

The reasons for these deaths differ from country to country but include lack of access to contraception, unsafe abortion and lack of primary care or transport facilities. Lack of basic obstetric care is important: only 55 per cent of deliveries within the developing world are attended by a trained attendant and only 37 per cent of deliveries occur within health facilities.

An important aspect of the problem is access to obstetric services, and the specialist staff and facilities available. Fundamentalist groups in the USA, which refuse all modern medical care, have maternal mortality rates higher than those in developing countries.

Trends in the UK

The maternal mortality rate in Britain has been recorded reliably since 1847, and its history over the last 150 years can be divided into three phases.

Phase 1

Throughout the period from 1847 until 1934 the rate remained virtually unchanged at around 400 per 100,000, or 1 in 250 births. Other indicators of public health, such as infant mortality, had begun to fall well before 1935 and the maternal mortality rate may have been kept artificially high through neglect of asepsis and excessive use of forceps under chloroform anaesthesia by general practitioner obstetricians.

Phase 2

A dramatic fall occurred between 1935 and 1985, when the rate halved every decade (Fig. 3.2). This fall is often seen as part of a general improvement in public health, but the timing suggests the effect of other factors besides improved social conditions. Indeed, as the fall began during the 1930s Depression and continued through the Second World War, improved social conditions may have been only a minor factor. Other improvements were as follows.

- Antibiotics: sulphonamides were introduced in 1937 and penicillin appeared during the Second World War. Death rates from puerperal sepsis quickly fell (Fig. 3.2).
- Blood transfusion became safe during the 1940s.
- Ergometrine, for the treatment and prevention of postpartum haemorrhage, was introduced in the 1940s.
- Better training of midwives and obstetricians: Midwives Acts were passed in 1902 and 1936, and the Royal College of Obstetricians and Gynaecologists was founded in 1929.
- Reduced parity: the average family size had already begun to fall before the pill was introduced in 1961.
- Legalisation of abortion in 1967 was followed by elimination of criminal abortion as a cause of maternal death (Fig. 3.3).

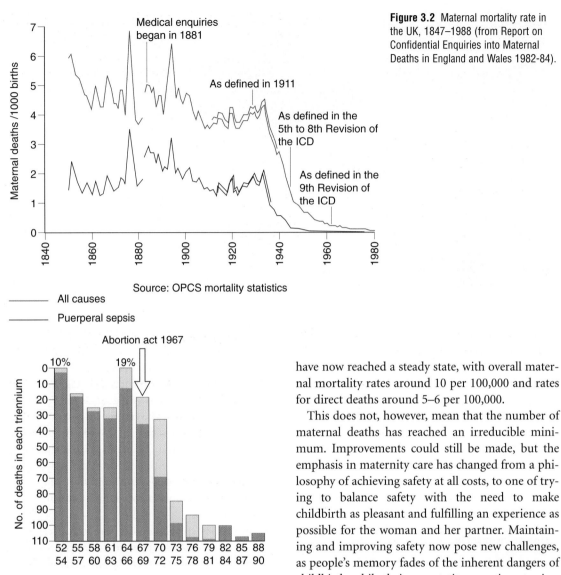

Figure 3.2 annotations: Medical enquiries began in 1881; As defined in 1911; As defined in the 5th to 8th Revision of the ICD; As defined in the 9th Revision of the ICD

Figure 3.2 Maternal mortality rate in the UK, 1847–1988 (from Report on Confidential Enquiries into Maternal Deaths in England and Wales 1982-84).

Source: OPCS mortality statistics

——— All causes

——— Puerperal sepsis

Abortion act 1967

Legal

Illegal

(Percentages within columns that of all direct maternal deaths in that triennium, 10% and 19% were caused by abortion)

Figure 3.3 Reduction in maternal deaths from abortion 1952–96.

Phase 3

Since 1985 there has been little change in the maternal mortality rate in the UK, and it is likely that we have now reached a steady state, with overall maternal mortality rates around 10 per 100,000 and rates for direct deaths around 5–6 per 100,000.

This does not, however, mean that the number of maternal deaths has reached an irreducible minimum. Improvements could still be made, but the emphasis in maternity care has changed from a philosophy of achieving safety at all costs, to one of trying to balance safety with the need to make childbirth as pleasant and fulfilling an experience as possible for the woman and her partner. Maintaining and improving safety now pose new challenges, as people's memory fades of the inherent dangers of childbirth, while their expectations continue to rise.

It may or may not be a coincidence that the rapid fall in maternal mortality began soon after the introduction of a system of enquiries into maternal deaths.

THE CONFIDENTIAL ENQUIRY

In 1928 the British Government set up a committee on maternal mortality and morbidity. This committee introduced the concept of a 'primary avoidable factor' in its reports. In 1951 a more thorough system of reviewing cases was started (Fig. 3.4a and b).

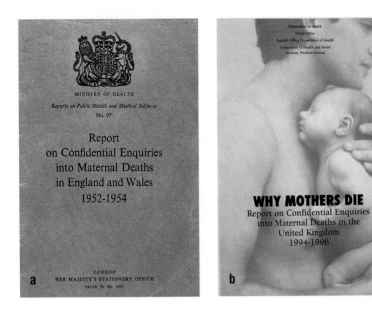

Figure 3.4 Maternal mortality reports from (a) 1952–54 and (b) 1994–96. (Crown copyright material is reproduced with the permission of the Controller of Her Majesty's Stationery Office.)

As noted above, the enquiries are conducted by clinicians: doctors and now midwives.

Method

When a woman dies during pregnancy or within a year after pregnancy, the Director of Public Health Medicine sends an enquiry form to the general practitioners, midwives, health visitors, obstetricians and any other staff involved in her care. The form requests full information about the case.

The completed form is then sent to Regional Assessors in obstetrics, midwifery, anaesthesia (if appropriate) and pathology. They add their comments and the form is sent to the Chief Medical Officer. It is made anonymous then passed to Central Assessors of the same disciplines to assess the causes of death and decide whether any aspects of the care were substandard.

Every three years a national report is published which collates all the cases, draws attention to areas of 'substandard care' and makes recommendations. The report excludes any details that might allow identification of individual cases.

This system originally applied to England though arrangements were similar in the rest of the UK. The last four national reports have covered the whole of the UK, again making it difficult for individual cases to be identified.

Causes of maternal mortality

In the triennium 1994–96 there were 376 maternal deaths, of which 268 were direct or indirect and the remainder were fortuitous or late deaths. The causes of the 133 direct and 134 indirect maternal deaths were:

Causes of maternal mortality

Direct deaths

Thrombosis and thromboembolism		48
Hypertensive disease		20
Amniotic fluid embolism		17
Early pregnancy deaths		15
Ectopic pregnancy	12	
Spontaneous miscarriage	2	
Legal termination	1	
Sepsis		14
Haemorrhage		12
Genital tract trauma		5
Other direct causes		2

Indirect deaths

Cardiac disease		39
Psychiatric disorder		9
Other indirect causes..................		86

The causes of maternal death are broadly similar in developed and developing countries, but the ranking is different. In the developing world, haemorrhage, sepsis and hypertensive disease are likely to be at the top of the list.

Thromboembolism

Pregnancy causes changes in the clotting factors and, labour and the puerperium may cause venous stasis, particularly after caesarean section. Death from thromboembolism can occur at any stage of pregnancy, even in the first trimester or after an ectopic pregnancy, and the risk continues throughout the puerperium.

Of the 48 deaths due to thromboembolism in 1994–96, 43 were cases of pulmonary thromboembolism, full details of which were available. Of these, 18 occurred before delivery and 25 after delivery. Two further deaths occurred more than 42 days after delivery and were counted as 'late deaths'.

Women at risk of postpartum thromboembolism are those over 35, very obese women and those who have had Caesarean Section. It is a striking feature in the report that in some cases complaints of leg pain in women, with all these known risk factors, are sometimes not taken seriously.

The risk of thromboembolism can be reduced by increased use of prophylaxis, for example with compression stockings, and by constant vigilance among GPs for suspicious symptoms during pregnancy and the puerperium, especially among women at high risk. Those at highest risk, women with a personal or family history of thromboembolism and those with thrombophilia, should receive heparin prophylaxis.

Hypertensive disorders

Of the 20 women who died of this cause in 1994–96, only one had pre-existing hypertension. The median gestation at the time of presentation with severe disease was 32 weeks' gestation, but four of the deaths occurred before 29 weeks' gestation. Only four deaths were due to intracranial haemorrhage. The immediate cause of death was acute respiratory distress syndrome in six cases and pulmonary or cerebral oedema in five cases. The others were ruptured liver, liver failure and pneumonia.

Eclampsia occurred in eight of the cases. Magnesium sulphate is now being recognised as the treatment of choice for eclamptic fits, but as few of the

cases in the Enquiry suffered multiple fits it remains uncertain whether widespread use of magnesium sulphate will reduce the mortality from this condition.

Substandard care was evident in 59 per cent of assessable cases, and this applied mainly to hospitals rather than GPs or midwives. When a woman has been admitted to hospital, pregnancy-induced hypertension is often managed at too junior a level, and symptoms are not taken seriously enough.

Amniotic fluid embolism

In this condition amniotic fluid enters the maternal circulation and causes an intense reaction in the lungs. Proof of the diagnosis is the finding of fetal squames in the maternal lungs at autopsy. It causes sudden collapse, usually during labour though cases have been reported after Caesarean Section, and it carries a high mortality. It was formerly thought to be associated with high parity but only three of the 17 cases reported in 1994–96 were of high parity. Many of the cases had had some form of obstetric intervention, such as induction of labour, but there was no clear pattern to link the condition with a specific intervention.

Early pregnancy deaths

Deaths occurring before 24 weeks' gestation are now included in this category (formerly the upper limit was 20 weeks). They include deaths due to ectopic pregnancy, spontaneous abortion and termination of pregnancy.

Ectopic pregnancy

Among the 12 deaths from ectopic pregnancy in 1994–96, the main problem was delayed diagnosis, particularly in socially disadvantaged women. Nowadays the diagnosis of ectopic pregnancy is a simple matter, but only if the possibility is constantly borne in mind. If abdominal pain is associated with a positive pregnancy test, the woman should be referred to hospital but even then diagnosis can be difficult, as ultrasound appearances can be deceptive in this condition.

Spontaneous abortion

Two deaths occurred from this cause in 1994–96, both due to infection.

Termination of pregnancy

It is now more than 10 years since the last maternal death from illegal abortion in Britain, but a small number of deaths from legal abortion continue to occur (see Fig. 3.3). In 1994–96 there was one such death, due to unrecognized bowel perforation during suction termination of a 15-week pregnancy.

Sepsis

Puerperal sepsis accounted for over 1000 deaths a year in Britain before 1937. The introduction of antibiotics has not quite eliminated it, and in 1994–96 there were 11 deaths from this cause. Other deaths were caused by sepsis after abortion, after caesarean section or before, or during, labour. Prophylactic antibiotics are recommended for Caesarean Section but not for normal vaginal delivery.

Haemorrhage

In general, obstetric haemorrhage is well-managed in the UK but deaths from bleeding still occur. They are approximately equally divided between antepartum and postpartum haemorrhage. Deaths from antepartum haemorrhage are equally divided between placenta praevia and abruptio placentae.

Placenta praevia

Three deaths from placenta praevia occurred in 1994–96. There is a particular risk when the placenta is implanted over a uterine scar. Caesarean Section for placenta praevia must be carried out by a consultant or senior registrar.

Abruptio placentae

Severe abruptio placentae is usually complicated by coagulopathy. In 1994–96 four deaths occurred from abruption. Two were in the middle trimester of pregnancy. Abruptio usually causes severe pain but the Report describes one woman who seemed well enough to wait in a cubicle in an Accident and Emergency Department: when the doctor saw her two hours later she was dead.

Postpartum haemorrhage

Of the five deaths from postpartum haemorrhage in 1994–96, four followed Caesarean Section and one followed vacuum extraction. There were no deaths from this cause after spontaneous vaginal delivery.

Although death rates from this cause are low, studies of 'near-misses' show that the incidence of life-threatening haemorrhage is around 1 in 1000 deliveries. This means that around 600 lives are saved by effective treatment in the UK every year. The risk of death increases with the woman's age, perhaps because older women are less able to cope with the effects of sudden haemorrhage.

Each hospital should have clear guidelines for the management of massive haemorrhage, and practice runs or rehearsals are advisable.

Genital tract trauma

Five deaths from this cause occurred in 1994–96. One was due to vaginal and uterine laceration after instrumental delivery. The other four were due to uterine rupture, and two of these cases followed induction of labour (one in a woman with a previous caesarean section scar). The other two uterine ruptures occurred during pregnancy (one associated with placenta percreta). Rupture of the uterus during pregnancy is extremely rare.

Anaesthesia

In 1994–96 there were 19 deaths associated with anaesthesia, but only one was due directly to the anaesthetic. Substandard care was present in that case. The safety of obstetric anaesthesia has improved dramatically over the last 20 years, and the risk of death is now around one in a million maternities. Reasons for this improvement include greater use of epidural rather than general anaesthesia, the exclusion of the most junior training grades from unsupervised work, and ready access to intensive care facilities.

Indirect deaths

Cardiac disease

For many years rheumatic heart disease was a major cause of maternal mortality in Britain, and it still is in many developing countries. In 1994–96, however, for the first time there were no deaths from rheumatic heart disease. Of the 40 maternal deaths from cardiac disease, 10 were from congenital disease, seven from myocardial infarction and 23 from other acquired conditions (mainly cardiomyopathy and aortic aneurysm).

The increased cardiac output of pregnancy puts a strain on a diseased heart. Patients with known heart disease should be managed by a cardiologist in co-operation with an obstetrician.

Psychiatric deaths

In the 1994–96 report, deaths from psychiatric causes are discussed separately for the first time. There were 28 deaths included in this category, almost all due to suicide — more than the number of deaths from hypertensive disease. Five of the deaths occurred during pregnancy, four before 42 days postpartum and the rest were late deaths. The report recommends screening at booking for psychiatric disorder, substance abuse or severe social problems, and a liaison service provided for patients identified as at-risk.

Other indirect deaths

Many diseases are exacerbated by pregnancy, but of the total of 86 deaths in 1994–96 the largest single cause was epilepsy, which caused 19 deaths. Relatives should be informed about the risks and educated to place patients in the recovery position once the fit is over. Pregnant women who are at risk of fits should not bathe alone, or use a shower.

Additional points in management

The pattern of maternal mortality is continually changing and the 1994–96 report produced some surprises. For example, the high proportion of deaths due to thromboembolism contrasts with the pattern in other countries and may be due in part to better awareness of these cases in the UK. The fall in deaths due to anaesthesia is not only a tribute to the quality of anaesthetic services, but is also relevant to discussions with women when caesarean section is being considered. The disappearance of rheumatic heart disease as a cause of maternal death is a cause for satisfaction.

There are also causes for concern. In 1994–96, for the first time, death rates were assessed by ethnic origin and were found to be higher among black women. Other countries have also found higher rates among non-Caucasians. The causes for these deaths are not clear and further research is needed.

The enquiries must not only gather accurate data but also interpret them intelligently. This involves regular reappraisal, particularly with a long-running enquiry. The recent realization that maternal suicide is now one of the major causes of mortality is an example of this, and highlights the need for better service provision.

'Near miss' enquiries

As the number of maternal deaths has declined in Britain, there have been suggestions that instead of looking only at deaths, enquiries should be widened to include 'near misses': incidents which might have resulted in a maternal death but for prompt and effective treatment. A 'near miss' is difficult to define, and national figures would probably be much less reliable than data on maternal deaths.

Nevertheless, 'near misses' have been examined on a local basis, using criteria such as admission to an intensive care unit. In a comprehensive survey in Pretoria, South Africa, a full list of criteria for 'near misses' has been developed. One of the main findings of these investigations is that haemorrhage is much more common among 'near misses' than in mortality enquiries.

New developments

Low maternal mortality rates in developed countries are now taken for granted and there is a tendency for people to forget what risks there are when care is not available. Practices that were introduced, often arbitrarily, in Phase 2 (page 21), when efforts were concentrated on improving safety, are now being questioned. The aim now is to remove unnecessary restrictions without compromising safety. It is unlikely that rates of maternal mortality will rise again while they are carefully monitored, but our aim should be to reduce them still further. This is quite a challenge, because as maternity care and maternal health improve, life-threatening events become even less common, and as a result staff are less practised in dealing with them.

PERINATAL MORTALITY

Perinatal death is about one hundred times more common than maternal death. Perinatal mortality rates therefore often seem more relevant to day-to-day practice, and because of the larger numbers of cases they perhaps give a clearer picture of the problems that may be encountered. However, analysis of individual cases at a national level is more difficult because of the large numbers.

As with maternal mortality data, the diagnosis of death is unequivocal. Furthermore, perinatal death is usually followed by a postmortem examination, which enables the cause of death to be accurately defined. One possible cause of difficulty, however, is that different countries may have different definitions of the dividing line between miscarriage and stillbirth. Definitions in this area can sometimes be confusing.

Definitions

The definitions that follow are those used by the Confidential Enquiry into Stillbirths and Deaths in Infancy (CESDI) (Fig. 3.5a and b) which is described below.

CESDI looks at all deaths from 20 weeks of pregnancy to the end of the first year of life, but only a proportion of these fulfil the definition of 'perinatal

deaths'. For example, death between 20 and 24 weeks of pregnancy is not counted in the perinatal mortality statistics.

Stillbirth
This is any fetus born with no signs of life, after 24 weeks' gestation.

(Note the British definition of stillbirth was changed in October 1992. Before that time only deaths after 28 weeks' gestation were included. The change in definition added nearly 30 per cent to the former official stillbirth rate.)

Early neonatal death
This denotes death in the first week after birth.

Perinatal deaths
All stillbirths, plus deaths in the first week after birth.

Perinatal Mortality Rate (PMR)
This term is used to define the number of perinatal deaths per thousand live births and stillbirths.

In addition to these cases, CESDI gathers data on deaths beyond the first week after birth. These definitions are given below.

Late neonatal death
Death from age 7 days to 27 completed days of life

Postneonatal death
Death at age 28 days and over, but under one year.

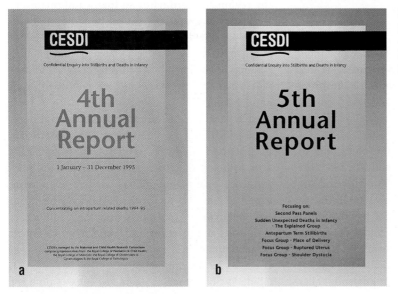

Figure 3.5 (a) Confidential Enquiry into Stillbirths and Deaths in Infancy 4th Annual Report; (b) Confidential Enquiry into Stillbirths and Deaths in Infancy 5th Annual Report.

Infant death

Death at age under one year.

Rates of neonatal and infant death are expressed as rates per thousand live births.

The worldwide picture

Across the world, there are wide differences in perinatal mortality rates. Overall life expectancy in some countries is less than half that in others, and this is largely due to high death rates in small children. For example, in much of southeast Asia, 40 per cent of children die by their fourth year, and in parts of central Africa infant mortality is ten times that in developed countries. The underlying reason is often malnutrition, which makes children more susceptible to infection and affects particularly those born into large and poorly spaced families. Promotion of breastfeeding is particularly important in developing countries. Not only does it provide appropriate nourishment for the newborn, but also it reduces the risk of infection from artificial feeding, provides passive immunity through maternal antibodies, and acts as a natural contraceptive to ensure adequate pregnancy spacing.

Amongst developed countries, comparisons of perinatal mortality rates can be misleading because different countries have minor variations in the definition.

History in the UK

Data on perinatal mortality have been collected in the UK for the last 60 years. During this time there has been a dramatic reduction in perinatal deaths. This has been mainly due to the improved health of the population, better nutrition and wider education, with an important but lesser role played by the medical professions.

Since 1963, stillbirth and neonatal death rates in England and Wales have fallen steadily. In 1963, the stillbirth rate was over 17 per 1000 births and the neonatal death rate was over 14 per 1000 births. In 1996 these rates were respectively 5.4 per 1000 total births and 4.1 per 1000 live births. The total perinatal mortality rate has remained stable from 1993 to 1996.

In 1996, according to the Fifth Annual CESDI Report, there were 677,758 births in England, Wales and Northern Ireland, and the total number of perinatal deaths was 5898, giving a perinatal mortality rate of 8.7 per 1000 total births. The numbers of deaths in the other categories were as follows:

Stillbirths	3688
Early neonatal deaths	2210
Neonatal deaths (total)	2785
Postneonatal deaths	1253

Method of the confidential enquiry

CESDI was set up in 1992 to improve understanding of how the risks of death from 20 weeks of pregnancy to one year after birth, might be reduced. CESDI attempts to identify risks that can be attributed to suboptimal clinical care.

In 1991 the Department of Health directed that the fourteen health regions of England undertake perinatal mortality surveys. Each region has a full-time co-ordinator with support staff. This network formed the basis of CESDI, with separate arrangements for Scotland, Wales and Northern Ireland. Much additional work is done by district co-ordinators, often working in their own time. The Department of Health still funds the Enquiry, but in 1996 its management was assumed by a consortium of Royal Colleges: those of Midwives, Obstetricians and Gynaecologists, Paediatrics and Child Health, and Pathology.

In the three countries there are some 10,000 deaths annually occurring between 20 weeks' gestation and one year of life. All deaths are notified to the regional co-ordinator so that a full picture of the causes of death is obtained. In addition, a specialist panel within each region reviews a sub-set of anonymous cases. The regional data and enquiry findings are collated by a central secretariat to provide a national overview and are published in an annual report.

Each panel consists of experts from several disciplines, including as a minimum, an obstetrician, paediatrician, midwife, specialist perinatal/paediatric pathologist, general practitioner and an independent chairman. Others with appropriate expertise may also be involved. Panel members are sent anonymous case-notes and they summarise their cases and meet for discussion. They comment on suboptimal care, grading each case as follows:

Grade 0 - No suboptimal care

Grade 1 - Suboptimal care, but different

management would have made no difference to the outcome

Grade 2 - Suboptimal care and different management might have made a difference to the outcome

Grade 3 - Suboptimal care and different management would reasonably have been expected to make a difference to the outcome.

Causes of perinatal mortality

The original classification proposed by Professor Wigglesworth has been extended as follows:

Category 1 – Congenital defect or malformation (lethal or severe)

Category 2 – Antepartum fetal death

Category 3 – Death from intrapartum asphyxia, anoxia or trauma

Category 4 – Immaturity

Category 5 – Infection

Category 6 – Other specific causes

Category 7 – Accident or non-intrapartum trauma

Category 8 – Sudden infant death, cause unknown

Category 9 – Unclassifiable (to be used as a last resort)

The commonest causes of perinatal mortality in 1996 are shown in Table 3.2

Thus 41 per cent of the total deaths up to the end of the first month of life were due to antepartum fetal death, 22 per cent to immaturity, 16 per cent to congenital malformations, and almost 10 per cent to intrapartum anoxia. Some of these conditions still cause death after the first month of life. Among the 1253 postneonatal deaths the common causes of death were Sudden Infant Death Syndrome (31.3 per cent), congenital malformation (29.1 per cent), infection (14.4 per cent) and immaturity (11.4 per cent).

Five causes of perinatal mortality in order of frequency of occurence

1. prematurity
2. congenital malformation
3. antepartum fetal death
4. birth asphyxia
5. infection

Table 3.2 – The commonest causes of perinatal mortality in 1996

Stillbirths: (total 3688)	
Antepartum fetal death	2666 (73%)
Congenital malformation	373 (10.1%)
Intrapartum anoxia	372 (10.1%)
Infection	80 (2.2%)

Early and Late Neonatal deaths: (total 2785)	
Immaturity	1390 (49.9%)
Congenital malformation	632 (22.7%)
Intrapartum anoxia	261 (9.4%)
Infection	197 (7.1%)

The individual causes will be discussed briefly in the order of the extended Wigglesworth classification.

1. Congenital malformation

Congenital abnormalities account for about 16 per cent of the perinatal deaths in the UK. Twenty years ago many of the malformations were neural tube defects (NTDs); spina bifida or anencephaly. However, the introduction of screening, first by serum alpha-fetoprotein and more recently by routine ultrasound, has resulted in the identification of the majority of NTDs at a gestation when the woman can be offered termination of pregnancy. This has resulted in a decrease in perinatal mortality but an increase in therapeutic termination for this condition. The Government has recently advised that all women should take periconceptual folic acid to reduce the incidence of NTDs: it remains to be seen whether this will be effective.

One of the most difficult structures to visualize adequately by ultrasound *in utero* is the cardiovascular system, and it is not surprising therefore that cardiovascular abnormalities now constitute the largest proportion of lethal congenital anomalies.

Biochemical screening for chromosomal abnormalities is now widely available through tests such as the 'triple test'. The commonest chromosomal abnormality, Down's syndrome, usually does not cause neonatal death and therefore this screening programme has little effect on perinatal mortality.

2. Antepartum fetal death

This category covers a heterogeneous group of causes. Fetal asphyxia may occur before labour as a result of premature separation of the placenta (placental abruption). Fortunately, the incidence of placental abruption appears to be on the decline. Another cause is inadequate placentation where the fetus is exposed to chronic hypoxia over a number of weeks. Asphyxia may then occur during labour, when a chronically starved fetus is subjected to the stress of labour.

Antepartum term stillbirth was the subject of a special study in the Fifth Annual CESDI Report. Cases were compared with controls and parents were interviewed in addition to the usual methods of gathering data. Of 86 cases studied, 27 were unexplained and 22 were associated with intrauterine growth restriction. Of the remainder, the two commonest conditions were placental abruption (nine cases) and and abnormal glucose tolerance (nine cases).

In the CESDI survey there was an excess of mothers of ethnic origin. It was also noted that many mothers had noticed a change in fetal movements or the occurrence of abdominal pain. These symptoms are very non-specific but may point the way towards further research in the future.

3. Intrapartum asphyxia

This cause was the subject of the Fourth Annual CESDI Report. In 1994 and 1995, of 19,348 deaths between 20 weeks and one year of age, 1266 (6.5 per cent) were of normally formed babies, of at least 1.5 kg in weight, dying after the onset of labour and before 28 days of life. The report looked at 873 cases of death from intrapartum related events. The risk of death in labour was 1 in 1561 births, and when the cases were looked at in detail, over 78 per cent were criticized for suboptimal care. Alternative management might (25 per cent) or 'would reasonably be expected to' (52 per cent) have made a difference to the outcome.

Although the risk of a baby dying in labour is less than 1 in 1000 it is very worrying that such a high

proportion of cases had suboptimal management. The main problem in antepartum care was failure to recognize risk factors, and the main problem in intrapartum care was inadequate assessment of the fetal condition by heart rate monitoring and fetal blood sampling. In 22 per cent of cases there was also criticism of the resuscitation of the newborn.

The report's recommendations, based on these findings, were radical. Three recommendations are particularly important:
1. 'The training, assessment, supervision and practice of obstetricians and midwives of all grades needs to be critically appraised by their parent bodies';
2. Professional bodies should 'look again at how level of practical competence of professionals of all grades caring for women in labour and for babies following delivery are achieved and maintained';
3. 'A multidisciplinary initiative at national level is needed to develop guidelines covering all aspects of fetal assessment before and especially during labour.'

The Royal Colleges of Midwives and of Obstetricians and Gynaecologists have responded to this recommendation by publishing guidelines for improved standards of care in labour, which recommend, among other things, more involvement of consultant obstetricians in the day-to-day running of delivery suites in Britain.

4. Immaturity

Although only 8 per cent of babies are born prematurely, this group contains 50 per cent of neonatal deaths. The immediate causes of death amongst this group include respiratory distress syndrome, infection, neurological causes and gastrointestinal causes. Advances in neonatal care have improved the survival of many premature infants but this has resulted in attempts to resuscitate even more premature fetuses.

From the obstetric point of view, there is clear evidence that giving the mother steroids before preterm delivery will reduce the baby's risk of developing respiratory distress syndrome, and reduce perinatal mortality. Steroids need to be given at least 24 hours before delivery, however, and sometimes it is impossible to delay delivery long enough to give them time to work.

Other categories

The other five categories of perinatal mortality are more relevant to postneonatal deaths.

Infection
This applies when there is clear microbiological evidence of infection, e.g. Group B streptococci.

Other specific causes
Some fetal, neonatal or paediatric conditions are not covered in the four main categories, e.g. hydrops fetalis, persistent transitional circulation or malignancy.

Accident or non-intrapartum trauma
This includes confirmed non-accidental injury.

Sudden infant death, cause unknown
This category includes all infants in whom the cause was unknown at the time of death. Information from postmortem may be added later.

Unclassifiable
This category may be used but only as a last resort.

Women's expectations

Most women are unwilling to take any risks with their baby's health. When attempts are made to quantify risks, the risks considered acceptable by doctors tend to be regarded as unacceptably high by mothers. If something goes wrong and a baby suffers death or handicap, the parents are now less inclined to think of this as an act of God and more likely to ask whether an error occurred in the clinical management. With some causes, such as antepartum stillbirth, death is often unavoidable but intrapartum asphyxia, in particular, is indeed associated with suboptimal practice in many cases. The high expectations of parents and professionals are major factors underlying the steady increase in the Caesarean Section rate in the UK.

Critical incident reporting

For many years it has been standard practice for hospitals to hold perinatal mortality meetings to review cases of perinatal death. The clinical features and the pathological findings are examined and the implications for management of similar cases are discussed. We are now beginning to recognize that this method should be extended to include 'near miss' incidents, and hospitals are introducing critical incident reporting. A critical incident is any event that a member of staff feels might put patients at risk. Such incidents are reported to a senior member of staff who decides that incidents should be discussed at staff meetings. Risk management committees are established in many UK obstetric units and assess 'near misses' and critical incidents leading to the implementation of recommendations.

New developments

Perinatal mortality could be reduced still further. Intrapartum management can be improved, with better training in the interpretation of electronic monitoring and more involvement of senior staff. Antepartum stillbirths remain a considerable challenge, and research is needed on the most effective way of detecting intrauterine growth restriction. A key part of reducing antepartum and intrapartum stillbirths will be the presence of more senior staff on labour wards and the appointment of new consultants.

COMPARISON OF MATERNAL AND PERINATAL MORTALITY

When comparing maternal and perinatal mortality rates, the denominators are more important than the numerators. Maternal mortality rates are expressed per hundred thousand births and perinatal mortality rates per thousand births. The risk to the baby around the time of childbirth is therefore about one hundred times higher than that to the mother. Every year in the UK there are about one hundred maternal deaths and about ten thousand perinatal deaths.

After its dramatic fall in the middle of the twentieth century the maternal mortality rate has reached a new steady state. It could be reduced further if substandard care was eliminated but this will require sustained effort by general practitioners as well as midwives and obstetricians. The main task is to maintain the excellent levels of safety that were achieved in the late 1980s.

Perinatal mortality continued to fall during the 1980s but rates have remained steady during the 1990s. The lowest rate of intrapartum-related stillbirth was in 1989, and there has been a slight rise since then. The perinatal mortality rate could be reduced substantially, by further research on antepartum stillbirth and, more urgently, by eliminating suboptimal care in labour.

References for further reading

Pittrof R. The sorry state of reproductive health of women: a global overview. *Contemporary Reviews in Obstetrics and Gynaecology* 1996; **8:** 93-7.

Kaunitz AM, Spence C, Danielson TS, Rochard RW, Grimes DA. Perinatal and maternal mortality in a religious group avoiding obstetric care. *American Journal of Obstetrics and Gynecology* 1994; **150:** 826-31.

Loudon I. *Death in childbirth: an international study of maternal care and maternal mortality 1800-1950.* Oxford: Clarendon Press, 1992.

Department of Health. R*eport on Confidential Enquiries into Maternal Deaths in the UK 1994-96.* London: HMSO, 1998.

Mantel GD, Buchmann E, Rees H, Pattinson RC. Severe acute maternal morbidity: a pilot study for a definition of a near-miss. *British Journal of Obstetrics and Gynaecology* 1998; **105:** 985-90.

Drife J. Management of primary postpartum haemorrhage. *British Journal of Obstetrics and Gynaecology* 1997; **104:** 275-7.

Schuitemaker N, van Roosmalen J, Dekker G, van Donger P, van Geijn H, Gravenhorst JB. Confidential enquiry into maternal deaths in the Netherlands 1983-1992. *European Journal of Obstetrics, Gynaecology and Reproductive Biology* 1998; **79:** 57-62.

Baskett TF and Sternadel J. Maternal intensive care and near-miss mortality in obstetrics. *British Journal of Obstetrics and Gynaecology* 1998; **105:** 981-4.

Confidential Enquiry into Stillbirth and Deaths in Infancy. Fifth Annual Report. London: Maternal and Child Health Research Consortium, 1998.

Confidential Enquiry into Stillbirths and Deaths in Infancy. Fourth Annual Report: concentrating on intrapartum deaths 1994-95. London: Maternal and Child Health Research Consortium, 1997.

Royal College of Obstetricians and Gynaecologists. *Report of the Working Party on Minimum Standards of Care in Labour.* London: RCOG, 1998.

Thornton JG. Measuring patients' values in reproductive medicine. *Contemporary Reviews in Obstetrics and Gynaecology* 1988; **1:** 5-12.

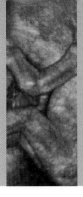

Chapter 4

Conception, implantation and embryology

OVERVIEW

It is becoming increasingly accepted that knowledge of the fundamental processes involved in conception, implantation and the early development of the human form will provide an understanding of the basic pathologies causing infertility, miscarriage, genetic disorders, abnormalities of fetal growth and placental function and even cardiovascular disease in later life. In the future, most of the important pioneering research will be focused on the earliest stages of human development.

Mitotic and meiotic division of primordial germ cells produce eggs and sperm cells.

Somatic versus germ cells

The human body has two types of cells: somatic cells and highly specialized germ cells. Somatic cells are diploid with the exception of sex chromosomes X and Y. Diploid cells have two copies of each chromosome described as homologues, one from the father and the other from the mother. These are found in cells, for example, from the brain, liver or heart. Prior to mitosis, each homologue is duplicated and the two copies remain together as sister chromatids. During mitosis, the sister chromatids are separated from each other and therefore each of the two daughter cells inherit one copy of each homologue (Fig. 4.1).

The mature germ cells (sperm or egg), unlike somatic cells, have only one copy of each chromosome and therefore are haploid. Following fertilization, fusion of the male and female pronuclei re-establish diploidy.

Mitosis and meiosis

Both mitosis and meiosis begin with diploid cells. However, the product of mitosis is two diploid daughter cells, whereas, a meiotic division leads to four haploid daughter cells. A diagram comparing mitotic and meiotic divisions is shown in Figure 4.1. Unlike mitosis, cell division occurs twice in meiosis. At the end of division 1, two haploid 2n daughter cells are produced. During the second division, no DNA replication occurs. Thus, 23 double-stranded chromosomes lined up in metaphase will separate as single-stranded chromosomes to form the nucleus of each daughter cell.

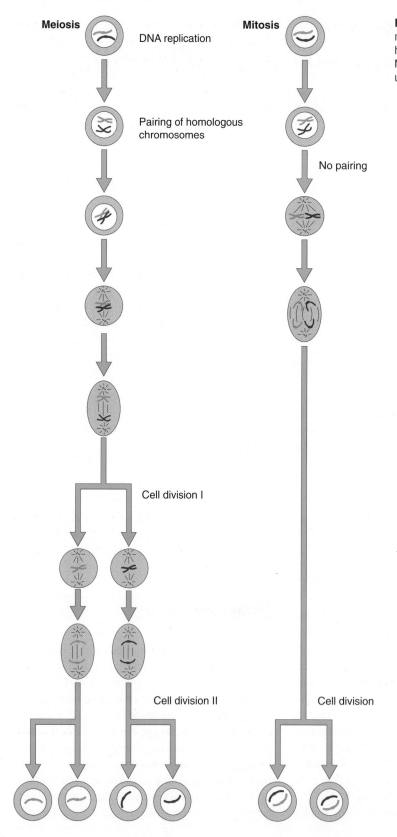

Meiosis

DNA replication

Pairing of homologous
chromosomes

Cell division I

Cell division II

Mitosis

No pairing

Cell division

Figure 4.1 A comparison of meiosis to
mitosis. To simplify, only one set of
homologous chromosomes is shown.
Note that pairing of homologues is
unique to meiosis.

Spermatogenesis and oogenesis in brief

Spermatogenesis: production of mature sperm

Spermatogenesis occurs in the seminiferous tubules of the testis. The primordial germ cells divide to produce spermatogonia, the precursors of mature sperm. The spermatogonia located at the basal lamina of the tubule begin to divide mitotically at the onset of puberty. Many of these daughter cells which are capable of undergoing further division are called primary spermatocytes. These spermatocytes undergo first meiotic division to produce the secondary spermatocytes. The diploid secondary spermatocytes further divide (meiotic division II) to produce the haploid spermatids (Fig. 4.2a).

The differentiation of round spermatids to motile spermatozoa is called spermiogenesis. Note that round spermatids appear like any other somatic cells with a distinct nucleus. During differentiation, a series of changes happen to produce a motile sperm. The most visible change is the reduction in size and formation of a tail, which allows the sperm cells to swim. The chromosomes in the sperm cells are almost crystallized by a special set of sperm-specific proteins called protamines. In fact, this protamine-induced condensation of the sperm chromosomes is so extensive that the size of the sperm nucleus is about one-thirtieth the size of a mature human egg. This compact structure of the sperm is important for its motility and we shall discuss below how these chromosomes are unpackaged during fertilization. In the human, it takes more than three weeks to complete meiosis and more than two months for a spermatogonia to divide into four mature sperm.

Oogenesis and maturation of eggs

In principle, the development of a mature egg from a primordial germ cell producing oogonia in the ovary is very similar to that of spermatogenesis in the testis. However there are some distinct cellular and biochemical differences. Following first meiotic division of primary to secondary oocytes, one of the two daughter cells, described as the first polar body, degenerates. Similarly, one of the two daughter cells produced after the second meiotic division, the second polar body, fails to survive. Therefore, one diploid oogonia after mitotic and meiotic divisions produces one haploid mature egg (Fig. 4.2b). In contrast, one diploid spermatogonia gives rise to four haploid mature spermatozoa.

Key Points

- In humans, most cells contain 46 chromosomes. These cells are in a diploid state
- Meiosis generates mature (haploid) eggs or sperm containing 23 chromosomes
- A diploid primary spermatocyte undergoes meiosis to produce 4 haploid mature sperm
- A diploid primary oocyte undergoes meiosis. It produces only one haploid mature ovum (containing one polar body)
- During the second meiosis, the primary oocyte remains in meiotic arrest. It will resume once fertilization has occurred

Conception

Conception is the consequence of several complex events that include the final maturation of the spermatozoa and oocyte, transport of the gametes in the female genital tract and, following the fusion of the male and female gametes, the assembly of a diploid number of chromosomes referred to as syngamy.

Key Points

- All mature eggs (ova) contain 23 chromosomes
- Mature sperm also contain 23 chromosomes
- One of the 23 chromosomes in all ova and sperm is a sex chromosome
- Unlike the female ovum which contains only X chromosomes, the sperm contain either X or Y chromosomes
- The resulting embryo contains 46 chromosomes, of which two will be sex chromosomes. A normal sex combination therefore will be either XX (female) or XY (male)
- The sperm determines the sex of a child

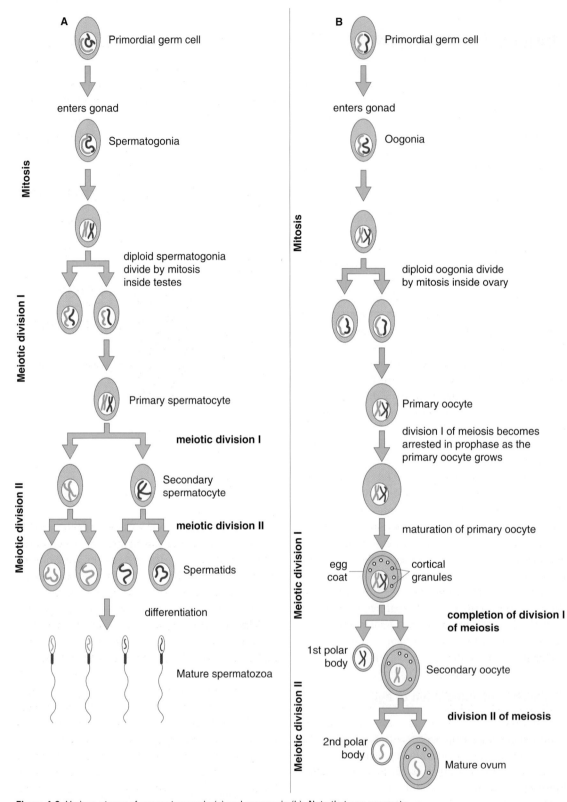

Figure 4.2 Various stages of spermatogenesis (a) and oogenesis (b). Note that one spermatogonia divides into four haploid mature spermotazoa whereas one oogonia produces only one haploid mature ovum or egg.

The sperm

Spermatozoa are produced at the onset of puberty in boys. Thereafter the seminiferous tubules of the testis will go on producing sperm daily until 60 years of age and beyond.

Following spermatogenesis, the spermatozoa pass through the seminiferous tubules to the rete testis, on to the vasa deferentia, the head of the epididymis and thence 12 days later to the tail of the epididymis. Transport of the mature sperm is via muscular activity within the epididymis and vas. The seminal fluid is made up from the secretions of a number of glands, such as the bulbo-urethral, seminal vesicles and the prostate, to all of which must be added the half a millilitre or so of epididymal fluid. During this time, the sperm acquires motility and undergoes the final biochemical changes that give them the ability to fertilize the ovum. The mature sperm containing a haploid number of chromosomes (22 + X or Y) is a few microns long. The mature sperm travels a distance of 30–40 cm in the female genital tract to fertilize the oocyte. Spermatozoa have a complex structure that provides motility and propulsion (tail), energy source (midpiece) and the acrosome for penetrating the oocyte (Fig 4.3).

Seminal fluid containing sperm coagulates immediately following ejaculation. Under normal circumstances it liquifies within 20 minutes. The basic pH of the seminal fluid protects the spermatozoa from the acidity of the vagina. Sometimes, when certain enzymes are missing in the seminal fluid, the coagulation persists and this could cause a type of infertility by restricting the sperm from accessing the cervix. Within minutes after ejaculation, sperm may be found in the cervix and are released constantly over a period of up to 72 hours.

During this time the sperm will move with great speed and direction towards the ampulla where fertilization of the mature, ovulated oocyte usually occurs. To achieve this, the sperm must undergo capicitation, which is oestrogen-dependent and calcium-dependent activation. During this process the inner membrane beneath the acrosome cap becomes primed for fusion with the inner membrane of the ovum.

The acrosome reaction exposes the inner membrane of sperm. This portion will fuse with the membrane of the ovum (Fig. 4.4).

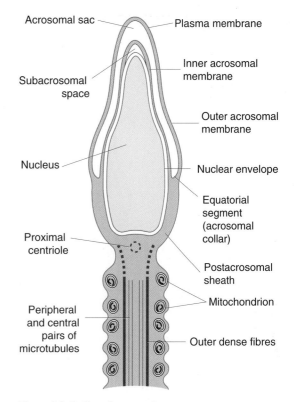

Figure 4.3 Outline of a spermatozoon.

The follicle

In the ovary, the primordial follicle is composed of primordial germ cells surrounded by mesenchymal cells derived from endodermal tissue. Having passed the first meiotic division, at birth, the primary oocyte is found arrested at metaphase of the second meiotic division until puberty. At the onset of puberty, a few follicles at a time recommence growth on a daily basis, the largest being 2–5 mm in the late luteal phase. It is from these follicles that the follicle destined for the next ovulation will be selected (Fig. 4.5), but it is important to note that in each cycle only one egg is usually ovulated. Antral follicles are surrounded by inner granulosa cells and outer theca cell layers. These cell layers are derived from mesenchyme. The granulosa cells synthesize oestrogens, whereas the theca cells produce androgens (Fig. 4.6). Meiosis is not resumed until after the leutinizing hormone (LH) surge.

Complex mechanisms ensure that only one dominant follicle becomes pre-ovulatory and the other follicles undergo degeneration or atresia within the first week of the follicular growth phase prior to ovulation. The biochemical interactions between the oocyte and the surrounding granulosa and thecal cells within the developing follicle are shown in Figure 4.6. The high oestrogen level in the follicle induces the pre-ovulatory surge of leutinizing hormone (LH), which then initiates the resumption of

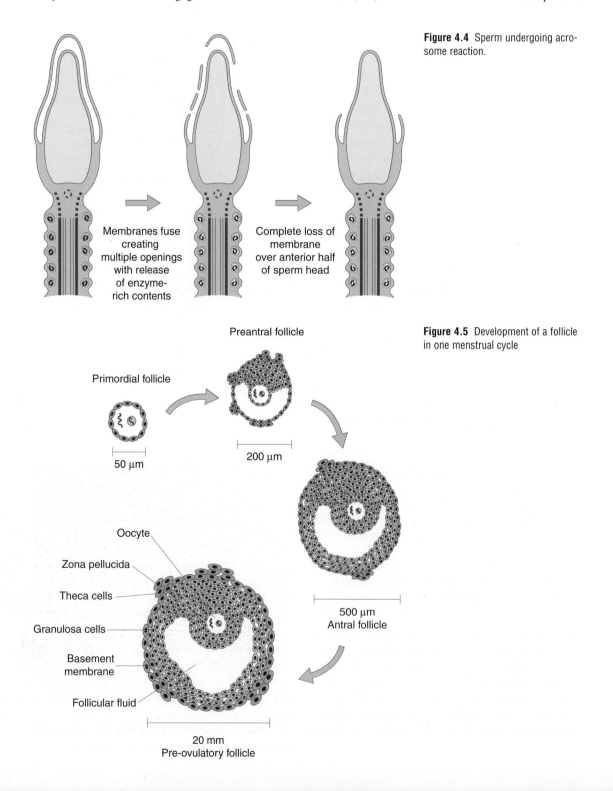

Membranes fuse creating multiple openings with release of enzyme-rich contents

Complete loss of membrane over anterior half of sperm head

Figure 4.4 Sperm undergoing acrosome reaction.

Preantral follicle

Primordial follicle

50 μm

200 μm

Figure 4.5 Development of a follicle in one menstrual cycle

500 μm
Antral follicle

Oocyte

Zona pellucida

Theca cells

Granulosa cells

Basement membrane

Follicular fluid

20 mm
Pre-ovulatory follicle

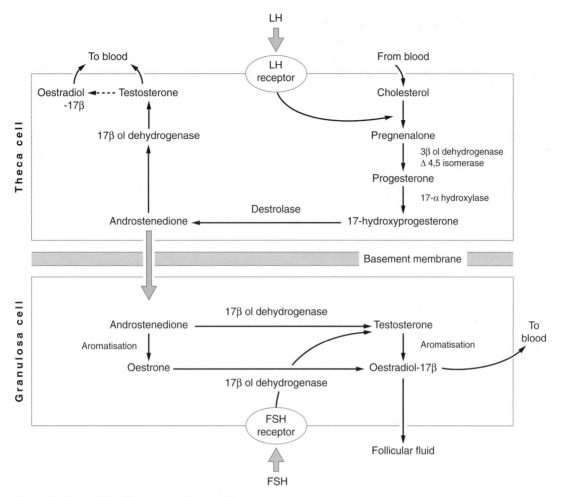

Figure 4.6 Biochemistry of hormone production in the ovary.

meiosis. The completion of first meiotic division results in the extrusion and release of the first polar body. The oocyte, now described as an ovum, has acquired the competence to be fertilized (metaphase II of the meiotic cycle, Fig. 4.7).

Fertilization: a zygote is formed by fusion of male and female pronuclei

At ovulation, the ovum is surrounded by a jelly-like protective coating, which predominantly consists of cumulus cells (Fig. 4.7). The ovulated egg is picked up by the fimbria of the Fallopian tube and then swept by ciliary action towards the ampulla where fertilization occurs. The sperm penetrates the cumulus cell layer and subsequently interacts with egg-specific surface

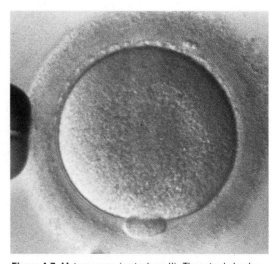

Figure 4.7 Mature ovum (metaphase II). The extruded polar body may be seen at 6 o'clock. (Kindly supplied by Dr S. Lee.)

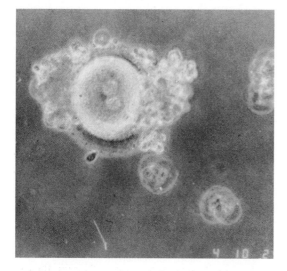

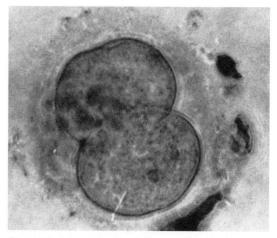

Figure 4.9 A two-cell embryo is formed after syngamy. (Kindly supplied by Dr S. Lee.)

Figure 4.8 Fertilized egg showing two pronuclei: one derived from the egg (containing 23 chromosomes); one derived from the sperm (containing 23 chromosomes). The fertilized egg is diploid containing 46 chromosomes in total. (Kindly supplied by Dr S. Lee.)

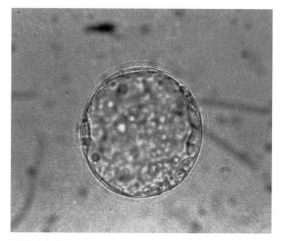

Figure 4.10 A blastocyst prior to hatching and implantation. (Kindly supplied by Dr S. Lee.)

receptors in the zona pellucida; a thick glycoprotein sheet covering the cytoplasmic membrane of the egg. This interaction triggers the sperm acrosome reactions necessary for penetration of the sperm into the egg cytoplasm. At this point, a series of complex macromolecular events must occur within the sperm head to transform it into a male pronucleus (see Fig. 4.4). Similarly, the egg must complete its meiotic division II to form the haploid female pronucleus and a second polar body, which is extruded.

As described earlier, the sperm chromosomes are almost crystallized and are uniquely glued together by sperm-specific basic protamines. One of the earliest events in male pronuclear formation is the decondensation of sperm chromosomes by releasing the protamines. Once the protamines are stripped from the sperm chromosomes, a new set of egg-specific proteins bind the sperm chromosomes. This process is known as chromosome remodelling. Subsequently, new cytoplasmic organelles and a nuclear envelope assemble around the remodelled sperm chromosomes to produce the male pronucleus. Finally, the fertilization ends with successful fusion of the male and female pronuclei (Fig. 4.8) resulting in a single cell called a zygote. In humans, fertilization is com-

pleted within 20 hours resulting in a return to a diploid genetic constitution of the embryo.

The coming together of the two haploid sets of chromosomes, called syngamy, is the final phase of fertilization. Soon after, anaphase and telophase are completed, and the one cell zygote becomes a two-cell embryo (Fig. 4.9).

Implantation

As soon as the zygote is formed, it begins dividing very rapidly and within five days a tiny mass of cells, the blastocyst is formed (Fig. 4.10). For a pregnancy to be established, the embryo must hatch. This means that the embryo has to escape from the zona pellucida and the outer covering of the original egg and then begin to 'burrow' into the decidua. To prepare for this, the endometrium undergoes complex cyclical changes. In particular, extensive proliferation occurs under the influence of oestrogen released from the ovarian follicles during maturation of the eggs.

Following ovulation, the corpus luteum grows near the surface of the ovary as it produces progesterone. Under this hormonal influence, the endometrium and its glands undergo rapid morphological changes leading them to a secretory phase. Factors other than gonadal steroids influence uterine receptivity for implantation when appropriately conditioned by oestrogen and progesterone. Assisting implantation are also local peptides, such as growth factors including epidermal growth factor (EGP), insulin-like growth factor-1 (IGF-I) and its binding protein (1GF-BP-I), prostaglandin (notably PGE2), plasminogen activators and possibly leukaemia inhibitory factor (LIF). Some of these have angiogenic properties.

The embryo remains in the Fallopian tube for 3–4 days until it reaches morula stage (8–32 cell stage), the embryo proceeds through the isthmus to the uterine cavity where it will float freely for up to 72 hours. By the sixth day, it orientates itself towards the decidua and begins to penetrate its epithelial surface by piercing its basement membrane. This is accomplished by generating metalloproteinases. Once inside the decidua it generates extracellular matrix (ECM) *de novo* which is thought to enhance the chances of implantation. This process facilitates one of the earliest embryo-maternal interactions such as secretion of human chorionic gonadotrophin by the trophoblastic cells leading to the maternal recognition of pregnancy. There appear to be many changes that involve modulation of the immune responses within the uterus.

The early steps of implantation involve numerous cell-cell interactions. For example, the binding to ECM (glycoproteins) with the basement membrane's (laminin and fibronectin) surface receptors. Also, there is activation of proteases and pericellular degradation of matrix components (matrix metalloproteinases). All these changes allow the invading cytotrophoblast easier access to the decidua for implantation. Indeed, *de novo* expression of the gene for gelatinases A and B is activated, causing breakdown of the basement membrane, which facilitates

cytotrophoblastic cells to make contact with the decidua's extracellular matrix through their fibronectin receptors (Fig. 4.11).

Endometrial cytokines modulate cytotrophoblastic proteolytic activity to control the depth of invasion. Twelve days after fertilization, the embryo is embedded within the decidual stroma, the trophoblast having already differentiated into cytotrophoblastic and invasive syncytiotrophoblast. The developing embryo at nine days is 500–600 μm in diameter, with predecidual cells surrounding the embryonic mass. Increased epithelial vasculature at the implantation site is observed due to oedema and localised hyperaemia. At 11–12 days, the implantation site can be seen as a 1 mm red spot on the mucosa due to maternal blood in lacunar spaces. By 14–21 days, the trophoblastic structure at the periphery of the embryo resembles the villi of the mature placenta as the inner cell mass has begun to undergo embryogenesis.

Embryology

In humans, following successful fertilization the differentiation of cells into specialized tissues, to form inter-related organ systems, is known as the embryonic period. It starts with the generation of the embryonic disk during the 2nd week post-fertilization (four weeks after the last menstrual period) and, conventionally, ends the last day of the 8th week (10 weeks after the last menstrual period). At this point, all organ systems are formed, but are not necessarily 'mature' or functioning. A brief account of the most important events during the embryonic period starting from the 3rd embryological week is given below.

3rd Week

On the dorsal aspect of the bilaminar germ disk a faint groove, the primitive streak, appears on the midline near its caudal end (Fig. 4.12a). This is an important event where a number of developmental landmarks are generated. For example, the primitive streak determines symmetry and defines the cephalic and caudal poles of the embryo. It follows, one can say, that ventrality as well as laterality are generated at the same time. Definition of symmetry, polarity and laterality at the outset of organogenesis is

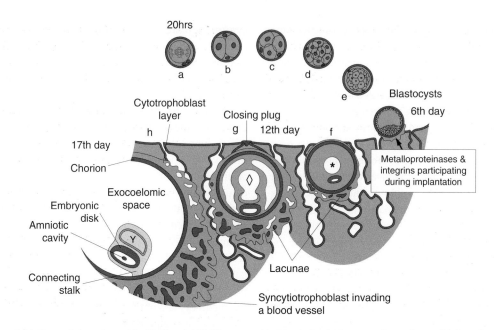

Figure 4.11 Sequential events post-fertilization. (a) Dividing zygote. (b) Two-cell embryo. (c) Four-cell embryo. (d) Eight-cell embryo. (e) Morula. (f) Implanting blastocyst: primary yolk sac (STAR), extra embryonic mesoderm (Diamond). (g) Implanted blastocyst: developing secondary yolk sac. (h) Gestational sac: the secondary yolk sac is broadly connected to the ventral aspect of the embryonic disk (Y). Note the expanded exo-coelomic space and the small amniotic sac.

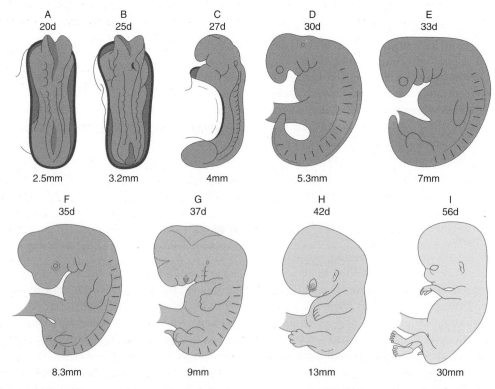

Figure 4.12 A–I Sequential changes during the development of the external form in a normal human embryo from day 20 (A) through to the 56th day (I) post-fertilization (add two weeks to consider the gestational time from the last menstrual period). The crown–rump length is expressed in mm.

fundamental for appropriate organ-system topology and a number of genes participate in this initial step. During the 3rd week two other structures become apparent on the embryonic disk; the neural plate and the somites which appear as symmetric eminences on either side of the midline.

Internally, the bilaminar embryo generates the mesodermal layer made up of cells which, from the primitive node, at the cephalic end of the primitive streak, migrate between the ectodermal and endo-dermal layers. The somites composed of paraxial mesodermal cells will appear on day 20, at a level corresponding to the future base of the skull.

Other structures intimately related to the embry-onic disk develop during this time. The primary yolk sac, which grows rapidly into the expanding exo-coelomic space. The yolk sac is an important organ for exchanging metabolites between the mother and the embryo at the time when there is no placenta but there are some chorionic villi undergoing vasculariza-tion. The life span of the yolk sac is limited, it attains full development by day 32 and its complex wall starts degenerating by the end of the 6th week. The amniotic membrane is another extraembryonic element, which by day 17 is closely apposed to the embryonic disk. There will be some time before the embryo is sus-pended in a well-expanded amniotic sac (Fig. 4.12h).

4th Week

During this week the embryonic disk folds into an embryonic cylinder (Fig 4.12b) within which is a cranio-caudal, blind-ending tube which has three segments, the foregut, the mid-gut opened to the developing yolk sac and the hindgut. This stage marks the start of organogenesis.

The first organ to become apparent is the primitive heart in the shape of a forward buckling loop (Fig. 4.12c). Cardiac activity is evident by day 22 post-fer-tilization.

Neurulation or, the development of the nervous system, takes place at this stage of development. Briefly, the neural plate becomes a deep groove on the dorsal aspect of the embryo, it sinks deeper and the opposing crests fuse, generating the neural tube. As closure takes place, the cephalic neuropore closes during day 26 and the caudal neuropore at the end of the 4th week. A special population of cells detach from the lips of the neural crest and migrate to several specific locations of the body. By the end of the 4th week, the central neural system has defined segments, the primary brain vesicles, the prosen-cephalon, mesencephalon and the rhombencephalon (Fig. 4.12d).

Towards the end of the 4th week, the foregut sep-tates along the midline into the respiratory and digestive primitive elements. The ventral pancreatic bud migrates posteriorly to fuse with the dorsal pan-creatic bud.

The lower respiratory system appears as septation of the foregut occurs. Two lung buds are evident at the end of the 4th week.

By day 26 the mesonephric duct and mesonephros differentiate. At 28 days the ureteric buds and the metanephric blastema are defined structures.

In summary it can be said that, by the end of the 4th week, almost all organ systems, albeit immature, can be readily identified.

Towards the end of the 4th week the body of the embryo is attached to the yolk sac by a broad vitelline duct and two connecting vitelline blood ves-sels. The yolk sac is placed within the exocoelomic space. The vitelline duct and the vitelline vessels are included within the umbilical cord just before the cord enters into the amniotic sac.

In the cephalic pole of the embryo, five pharyngeal arches appear in succession. Towards the end of the 4th week, the buccopharyngeal membrane perforates.

Changes in the external appearance

During the ensuing three weeks the outer aspect of the human embryo changes dramatically. The head starts to grow faster than the rest of the body and is bent forward until the end of the 7th week (Fig. 4.12g and h). The face is formed by a series of trans-formations of the pharyngeal arches. The eyes are in a lateral position and after the 34th week they appear pigmented. As the embryo grows bigger the eyes appear to 'migrate' towards the midline of the face. The eyelids develop after the 6th week and by the end of the 8th week the eyes are closed by the eyelids, which fuse with one another. The eyelids will sepa-rate after the 20th week of gestation.

The ears differentiate at either side of the neck, early during the 5th week of gestation and appear to be displaced upwards, as the body of the embryo gains length.

The nose is present early during the 6th week and the nostrils will be plugged with keratin until after the 20th week of gestation. The mouth can be recognized after the 6th week of gestation. However, the palatal shelves will only fuse during the 8th week. The uvula remains bifid for a week or so after which it assumes the shape observed later in gestation or after birth.

During the 4th week, the thorax is largely occupied by the heart. As embryonic growth proceeds, the lungs develop within the thorax.

The development of the upper limbs precedes that of the lower limbs. The upper limb buds appear at about the 27th day. The lower limb buds become evident a day later. Early during the 6th week the hand plate presents lobulations which anticipate digit differentiation. The lower limbs lag behind. However, by the end of the 8th week, both the upper and lower limbs are fully differentiated, the head is slightly up-right and the embryo has a distinct human appearance (Fig. 4.12i).

Key Points

- Embryos must synthesize integrins (cell adhesion molecules, CAMs)
- The decidua must synthesise fibronectin and other extracellular matrix (ECM) components
- The above-mentioned activities are likely to be mediated by growth factors and cytokines. Both the decidua and the embryo are likely to make and release these factors
- The embryo must produce cytotrophoblastic and synctiotrophoblastic tissue in order to successfully infiltrate the endometrial stroma
- It is now thought that cytokines are involved in initiating a localised immunosuppression, which would allow the developing embryo to avoid a rejection-like response from the womb
- Leukocyte infiltration of the implantation site has been observed. Most of these seem to be T-suppressor cells

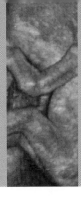

Chapter 5

Physiological changes in pregnancy

OVERVIEW

Textbooks of physiology conventionally present data obtained from young adult males. The norms for young adult females, particularly when pregnant, often differ significantly from these. Lack of appreciation of these differences may lead to inappropriate management of clinical problems in obstetrics.

   This chapter will outline the major maternal physiological adaptations to pregnancy, indicating the potential for misinterpretation of clinical signs. Where possible, explanations for the changes will be provided. Where no explanation is universally accepted speculation will be acknowledged. In a few instances, information obtained from cell or molecular biology is beginning to provide new insights into the mechanisms underlying these processes: this is a fruitful field for future research.

Systemic changes

Volume homeostasis

One of the most fundamental systemic changes of normal pregnancy is fluid retention, which accounts for between 8 and 10 kg of the average maternal weight gain of 11–13 kg. There is probably some increase in intracellular water but the most marked expansion occurs in extracellular fluid volume, especially in circulating plasma volume (Fig. 5.1). This change is central to a series of other physiological adaptations, notably increases in cardiac output and in renal blood flow. It also has important consequences for the

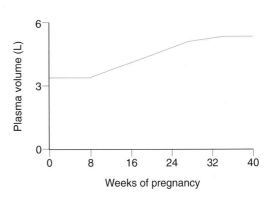

Figure 5.1 Changes in plasma volume during normal human pregnancy. There is an increase in mean values from 3L in the non-pregnant state to between 4 and 4.5L during late pregnancy.

interpretation of haematological indices in normal pregnancy (Fig. 5.2). Relative increases in plasma volume have been reported in women taking regular exercise during pregnancy and relative decreases occur in the pregnancy complications of intrauterine growth restriction (IUGR) and pre-eclampsia.

The precise mechanisms responsible for this important adaptation remain uncertain. In the non-pregnant situation, sodium is the most important determinant of extracellular fluid volume. There is a net retention of sodium during normal pregnancy, amounting to a total of 900 mmoL (or 3–4 mmoL per day). In keeping with this finding are the very marked increases in the concentration of the antinatriuretic hormones, aldosterone and deoxycorticosterone, observed during pregnancy. However, natriuretic factors, such as atrial natriuretic peptide and progesterone, also increase during pregnancy. Furthermore, a substantial proportion of the retained sodium must be sequestered within fetal tissues (including placenta, membranes and amniotic fluid). Maternal plasma sodium concentration actually decreases slightly during pregnancy and it is therefore possible that other factors, such as alterations in intracellular metabolism, may also contribute to the fluid retention.

One noteworthy feature of this change in fluid homeostasis is that plasma osmolality decreases by about ten milliosmoles per kilogram. In the non-pregnant state such a marked decrease would be associated with a rapid diuresis in order to maintain volume homeostasis. However, the pregnant woman appears to accept this new level of osmolality as evidenced by infusion experiments where urinary concentration is regulated in order to maintain the new equilibrium. Interestingly, there is also evidence of a decrease in the thirst threshold in that pregnant women feel the urge to drink at a lower level of plasma osmolality than they do in the non-pregnant state.

Not only does plasma osmotic pressure decrease during pregnancy but oncotic pressure (otherwise known as colloid osmotic pressure) is also markedly reduced. Plasma oncotic pressure is predominantly determined by the concentration of albumin which decreases by about 20 per cent during normal pregnancy to levels that would be considered pathological in a non-pregnant person. The significance of this change is that plasma oncotic pressure is a major contributor to the Starling equilibrium which determines the degree to which fluid passes into and out of capillaries (including glomerular capillaries). Thus the decrease in plasma oncotic pressure is one of the factors responsible for the marked increase that occurs in glomerular filtration rate during normal pregnancy (see page 52). It is also likely to contribute to the development of peripheral oedema which is now known to be a feature of normal, uncomplicated pregnancy.

🔑 Key Points

The factors contributing to fluid retention are

- Sodium retention
- Resetting of osmostat
- Decrease in thirst threshold
- Decrease in plasma oncotic pressure

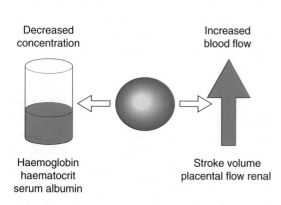

Decreased concentration

Increased blood flow

Haemoglobin haematocrit serum albumin

Stroke volume placental flow renal

Figure 5.2 The consequences of fluid retention during pregnancy. The concentrations of certain substances in the circulation decrease while there are marked increases in haemodynamics.

🔑 Key Points

Consequences of fluid retention are

- Haemoglobin concentration falls
- Haematocrit falls
- Serum albumin concentration falls
- Stroke volume increases
- Renal blood flow increases

Blood

The marked increase in plasma volume associated with normal pregnancy causes dilution of many circulating factors. Of particular note is the haemodilution of red blood cells. Although pregnancy is associated with an increase in the production of erythrocytes, this increase is outstripped by the relative increase in plasma volume. Thus haematological indices which depend upon the proportion of plasma in a measured blood sample tend to decrease. Such indices include red cell count, haematocrit and haemoglobin concentration.

The mean haemoglobin concentration falls from 13.3 g/dL in the non-pregnant state to 10.9 g/dL at the 36th week of normal pregnancy. This physiological change has been mistaken in the past for the development of pathological anaemia and pregnant women have often been given 'prophylactic' haematinics, notably oral iron. This drug can cause unpleasant side effects including nausea and constipation. Pregnant women are already predisposed to these symptoms, thereby explaining the non-compliance with oral iron therapy well-recognized in studies involving pregnant women. On the other hand, there is no doubt that a pregnant woman's need for iron increases substantially: she compensates for this by absorbing a dramatically larger proportion of dietary iron from the gut. Even so, women who do not take supplementary iron during pregnancy do show a reduction in stainable iron in the bone marrow as well as a progressive reduction in mean cell volume.

Many obstetricians now feel that women who are likely to have an adequate dietary intake of iron should be monitored by assessing serial changes in haemoglobin concentration and in mean cell volume. However, they do not need to be given supplementary oral iron unless measurements fall below pre-determined arbitrary levels, such as a haemoglobin concentration of 10 g/dL. Another method of monitoring is by assessing iron stores (ferritin and iron-binding capacity). It should, of course, be remembered that iron deficiency is endemic in certain parts of the world and that there are women living in other communities who may for personal or cultural reasons take a diet which is relatively deficient in iron. Furthermore, certain pregnant women,

such as those with multiple gestations, may have a greater than normal dietary iron requirement. Iron supplementation should not be unreasonably withheld in such cases.

Folic acid supplementation has also been widely advocated in the past to prevent macrocytic anaemia. It is certainly true that the renal clearance of folic acid increases substantially during normal pregnancy and that plasma folate concentrations fall. However, red cell folate concentrations do not decrease to the same extent as plasma folate concentrations and there does not seem to be a strong case for routine folate supplementation for haematinic purposes in women eating an adequate diet and carrying a single fetus. On the other hand, there is now clear evidence that supplementation with folic acid over the time of conception and during the first trimester of pregnancy can reduce the frequency of neural tube defects and women in the UK have therefore been advised to take the vitamin at this time.

Unlike red blood cells, white cell concentrations do not show a dilutional decrease during normal pregnancy. Indeed, the total white cell count increases, the average value during the third trimester being 9×10^9 per litre. The predominant reason for this change is a marked increase in the numbers of polymorphonuclear leucocytes. This phenomenon is even more marked during the early days of the puerperium, when values of greater than 20×10^9 per litre have been found in apparently entirely healthy women. Alterations in the concentrations of other circulating white cells, including both T and B lymphocytes, are relatively slight in comparison with these changes in neutrophils. There is, however, a slight reduction in the platelet count, with an increased proportion of larger, younger platelets.

There are also substantial changes in coagulation during normal human pregnancy, which may be regarded as a hypercoagulable state. There are significant increases in the production of several procoagulant factors and a reduction in plasma fibrinolytic activity. One of the most noteworthy changes is a marked increase in plasma fibrinogen concentration which, incidentally, is thought to be responsible for the substantial augmentation of erythrocyte sedimentation rate which occurs during pregnancy, since it enhances rouleaux formation. The need for relative hypercoagulability is particularly apparent at the time of placental separation. At term, about 500 mL of blood flows through the placental bed per minute. Without effective and rapid haemostasis a woman could die from exsanguination within a few minutes. Myometrial contraction is the first line of defence, compressing the blood vessels supplying the placental bed (see Fig. 5.5). Almost immediately fibrin begins to be deposited over the placental site and ultimately between 5 and 10 per cent of all of the fibrinogen in the circulation is used up for this purpose. Factors that impede this haemostatic process, such as inadequate uterine contraction or incomplete placental separation, can therefore rapidly lead to depletion of fibrinogen reserve. There is, however, a disadvantage to the potentially life-saving physiological adjustment of hypercoagulation as pregnancy and the puerperium are associated with substantially increased risks of thromoembolic problems and these remain the largest single group of causes of maternal death in the UK.

Cardiovascular system

Early pregnancy is characterized by peripheral vasodilatation. The precise cause of this phenomenon is still, to some extent, speculative but there is evidence to implicate vasoactive factors derived from the endothelium, such as nitric oxide. Initially, the vasodilatation appears to be perceived centrally as circulatory underfill, similar to that which might occur following haemorrhage. A significant increase in heart rate can be demonstrated as early as the 5th week of pregnancy (three weeks after conception) and this contributes to an increase in cardiac output at this time. However, no increase in stroke volume can be detected for several weeks: this presumably occurs when plasma volume expands, following the activation of mechanisms of fluid retention such as those described above.

Further changes in the factors regulating cardiac output continue as pregnancy advances (Table 5.1 and Fig. 5.3). A progressive increase in heart rate continues until the third trimester of pregnancy, when rates are typically 10–15 beats per minute greater than those found in the non-pregnant state. There is also a progressive augmentation of stroke volume (10–20 mL) during the first half of pregnancy, probably related to the incremental changes in plasma volume at this time. As a consequence of

Table 5.1 – Changes in cardiac output with labour

	Increase in cardiac output (%)
Latent phase (cervix <3 cm dilated)	17%
Active labour	23%
Late 1st stage/2nd stage	34%

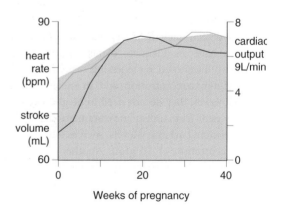

Figure 5.3 There is a marked increase in maternal cardiac output during pregnancy. Increases in both heart rate and stroke volume contribute but changes in these components are not synchronous.

Normal changes in heart sounds during pregnancy

- Increased loudness of both s1 and s2
- Increased splitting of mitral and tricuspid components of s1
- No constant changes in s2
- Loud s3 by 20 weeks' gestation
- <5% with s4
- >95% develop systolic murmur which disappears after delivery
- 20% have a transient diastolic murmur
- 10% develop continuous murmurs due to increased mammary blood flow

Key Points

Cardiovascular changes
- Heart rate increases (10–20%)
- Stroke volume increases (10%)
- Cardiac output increases (30–50%)
- Mean arterial pressure decreases (10%)
- Peripheral resistance decreases (35%)

these changes cardiac output increases from an average of under 5 L/min before pregnancy to approximately 7 L/min at the 20th week of pregnancy. Thereafter changes are less dramatic and there is inconsistency among the reports of investigators. It is important to be aware that the techniques of investigation may influence results, especially during the third trimester of pregnancy, when the large gravid uterus impairs venous return to the heart in the supine position. A proportion of women will in consequence develop significant

supine hypotension and may even lose consciousness. By rolling over on to her left side cardiac output will almost instantly be restored.

Despite the marked increases in circulating plasma volume and in cardiac output described above, the greater part of normal pregnancy is characterized by a reduction in arterial blood pressure (Fig. 5.4). This implies that there must be very substantial decreases in total peripheral vascular resistance during pregnancy and the mechanisms responsible for this dramatic alteration are currently under active investigation. Peripheral arterial tone is the result of a balance of opposing vasoconstrictor and vasodilator influences and, since substantial alterations have been reported in the production of both types of agents, it is unlikely that a single simple unifying hypothesis will be sufficient to explain this remarkable physiological phenomenon.

High blood pressure is a major contributor to maternal and perinatal disease and death. The accurate measurement of maternal blood pressure is therefore of critical importance in the assessment of pregnancy. It will be noticed from Figure 5.4 that the decrease in diastolic blood pressure is more marked during the antenatal period than the decrease in systolic pressure. Thus early pregnancy is associated with a relative increase in pulse pressure. Later, however, diastolic blood pressure increases significantly to levels that are at least equivalent to those found in the non-pregnant state. The precise determination of diastolic pressure is therefore critically important. Recent studies have demonstrated that more reproducible and accurate measurements are obtained when the fifth Korotkoff sound (disappearance of sounds) is used rather than the fourth (muffling). This has long been standard practice in the USA and is now being to be adopted in the UK.

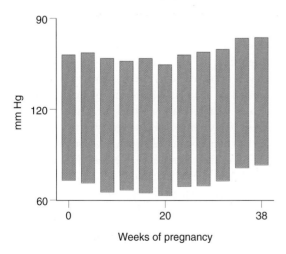

Figure 5.4 Arterial blood pressure decreases during the first half of pregnancy but gradually increases during the third trimester. This has major implications for the management of hypertensive disorders during pregnancy.

CASE HISTORY

A 21-year-old Bangladeshi woman presents to the Accident and Emergency Department. She arrived in the UK four months earlier. She is so short of breath that she is unable to give a history, but her partner tells you that she is two months' pregnant and was well until three days ago. On examination you find that her pulse is 100 bpm, her blood pressure is 90/60 mmHg and she has a respiratory rate of 36. Examination of her chest reveals signs of pulmonary oedema.

What is the diagnosis?

Sudden onset of breathlessness could be due to chest infection, pulmonary embolism, or pulmonary oedema. This patient had no temperature, and a careful cardiovascular examination revealed a facial rash; a tapping, undisplaced apex beat, atrial fibrillation and a low-pitched, mid-diastolic murmur, consistent with the diagnosis of mitral stenosis.

Why has the woman presented at this time?

Early pregnancy is associated with hormonal changes resulting in fluid retention and expansion of the plasma volume. This, with increased cardiac rate and stroke volume (Starling's law of the heart) causes an increase in cardiac output early in the first trimester of pregnancy. With stenosis of the mitral valve, the increased blood flow through the heart cannot be accommodated, there is a rise in pulmonary venous pressure and pulmonary oedema results. Thus a person who normally has few symptoms unless very active can be made very unwell by not coping with the physiological changes of pregnancy.

What is the treatment?

The pulmonary oedema should be treated with oxygen and diuretics. In extreme cases venesection is sometimes necessary to rapidly reduce the circulating volume, and therefore the pulmonary venous pressure. As left ventricular filling is limited by the stenosis, beta-blockers will reduce cardiac rate and allow more time for filling to occur. Balloon valvotomy, or closed mitral valvotomy have good results in pregnancy and there is an increasing postgraduate literature on full cardiopulmonary by-pass in pregnancy. For many couples termination of pregnancy, reversing the physiological changes which have precipitated the acute problem, will be an option allowing definitive treatment (valve replacement) to occur before a subsequent pregnancy is planned.

Reproductive organs

The uterus

Changes in circulating hormone concentrations also markedly affect the tissues of the genital tract. The uterus is formed from fusion of the two Mullerian ducts in the midline, which gives rise to the adult structure of the uterus comprising three layers. These are a thin, inner layer of circular muscle fibres; a thin, outer layer consisting predominantly of longitudinal muscle fibres, and a thicker, central layer of interlocking fibres. In addition the ratio of muscle to connective tissue increases from the lower part of the uterus towards the fundus. The high levels of maternal oestradiol and progesterone stimulate both hyperplasia and hypertrophy of the myometrial cells, increasing the weight of the uterus from 50–60 g prior to pregnancy, to 1000 g by term. In early pregnancy uterine growth is a result of both hyperplasia and hypertrophy. At this stage it is independent of the growing fetus, and occurs equally rapidly with an ectopic pregnancy. As gestation increases myometrial cell division is less important and hypertrophy of individual cells accounts for most of the increase in uterine size. The growing size of the uterine contents is an important stimulus at this stage, with individual muscle fibres increasing in length by up to fifteen-fold. In the second half of pregnancy a growth restricted fetus (see Chapter 11) may be detected on abdominal palpation, by finding a uterine size smaller than expected for gestational age. The uterine arteries also undergo hypertrophy in the first half of pregnancy, although in the second half of gestation the increasing uterine distension is matched by arterial stretching.

As well as changes in the size and number of myometrial cells, specialized cellular connections also develop with increasing gestation. These intercellular gap junctions allow changes in membrane potential to spread rapidly from one cell to another, facilitating the spread of membrane depolarization, and subsequent myometrial contraction. As these junctions mature, uterine contractions become more frequent. These are apparent initially as Braxton-

Hicks contractions, these are painless contractions that are increasingly apparent to the woman in the second half of pregnancy. Subsequently these allow the pacemaker activity of the uterine fundus to promote the coordinated, fundal-dominant contractions necessary for labour.

Conventionally the uterus is divided into the lower and upper segments. The lower segment is the part of the uterus and upper cervix which lies between the attachment of the peritoneum of the uterovesical pouch superiorly and the level of the internal cervical os inferiorly. This part of the uterus contains less muscle and blood vessels, is thinner, and is the site of incision for the majority of caesarean sections.

Immediately after the placenta has separated from the wall of the uterus, the interlocking muscle fibres of the uterus contract (Fig. 5.5). This occludes the blood vessels that were supplying the placenta and reduces blood loss. If the placenta has been attached to the lower uterine segment, the relative lack of muscle in this part of the uterus makes the haemostatic mechanism less efficient, and postpartum haemorrhage can occur.

The cervix

Under the influence of oestradiol and progesterone the cervix becomes swollen and softer during pregnancy (Fig. 5.6). Oestradiol stimulates growth of the columnar epithelium of the cervical canal that

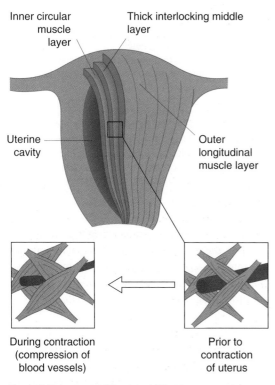

Figure 5.5 Anatomy of the uterus. The uterus comprises three muscle layers, derived from the layers of the Mullerian ducts. The muscle fibres in the inner layer are arranged in a predominantly circular pattern. The thicker, intermediate layer comprises interlocked muscle fibres. The outer layer of muscle fibres runs longitudinally, over the fundus.

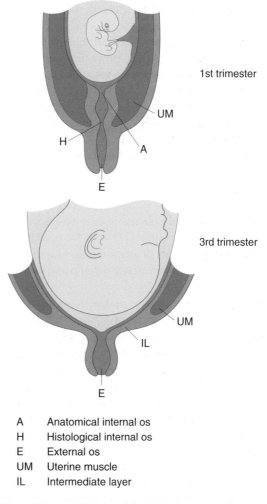

A   Anatomical internal os
H   Histological internal os
E   External os
UM   Uterine muscle
IL   Intermediate layer

Figure 5.6 Formation of the lower uterine segment. With increasing gestation uterine stretch occurs. This has the effect of drawing the anatomical internal cervical os (A) further from the histological internal cervical os (H). The retraction of the thick, intermediate layer (IL) of muscle with increasing gestation thins the lower segment.

becomes visible on the ectocervix, and is called an ectropion. This is of significance as it is a less robust epithelium and is prone to contact bleeding. The cervix is often described as looking 'bluer' during pregnancy. This is a function of increased vascularity. In addition to these changes the mucus glands of the cervix become distended and increase in complexity. Prostaglandins induce a remodelling of cervical collagen, particularly towards the end of gestation, whilst collagenase released from leukocytes also aids in softening the cervix.

Under the influence of oestrogens the vaginal epithelium becomes thicker during pregnancy, and there is an increased rate of desquamation resulting in increased vaginal discharge during pregnancy. This discharge has a more acid pH than non-pregnant vaginal secretions (4.5–5.0) and may protect against ascending infection. The vagina also becomes more vascular with increasing gestation.

Breasts and lactation

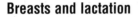

Cyclical changes are seen in breast tissue in response to the menstrual cycle and during pregnancy these changes are amplified. There is considerable deposition of fat around the glandular tissue. The number of glandular ducts is increased by oestrogen, whilst progesterone (and human placental lactogen [hPL]) increases the number of gland alveoli. hPL may also stimulate alveolar casein, lactoglobulin and lactalbumin synthesis.

Although the serum prolactin concentration increases throughout pregnancy it does not result in lactation as its effect is antagonized at an alveolar receptor level by oestrogen. It is the rapid fall in oestrogen concentration over the first 48 hours after birth that removes this inhibition and allows lactation to begin. Towards the end of pregnancy, and in the early puerperium the breasts produce colostrum, a thick, yellow secretion rich in immunoglobulins.

Lactation is promoted by early, frequent suckling which stimulates both the anterior and posterior pituitary to release prolactin and oxytocin respectively. Stress and fear reduce the synthesis and release of prolactin through increased dopamine (prolactin inhibitory factor) synthesis. During the first two or three days of the puerperium prolactin promotes breast engorgement, as the alveoli become distended with milk. Oxytocin released from the posterior

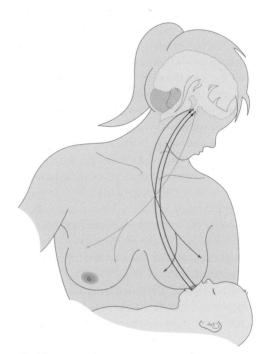

Suckling causes:
Afferent signals to posterior pituitary increasing oxytocin release, inducing myoepithelial cells to contract and express milk.
Afferent signals to anterior pituitary increasing prolactin release, thus increasing milk synthesis.

Figure 5.7 Schematic representation of lactation. Suckling induces afferent signals to the anterior and posterior pituitary. This results in the release of prolactin and oxytocin. Prolactin induces milk production by the glandular tissue of the breast. Oxytocin causes contraction of the myoepithelial cells surrounding the glandular ducts, squeezing milk towards the nipple.

pituitary causes contraction in myoepithelial cells surrounding the alveoli and small ducts. This squeezes milk into the larger ducts and subareolar reservoirs. In addition oxytocin may inhibit dopamine release, further promoting successful lactation (Fig. 5.7).

The urinary tract and renal function

Vasodilatation, such as occurs in pregnancy, results from the relaxation of vascular smooth muscle. Other organs that have a significant component of smooth muscle also exhibit a change in function during pregnancy. Thus, in the alimentary tract there is delay in gastric emptying (important in the management of women requiring general anaesthesia) and reduced colonic motility (contributing to constipation). Similarly, the urinary tract becomes dilated during pregnancy. By the third trimester about 97 per cent of women have been shown to have some evidence of stasis or hydronephrosis. This physical change, together with certain alterations in the composition of the urine itself (see later) predispose pregnant women to ascending urinary tract infection, a common and important complication of pregnancy.

One consequence of vasodilatation, reduction in blood pressure, has already been discussed. Another important consequence is increase in blood flow. There is evidence that pregnant women increase blood flow to many organs, notably the uterus, breasts and skin (hence the glow of health with pregnancy). There is also a marked (60–75 per cent) increase in renal blood flow. One major result of this increase is substantial augmentation of glomerular filtration rate, by about 50 per cent (Fig. 5.8). Since filtration of the plasma is of critical importance in the maintenance of fluid balance, the excretion of waste products and the regulation of essential nutrients, such a major re-adjustment has far-reaching consequences for the other physiologi-

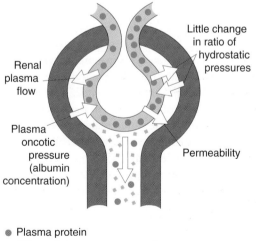

- ● Plasma protein
- ✳ Other solute

Figure 5.8 Factors contributing to enhanced glomerular filtration during pregnancy. The marked increase in renal blood flow is the major factor but there are significant contributions from the decrease in plasma oncotic pressure and enhanced permeability. Although systemic arterial pressure decreases during pregnancy, it seems likely that there is little difference in the relative pressures at either end of the glomerular capillary loop nor in intrarenal pressure.

> ### 🗝 Key Points
>
> **Renal changes**
> - Blood flow increases (60–75%)
> - Glomerular filtration increases (50%)
> - Clearance of most substances is enhanced
> - Plasma creatinine, urea and urate are reduced
> - Glycosuria is normal

cal mechanisms by which the kidney contributes to these processes.

Of clinical importance is the fact that the increase in glomerular filtration rate is responsible for an increase in the clearance of a number of substances from the bloodstream. Thus the plasma concentrations of chemicals which are conventionally used as markers for the severity of renal disease, such as urea and creatinine, are reduced during normal pregnancy and it is important to use appropriate pregnancy-specific norms when managing the pregnancies of women with major renal diseases. There is also an increase in total protein excretion (particularly microalbuminuria) during pregnancy, a factor making the interpretation of disordered renal function more difficult.

Of all of the solutes present in urine, the one most commonly tested during pregnancy has conventionally been glucose. By this means obstetricians have sought to identify women with disordered carbohydrate metabolism, which may have adverse consequences for both mother and baby. However, it is now clear that glycosuria, which is rarely present in the non-pregnant state, is so common during pregnancy as to be considered physiological. Furthermore, the phenomenon varies substantially from time to time during any given pregnancy and does not relate reliably to disorders of carbohydrate metabolism. The increase in glomerular filtration rate may be partially responsible for this glycosuria and it used to be believed that a reabsorptive mechanism in the proximal renal tubule thus became saturated so that the 'renal threshold' was exceeded. It is now known that this explanation is simplistic and that glucose reabsorption occurs secondarily to the absorption of sodium. It is therefore likely that other factors contributing to volume homeostasis and sodium retention are involved in the process. Whatever the true explanation, most obstetricians now accept that the routine testing of urine for glucose is of much less value than was previously believed.

Respiratory tract

Increases in cardiac output affect both sides of the heart and thus it will be readily appreciated that human pregnancy must be associated with very substantial increases in pulmonary blood flow. There is also a significant increase in tidal volume (see below) and the lungs are therefore able to function more efficiently, facilitating gas transfer. In consequence, there is a very marked decrease (15–20%) in the partial pressure of carbon dioxide, PCO_2. Furthermore, there is a slight increase in the partial pressure of oxygen, PO_2. These changes clearly facilitate gas transfer to and from the fetus (Fig. 5.9).

In fact the situation is rather more complex than these data would imply. During pregnancy there is an increase in 2,3-diphosphoglycerate (2,3-DPG) concentration within maternal erythrocytes. This anion, which binds preferentially to deoxygenated haemoglobin, should therefore predispose to the release of oxygen from the red cell at relatively lower levels of haemoglobin saturation (i.e. shifting the oxygen haemoglobin dissociation curve to the right). This would therefore increase the availability of oxygen within the tissues. Furthermore, the fetus is also adapted to take the maximum advantage from this alteration in maternal physiology. Fetal haemoglobin differs from adult haemoglobin in that the two beta-chains are replaced by gamma-chains. Binding of 2,3-DPG to haemoglobin occurs preferentially to beta-chains, with the result that in the fetus the oxygen haemoglobin dissociation curve is shifted to the left relative to the maternal state. This situation therefore considerably facilitates oxygen transfer from mother to fetus.

The marked reduction in PCO_2 could also have dramatic implications for maternal homeostasis. Since carbon dioxide forms carbonic acid in the presence of water, it is a major factor in acid-base balance. There is an elaborate system of buffering which compensates for fluctuations in acid production. Clearly large reductions in PCO_2 will activate these mechanisms in order that potentially hazardous alkalosis can be prevented. Compensation for such a respiratory-induced alkalosis classically involves the activity, predominantly within the erythrocytes, of the enzyme carbonic anhydrase, which converts carbonic acid to bicarbonate, thus releasing hydrogen ions to restore pH. The bicarbonate thus formed is excreted by the kidney. In human pregnancy there is indeed evidence of such compensation, renal excretion of bicarbonate increases significantly and maternal arterial pH changes very little. Furthermore, there is evidence of an increase in the concentration of carbonic anhydrase within maternal erythrocytes, but whether this is a primary event (contributing directly to the reduction in PCO_2), or a secondary adaptation is at present uncertain.

There are significant changes in the mechanical

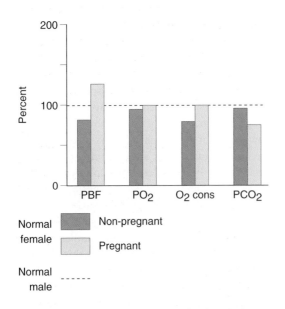

Figure 5.9 Human pregnancy is associated with marked changes in respiratory physiology. This diagram illustrates percentage changes in normal values found in non-pregnant and pregnant women in comparison with typical male values for pulmonary blood flow (PBF), partial pressure of oxygen (PO_2), oxygen consumption (O_2 cons), and partial pressure of carbon dioxide (PCO_2).

🔑 Key Points

Blood gas and acid-base changes
- PCO_2 decreases (15–20%)
- PO_2 increases (slight)
- Tissues and oxygen availability to placenta improves
- pH alters little
- bicarbonate excretion increases

aspects of ventilation during pregnancy. These are of particular importance in the management of women with chronic respiratory diseases. Dyspnoea is a common symptom during pregnancy but there is no evidence to suggest the involvement of any pathological process in most cases. Even in dyspnoeic women, the enhanced ventilation of pregnancy appears to result from increased tidal volume rather than from an increase in respiratory rate. The changes in lung volumes are demonstrated graphically in Figure 5.10. The enhanced tidal volume contributes to an increase in inspiratory capacity and there is a slight increase in vital capacity, which represents the total functional capacity of the lungs. As a result, there is a relative decrease in the non-inspiratory fraction of vital capacity, the expiratory reserve. There is also a reduction in the non-ventilated part of the lung volume, the residual volume, so that there is a fairly substantial reduction in the sum of these two volumes, known as functional residual capacity. The main reason for this reduction is thought to be an alteration in thoracic anatomy during pregnancy when the ribcage is displaced upwards and increases in transverse diameter. Such changes should improve airflow along the bronchial tree and indeed it is generally noticeable that women with respiratory problems tend to deteriorate somewhat less during pregnancy than those with other chronic disorders. These changes do not adversely affect the interpretation of such tests of ventilation as forced expiratory volume in one second (FEV_1)

Key Points

Ventilatory changes
- Thoracic anatomy changes
- Tidal volume increases
- Vital capacity decreases
- Functional residual capacity decreases

and peak expiratory flow rate. Thus these tests may continue to be used in the management of pregnant asthmatics and women with other obstructive pulmonary disorders.

Endocrinological changes

Understanding of the complex endocrinological changes of pregnancy remains incomplete. It is now clear that many of the peptide and steroid hormones, which are produced by the endocrine glands in the non-pregnant state, can also be produced by intrauterine tissues during pregnancy (Table 5.2). The precise contributions of these alternative sources to circulating concentrations of hormones, as well as their possible feedback activities, is as yet poorly understood. It is now clear that many hormones exert their actions indirectly, by interacting with cytokines and chemokines. The production and activity of many of these substances are also significantly altered

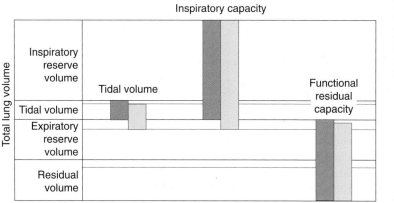

Figure 5.10 Typical changes in the volumes of selected lung compartments during pregnancy. There is a general augmentation of inspiration at the expense of functional respiratory capacity.

 Non-pregnant

Pregnant

Table 5.2 – Hormones produced within the pregnant uterus

(Note that this list is not exhaustive)
Pregnancy-specific
　　Human chorionic gonadotrophin (hCG)
　　Human placental lactogen (hPL)
Hypothalamus-related
　　Gonadotrophin-releasing hormone (GnRH)
　　Corticotrophin-releasing factor (CRF)
Pituitary-related
　　Prolactin
　　Human growth hormone (hGH)
　　Adrenocorticotrophic hormone (ACTH)
Other peptides
　　Insulin-like growth factor I and II (IGF)
　　1,25-Dihydroxycholecalciferol
　　Parathyroid hormone-related peptide
　　Renin
　　Angiotensin II
Steroids
　　Oestradiol
　　Progesterone

---

during human pregnancy. Other factors that may influence circulating concentrations may also change during pregnancy. Thus metabolic clearance rates and protein binding characteristics frequently differ from those characteristic of the non-pregnant state.

Hormones produced predominantly within the uterus

Many pregnancy-specific peptides are produced within the uterus but not all have yet been shown to have definite endocrine roles. Of those that have, the best known is human chorionic gonadotrophin (hCG). This hormone is composed of a and b subunits and the b subunit is pregnancy-specific, being widely used in modern practice as a sensitive pregnancy test. The hormone is produced by trophoblast cells and is detectable within the maternal circulation in small quantities within days of implantation. There is now evidence to suggest that production of this hormone is influenced both by the cytokine

leukaemia inhibitory factor (LIF) and by an isoform of gonadotrophin-releasing hormone (GnRH), which is also probably produced within the placenta. It seems that hCG has a major role during early pregnancy in maintaining the function of the corpus luteum. When the importance of this ovarian source of maternal progesterone diminishes (as placental production of progesterone becomes dominant during the later weeks of the first trimester) concentrations of circulating hCG decrease from peak values around the 10th week of pregnancy to plateau after the 12th week (Fig. 5.11).

The a subunit of hCG is not unique to this hormone. It differs only slightly from the a subunits of the hormones luteinizing hormone (LH), follicle-stimulating hormone (FSH) and thyroid-stimulating hormone (TSH) and can probably interact with receptors for at least some of these hormones. For example, hCG is widely used clinically by those involved in the practice of assisted reproduction to mimic the physiological LH surge in order to induce ovulation from stimulated ovarian follicles. It also seems likely that during normal pregnancy hCG suppresses secretion of FSH and LH by the gonadotrophs of the anterior pituitary gland, perhaps by similar hormone/receptor interaction at the hypothalamic level.

Another peptide that is produced from the placenta and which is thought to have endocrine activity also shares structural characteristics with hormones produced in the non-pregnant state. This peptide is

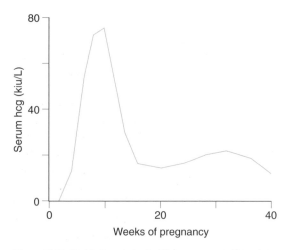

Figure 5.11 Serial changes in the plasma concentration of human chorionic gonadotrophin during pregnancy. Note the marked increment during the first trimester.

known as human placental lactogen (hPL) and it has partial homology with both prolactin and with hGH. It is likely that hPL has major effects upon maternal production of these hormones (see later). No doubt there are many other substances produced by the uterus, placenta and fetus which affect maternal endocrine status. This is a fascinating area for further research.

Sex steroid hormones are also produced in very large quantities by the placenta and fetus. Concentrations of oestrogens, including the active hormone oestradiol, and progesterone increase very substantially from the earliest weeks of pregnancy, then plateau for the remainder of the pregnancy. These hormones were at one time used to assess fetal well-being but the advent of more specific biophysical methods for this purpose has made this practice unnecessary. It is known that both oestrogen and progesterone have effects upon the myometrium (oestrogen encourages cellular hypertrophy whereas progesterone discourages contraction) and, together with prolactin, the tissues of the breast (see the breast, page 148). It is likely that they exert effects upon many other target tissues during pregnancy, such as the smooth muscle of the vascular tree and of the urinary and gastrointestinal tracts. Rather surprisingly, however, the precise roles of these hormones have not been unequivocally defined. Much research is still needed in this area.

Prolactin and growth factors

Hormones produced by uterine tissues understandably increase dramatically during pregnancy. However, the production of several other hormones is also substantially increased. One of the most outstanding examples of this phenomenon is prolactin, which reaches plasma concentrations during pregnancy that would be considered pathological in a non-pregnant woman. There is evidence to suggest that oestrogen has a stimulatory role in this process but that hPL may be inhibitory. Of importance is the fact that those endocrinological mechanisms that regulate prolactin production in the non-pregnant state, such as sleep (which increases prolactin concentrations) and dopamine agonists (which reduce them) remain effective during pregnancy. This implies that prolactin continues to be produced by the lactotrophs of the anterior pituitary gland. This is important because there is now clear

evidence of intrauterine production of prolactin, especially from cells within the decidua. Interestingly, receptors for prolactin are present on trophoblast cells and within the amniotic fluid. It therefore seems possible that there is an interaction between the maternal uterine tissues and the fetus but the details of any such relationship remain speculative at present. The increased prolactin production is essential for lactation and this is discussed in Chapter 10.

In marked contrast to the situation with prolactin, there is evidence that hGH production by the anterior pituitary gland is suppressed during pregnancy. A reduction has been reported in the number of pituitary somatotrophs and responses to conventional provocation tests are blunted. Circulating concentrations of hGH are also reduced during pregnancy. It is likely that hPL suppresses GH release by the maternal pituitary: in women who have a pregnancy in which hPL is deficient (for example in trophoblastic disease) it appears that pituitary growth hormone production is not suppressed.

Fetal growth does not appear to be regulated primarily by hGH. A major role appears to be played by insulin and the insulin-like growth factors (IGFs). There are two major types of these somatomedins and the relative concentrations of each vary from site to site and from time to time during pregnancy. It is IGF-II that predominates in the fetal circulation throughout pregnancy. However, both IGF-I and IGF-II are produced not only by fetal cells (in the liver) but also by maternal cells (in the uterus). The relative proportions of maternal IGFs and of the specific binding proteins that regulate their activity appear to vary during the menstrual cycle and during the early part of pregnancy. Fetal growth is now known to be of major importance in determining an individual's susceptibility to several disorders later in life. The control of fetal growth is therefore the subject of intensive research at present.

Factors controlling carbohydrate metabolism

During the first half of pregnancy, fasting plasma glucose concentrations are reduced but there is relatively little change in plasma insulin levels. A standard oral glucose tolerance test at this time shows an enhanced response compared to the non-pregnant state, with a normal pattern of insulin release but reduced blood glucose values. This pattern changes during the second half of pregnancy, at least in women who take a Western-style diet. Now there is a delay in reaching peak glucose values and an increase in these values throughout the test despite significant increases in plasma insulin concentrations, a pattern suggestive of relative insulin resistance. It has been suggested that the mechanism responsible for this change may once again involve the activity of hPL or other growth-related hormones, which can be shown to reduce peripheral insulin sensitivity. An even more intriguing suggestion is that there are alterations in the characteristics of insulin binding to its receptor, similar to those that have been described in non-pregnant women who are obese or have non-insulin-dependent diabetes mellitus. If such women become pregnant, interestingly, they are liable to have babies of higher mean birthweight than normal women. Whether this phenomenon results from increased transplacental transfer of glucose or from the growth promoting characteristics of insulin and somatomedins (see above) remains to be established.

Thyroid function

It has been suggested that hCG has a thyrotrophic function (perhaps as a result of a subunit homology with TSH) and that maternal TSH production may be suppressed during the first trimester of pregnancy, when hCG levels are maximal. The TSH response to injection of thyrotrophin-releasing hormone (TRH) is blunted during the first trimester but later returns to normal. Isolated cases of thyroid malfunction have also been reported at this time and some authors have suggested that there may be an association with the marked increase in nausea and vomiting which is often experienced by normal women and which usually improves after the first trimester. In general, however, thyroid function is considered to remain normal throughout the remainder of pregnancy. Some features previously thought to be physiological during pregnancy, such as increase in the size of the thyroid gland, are now felt to have been observed in populations of women who were relatively iodine deficient and these increases have not been confirmed in women from Iceland and the Netherlands,

where iodine intake is greater. Pregnancy is associated with a marked increase in thyroid-binding globulin and also in the bound forms of thyroxine (T_4) and tri-iodothyronine (T_3) but the circulating concentrations of unbound (and therefore active) forms of these hormones are essentially unaltered. Thus there is no evidence to support a direct role for the thyroid gland in the development of such features of normal pregnancy as increases in basal metabolic rate, body temperature and heart rate.

Factors controlling calcium metabolism

In the circulation, about 40 per cent of calcium is bound to albumin. Since plasma albumin concentrations decrease markedly during pregnancy (see above), total plasma calcium concentrations also decrease. There appears to be relatively little change in the circulating concentration of unbound, ionised calcium. It is therefore tempting to speculate that, as in the case of thyroid function, calcium homeostasis is little altered in the pregnant woman. This is not true. There is a very substantial fetal demand for calcium and transplacental flux rates of about 6.5 mmoL per day have been calculated. Such a quantity would represent about 80 per cent of the net amount absorbed from the upper gastrointestinal tract in a non-pregnant woman. However, the pregnant woman substantially increases absorption and slightly decreases excretion, thereby coping with little net change in transfer rates into and out of bone stores. Nevertheless, this new equilibrium is finely poised: women who are unable to sustain this level of fetal transfer from dietary sources alone may develop osteopenia during and after pregnancy.

The mechanism responsible for the marked increase in calcium absorption appears to result directly from increased production of one metabolite of vitamin D_3, 1,25 dihydroxycholecalciferol (1,25-[OH]$_2$D$_3$). Production of 1,25-(OH)$_2$D$_3$ appears to be partly under the influence of parathyroid hormone (PTH) which increases by about one-third during human pregnancy. Consistent changes have not, however, been reported in circulating concentrations of other agents with roles in calcium metabolism, notably calcitonin and other metabolites of vitamin D_3. It is of interest to note that the fetus has higher plasma concentrations of calcium than the mother, although hormones such as PTH and calcitonin appear to be independently regulated by mother and fetus and are not thought to cross the placenta. Once again, the mechanism by which this phenomenon is regulated appears to reside within the uterus. Placental sources of $1,25\text{-}(OH)_2D_3$ and of a PTH-related peptide have been identified.

Placental CRF and the onset of human labour: the Placental Clock theory

From mid-pregnancy onwards the trophoblast is able to synthesize CRF. CRF stimulates the fetal pituitary to increase fetal ACTH and thereby fetal dihydroepiandrosterone (DHEA) production by the fetal adrenal is increased. DHEA is the main precursor for placental oestrogen secretion. The high levels of oestrogens towards the end of pregnancy increase gap junction synthesis between uterine myometrial cells, aiding conduction and therefore regular uterine contractions. CRF synthesis is regulated in a positive feedback loop by oestrogens.

The potential mechanism by which the placenta regulates its own metabolism by effects on the fetus, which has subsequent effects on maternal uterine physiology, and possibly the onset of labour, has been christened the Placental Clock.

Corticosteroids and the renin-angiotensin system

Trophoblast cells are now known to produce both corticotrophin-releasing factor and ACTH. It is thought that these placental hormones have roles in regulating the activity of the fetal adrenal glands and the myometrium but it is not clear what influence, if any, they exert upon the mother. There is a progressive increase in maternal circulating concentrations of cortisol throughout pregnancy, despite a relative decrease in the concentration of ACTH during the later weeks. Much of the cortisol is bound to cortisol-binding globulin, which doubles in concentration during pregnancy, but there appears nevertheless to be a slight increase in unbound cortisol. Interestingly, the lack of diurnal fluctuation of cortisol and the attenuated response to dexamethasone suppression suggest that placental ACTH may have a greater role than was previously suspected.

It has already been noted that there are marked increases during pregnancy (up to tenfold) in the circulating concentrations of the antinatriuretic hormones, aldosterone and deoxycorticosterone. At one time this change was attributed entirely to progesterone, which has natriuretic properties, and it was noted that the progressive changes in circulating levels of aldosterone and progesterone were similar. However, it is now clear that other factors that may influence aldosterone production, notably atrial natriuretic peptide and angiotensins, are also produced in increased amounts during pregnancy. The increased production of angiotensins, including the vasoactive angiotensin II, is known to be the result of an augmented production of the enzyme renin and its substrate angiotensinogen. However, it is now becoming clear that intrauterine tissues, both maternal and fetal in origin, also produce the elements of this system. The precise roles of these intrauterine hormones have yet to be elucidated.

🔍 Key Points

Endocrine changes
- Prolactin concentration increases markedly
- Human growth hormone is suppressed
- Insulin resistance develops
- Thyroid function changes little
- Transplacental calcium transport is enhanced
- Corticosteroid concentrations increase

New Developments: mechanisms of change

Maternal homeostasis
It will be obvious from the preceding sections that pregnancy results in marked changes in homeostatic equilibria. Many of these changes occur early in pregnancy, when the embryo is little more than microscopic and would not appear to need to induce such violent alterations in maternal physiology. It is becoming increasingly clear that these changes are underpinned by alterations in gene expression. For example, the gene for leukaemia inhibitory factor (LIF), which is known to be involved in

implantation of the blastocyst in mice, is expressed in human endometrial tissue and decidua at the appropriate stage of human pregnancy. LIF is thought to stimulate the production of hCG by trophoblast cells and there is now evidence that a receptor for LIF is expressed by trophoblast cells early in pregnancy.

Uterine activity

Much research is currently directed towards understanding the mechanisms by which the myometrium remains quiescent for most of pregnancy but is able to function in a coordinated manner to enable normal parturition to take place. Variations in gene expression, probably modulated by hormones and cytokines, are of fundamental importance in permitting the expression of anti-contractile factors early in pregnancy and of factors encouraging contraction and intercellular communication later.

It seems certain that most of the maternal physiological changes which have been described in this chapter result from similar changes in gene expression. Work in this fundamentally important area is as yet rudimentary. Here is a major research challenge for the new millennium.

CASE HISTORY

A 34-year-old woman had an uncomplicated first pregnancy. She was admitted to the Delivery Suite at term and had a slow labour with a first stage lasting 16 hours and a three hour second stage, prior to assisted vaginal delivery with forceps. She subsequently had hypotension and a significant postpartum haemorrhage, losing 1500 mL of blood. After resuscitation she went to the postnatal ward and despite a desire to breastfeed her son, this proved unsuccessful. When seen by her GP at eight weeks after the delivery she felt tired and lethargic. The GP initially ascribed these symptoms to the new arrival, however when they persisted two months later, and she still had not had a period, he referred the patient back to the obstetrician.

What investigations will help with the diagnosis?

Whilst it is not unreasonable to blame postpartum tiredness on the arrival of a new baby, the inability to establish lactation in a well-motivated mother and the lack of menstruation after a postpartum haemorrhage require that pituitary infarction (Sheehan's syndrome) is excluded. The anterior pituitary increases markedly in size during pregnancy and is particularly vulnerable to hypotension. The diagnosis of hypopituitarism can be made by finding reduced plasma concentrations of thyroxine, TSH, cortisol, ACTH, FSH, LH and GH. The secretion of ACTH, GH and prolactin in response to hypoglycaemia (an insulin stress test) is reduced. The differential diagnosis of the cause for the hypopituitarism includes lymphocytic hypophysitis and tumour. CT or MRI of the pituitary fossa is therefore a mandatory investigation.

What is the management?

Cases of Sheehan's syndrome have resolved spontaneously. This patient did not present acutely, suggesting some pituitary function was retained. In general, patients will require thyroid and glucocorticoid hormone replacement. A lack of FSH and ovulation will require oestrogen replacement therapy to prevent cardiovascular disease and osteoporosis. As the woman still has a uterus, progestogen therapy to induce a withdrawal bleed will also be required.

How will Sheehan's syndrome affect future pregnancies?

Spontaneous pregnancies have been reported after confirmed diagnosis of Sheehan's syndrome. However, for most women it is likely that ovulation induction with exogenous gonadotrophins would be required to induce ovulation. If hormone replacement is inadequate an increased risk of miscarriage, stillbirth and maternal morbidity (hypotension and hypoglycaemia) have been reported. Where hormone replacement is adequate prior to, and during, pregnancy outcome is normal.

References for further reading

De Swiet M. *Medical disorders in obstetric practice, 3rd edition.* Oxford: Blackwell Science.

Dunlop W. Normal pregnancy: physiology and endocrinology. In: Dewhurst's *Textbook of Obstetrics and Gynaecology, 6th edition.* Oxford: Blackwell Science, in press.

Chamberlain G, Broughton Pipkin F. *Clinical physiology in obstetrics, 3rd edition.* Oxford: Blackwell Science, 1991.

Chapter 6

Normal fetal development and growth

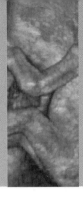

OVERVIEW

An appreciation of normal development, growth and maturation is important for understanding complications that may arise in pregnancy.

At the end of embryogenesis, organogenesis is complete and the fetus is completely formed. The ensuing six months *in utero* will be devoted to maturation and growth.

Fetal growth and maturation

Fetal growth is dependent on adequate transfer of nutrients and oxygen across the placenta. This in itself is dependent on appropriate maternal nutrition and placental perfusion. Factors affecting these are discussed in Chapter 11. Other factors are important in determining fetal growth. For example, fetal hormones are essential for normal fetal growth and development. They affect the metabolic rate, growth of tissues and maturation of individual organs. In particular, insulin growth factors (IGF) coordinate a precise and orderly increase in growth throughout late gestation. Insulin and T4 are required through late gestation to ensure appropriate growth in normal and adverse nutritional circumstances. Fetal hyperinsulinaemia, which occurs in association with maternal diabetes mellitus, results in fetal macrosomia with, in particular, excessive fat deposition.

Conversely in growth restricted fetuses, fetal insulin levels are low, thus further reducing fetal tissue accretion. Lack of thyroid hormone produces deficiency in skeletal and cerebral maturation, characteristic of cretinism, and surfactant production is delayed. Cortisol has a limited role in stimulating growth, but is essential for the structural and functional development of a wide variety of individual fetal tissues. In the lung, it increases compliance and surfactant release, which ensures that spontaneous breathing can occur at birth. In the fetal liver, cortisol induces beta-receptors and glycogen deposition to maintain a glucose supply to the neonate immediately after birth. In the gut, cortisol is responsible for villi proliferation and induction of digestive enzymes, which enable the neonate to switch to enteral feeding at birth.

In developed countries, the average birth weight is about 3.5 kg at the end of a normal pregnancy lasting an average of 40 weeks. About one-third of the eventual birth weight is reached by 28 weeks, half by 31 weeks, and two-thirds by 34 weeks. Fetal weight gain continues and does not flatten at term. In an average normal pregnancy, the baby gains about 25 g a day before birth. The slope of the curve or the fetal growth trajectory depends on the birth weight end-point which is to be reached, i.e. the curve of a baby which is expected to have a weight of 3700 g is steeper than one which is expected to weigh say 3200 g at term.

New developments

Variables affecting fetal growth and size at birth

Each baby has its own optimal growth potential, which is, to a degree, predictable from physiological characteristics known at the beginning of pregnancy. The principal known factors are maternal weight and height, parity, race or ethnic group, and the baby's sex. Maternal age is also a factor, but the variation is mostly accounted for by parity. Of paternal characteristics, height is associated with birth weight, but to a lesser extent than any of the maternal variables. The main coefficients are listed in Table 6.1. The physiological variation in normal birth weight in any heterogeneous maternity population can be considerable. For example, a mother from India who weighs 5 kg less and is 5 cm shorter than the population average, would be expected to have a baby that weighs [185 g (ethnic group) + 45 g (weight) + 40 g (height)] 290 g less at 40 weeks. However, a European mother of average size, but in her third pregnancy, would have a baby that is approximately 150 g heavier than a mother with the same characteristics but in her fifth pregnancy (Table 6.2). Such differences become magnified when trying to determine, on the basis of birth weight alone, what is abnormally small. In an average birth weight distribution, a 150 g adjustment at the tenth centile cut-off for small for gestational age (SGA) is enough for 50 per cent of babies being reclassified in either direction between the SGA/non-SGA categories.

It is important to exclude the known pathological influences on birth weight when calculating the optimal weight that a baby can reach. Most of those listed in Chapter 11 are too rare and/or too heterogeneous in their effect to result in a statistically significant value in multivariate analysis of birth weight in a maternity population. However, smoking has an all too high prevalence in an average NHS population: about 25 per cent of mothers admit to being smokers

Table 6.1 – Physiological variables affecting normal fetal growth

Pre-pregnancy weight and maternal booking weight
Maternal height
Maternal age and parity
Ethnic group
Fetal sex
Paternal height

Table 6.2 – Optimal birth weight

Approximate coefficients used for individually adjusting the predicted birth-weight at the end of a normal pregnancy, i.e. pathology-free birth-weight. The baseline birth weight for a baby of a non-smoking Anglo-European mother in her first pregnancy, of average height (163 cm) and booking weight (64 kg), is about 3480 g at 40.0 weeks

Maternal weight		9 g/kg
Maternal height		8 g/cm
Parity	- para 1	+ 110g
	- para 2+	+ 150g
Ethnic group		
	South Asian (India, Pakistan)	- 185 g
	Afro-Caribbean	- 130 g
Baby's gender		
	Male>female	+/- 60 g

at the time of the booking visit, and most of them continue to smoke throughout pregnancy. The effect of smoking on birth weight is significant, consistent and dose-dependent (Fig. 6.1).

Cardiovascular system

The fetal circulation is quite different from that of the adult (Fig. 6.2). Its distinctive features are:

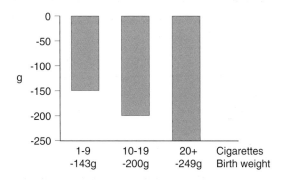

Figure 6.1 Deficit in birth weight due to smoking as recorded in early pregnancy (adjusted for other variables listed in Table 6.2).

- Oxygenation occurs in the placenta.
- The right and left ventricles work in parallel rather than in series.
- The heart, brain and upper body receive blood from the left ventricle, while the placenta and lower body receive blood from both right and left ventricles.

Three modifications in fetal vascularity ensure that the best, oxygenated blood from the placenta is delivered to the fetal brain. These are the ductus venosus, the foramen ovale and the ductus arteriosis. Oxygenated blood from the placenta returns to the fetus through the umbilical vein. This vein divides into two main branches, one that supplies the portal vein in the liver, and another narrow vessel called the ductus venosus, which joins the inferior vena cava as it enters the right atrium. Fifty per cent of the blood will pass to the portal system and 50 per cent to the ductus venosus. The ductus is a narrow vessel and high blood velocities are generated in this vessel. This streaming of the ductus venosus blood, together with a membranous valve in the right atrium (the crista dividens) prevents mixing of the well-oxygenated blood from the ductus venosus with the desaturated blood of the inferior vena cava. The ductus venosus stream passes across the right atrium through a physiological defect in the atrial septum, called the foramen ovale, to the left atrium; from here blood passes through the mitral valve to the left ventricle and hence to the aorta. About 50 per cent goes to the head and upper

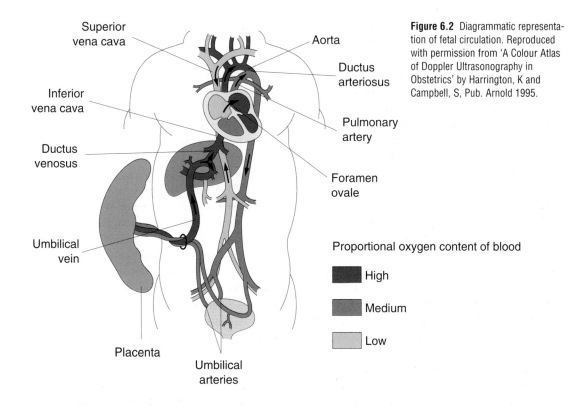

Figure 6.2 Diagrammatic representation of fetal circulation. Reproduced with permission from 'A Colour Atlas of Doppler Ultrasonography in Obstetrics' by Harrington, K and Campbell, S, Pub. Arnold 1995.

extremities, the remainder passes down the aorta to mix with blood of reduced oxygen saturation from the right ventricle.

Blood from the inferior vena cava and the superior vena cava is directed across the tricuspid valve to the right ventricle. Only a small portion of blood from the right ventricle passes to the lungs as they are not functional. Most of the blood is directed through a narrow vessel called the ductus arteriosus into the descending aorta below the origin of the head and neck vessels from the aortic arch. By this means, the desaturated blood from the right ventricle passes down the aorta to enter the umbilical arterial circulation and thence to the placenta.

At birth, the cessation of umbilical blood flow causes cessation of flow in the ductus venosus, a fall in pressure in the right atrium and closure of the foramen ovale. Ventilation of the lungs opens the pulmonary circulation and the ductus arteriosus closes as a direct effect of increasing PO_2. Prior to birth, the ductus remains patent due to the reduction of prostaglandin E2 and prostacyclin, which act as local vasodilators. Premature closure of the ductus has been reported with the administration of cyclo-oxygenase inhibitors.

Fetal blood

The first fetal blood cells are formed on the surface of the yolk sac. During the 6th week of embryonic life, extra medullary haemopoesis begins in the liver and to a lesser extent in the spleen. The bone marrow starts to produce red cells at 16 weeks and is the predominant source of red cells from 26 weeks' gestation.

Most haemoglobin in the fetus is fetal haemoglobin (HbF), which is two gamma chains (alpha 2, gamma 2) in place of the adult haemoglobins HbA (alpha 2, beta 2) and HbA2 (alpha 2, delta 2). Ninety per cent of fetal haemoglobin is HbF between 10 and 28 weeks' gestation. From 28 to 34 weeks, a switch to HbA occurs and at term the ratio of HbF to HbA is 80:20 and by six months of age, only 1 per cent of haemoglobin is HbF. HbF is resistant to denaturation by acid and alkali and there is a higher affinity for oxygen than HbA. At birth, the mean capillary haemoglobin is 18 g/dL. The higher haemoglobin concentration in the fetus and the greater affinity of HbF for oxygen, enhances transfer of oxygen across the placenta.

Fetal lung

Full differentiation of capillary and canalicular elements of the fetal lung is apparent by 20 weeks' gestation. Alveoli develop after 24 weeks. Numerous, but intermittent, fetal breathing movements occur *in utero*, especially during REM sleep and appear to be necessary for lung maturation. Fetal breathing occurs for 15 per cent of the observation time in the second trimester, rising to 30 per cent in the third trimester. Lung alveoli are lined by a group of phospholipids, known collectively as surfactant. Surfactant prevents collapse of small alveoli during expiration by lowering surface tension. The surfactant is continually replaced by synthesis from type 2 alveolar cells. These cells make up 10 per cent of lung parenchyma. The predominant phospholipid (80 per cent of the total) is phosphatidyl choline (lecithin). The production of lecithin is enhanced by cortisol, growth restriction and prolonged rupture of the membranes and is delayed in diabetes. Other phospholipids may be more potent in reducing surface tension. For example, levels of phosphatidyl glycerol in the amniotic fluid are more predictive of respiratory distress syndrome especially in diabetic fetuses.

Immune system

The fetus requires an effective immune system to resist intrauterine and perinatal infections. Lymphocytes appear from 8 weeks, and by the middle of the second trimester all phagocytic cells, T and B cells and complement are available to mount a response. Early infection with any of the TORCH organisms (toxoplasmosis, rubella, cytomegalovirus, herpes) will affect a number of systems including the immune defences themselves. Immunoglobulin (IgG) originates mostly from the maternal circulation. The fetus normally produces only small amounts of IgM and IgA, which do not cross the placenta. Its detection in the newborn without IgG is indicative of fetal infection.

General immunological defences include the amniotic fluid (lysosymes, IgG), the placenta (lymphoid cells, phagocytes, barrier), granulocytes from liver and bone marrow and interferon from lymphocytes.

Skin and homeostasis

Fetal skin protects and facilitates homeostasis. The thickness of the skin increases progressively from the first month of gestation until birth. A stratum corneum forms in the fifth month. During the last weeks, skin is covered by vernix which consists of desquamated skin cells, cholesterol and glycogen. Preterm babies have no vernix and thin skin, which allows a proportionately large amount of insensible water loss.

Thermal control in cool, ambient temperatures is limited by a large surface-to-body weight ratio and poor thermal insulation. Heat may be conserved by peripheral vasoconstriction and can be generated by brown fat catabolism, but this is deficient in preterm or growth restricted babies. The response to warm ambient temperatures is also poor, as the development of sweat glands is delayed.

Alimentary system and energy stores

The rotation of the gut is complete by 12 weeks. From the time that the gastrointestinal tract is fully formed its lumen is patent. The swallowing reflex develops and matures gradually. The fetus continually and increasingly swallows amniotic fluid, up to approximately 20 mL/hr at term.

Peristalsis in the intestine occurs from the second trimester. The large bowel is filled with meconium at term. However, defecation *in utero*, and hence meconium in the amniotic fluid, is unusual unless there is fetal anoxia.

While body water content gradually diminishes, glycogen and fat stores increase about five-fold in the last trimester.

Preterm infants have virtually no fat, and a severely reduced ability to withstand starvation. This is aggravated by an incompletely developed alimentary system, which may manifest in a poor and unsustained suck, uncoordinated swallowing mechanism, delayed gastric emptying, and poor absorption of carbohydrates, fat and other nutrients.

Kidney and urinary tract

After regression of the mesonephros or Wolffian duct, the metanephros forms the renal collecting system (ureter, pelvis, calyces and collecting ducts) and induces the formation of the renal secretory system (glomeruli, convoluted tubes, loops of Henle) from the mesenchyme of the nephrogenic cord. Nephrogenesis is complete by 36 weeks, but the maturation of excretory and concentrating ability of the fetal kidneys is gradual. It is immature in the preterm infant, and may lead to abnormal water, glucose, sodium or acid-base homeostasis.

Fetal urine forms much of the amniotic fluid, which is a protein- and sugar-free hypotonic ultrafiltrate of fetal plasma. Fetal urine production rises gradually with fetal maturity, from about 12 mL per hour at 32 weeks to 38 mL per hour at 40 weeks.

Fetal behaviour

Fetal movement can be first perceived by the mother by about 18 weeks in primipara and several weeks earlier in multipara ('quickening'). Self-monitoring or formal counting of fetal movements are an important method of monitoring fetal wellbeing. A sensation of diminished fetal activity may be associated with chronic hypoxia and growth failure, and may be a precursor of fetal death. Reduced fetal movements are an important screening tool for further investigation.

With maturation of the central nervous system, the fetus develops more complex patterns and well-defined behavioural states that have been named 1F to 4F. State 1F is similar to quiet (non-REM) sleep, with absence of eye and body movements. In state 2F, periodic eye and body movements are present (REM sleep). State 3F has eye movements but no body movements, i.e. equivalent to quiet wakefulness; while 4F is an active phase with ongoing eye movements and fetal activity. For most of the time (>80 per cent), the fetus alternates between the sleep cycles 1F and 2F.

Amniotic fluid

By 12 weeks' gestation, the amnion comes into contact with the inner surface of the chorion and obliterates the extraembryonic coelom. The two membranes become adherent, but never intimately fused. Neither the amnion nor chorion contains vessels or nerves, but contain a significant quantity of phospholipids as well as enzymes involved in phospholipid hydrolysis. The choriodecidual function is thought to play a pivotal role in the initiation of labour through the production of prostaglandins E2 and F2a.

The amniotic fluid (AF) initially is secreted by the amnion, but by the 10th week it is mainly a transudate of the fetal serum via the skin and umbilical cord. From 16 weeks' gestation, the fetal skin becomes impermeable to water and net increase in AF is through a small imbalance between the contributions of fluid through the kidneys and lung fluids and removal by fetal swallowing. AF volume increases progressively (10 weeks: 30 mL; 20 weeks: 300 mL; 30 weeks: 600 mL; 38 weeks: 1000 mL), but post-term, there is a rapid fall in volume (40 weeks: 800 mL; 42 weeks: 350 mL). The reason for the late reduction in AF volume has not been explained.

The function of the AF is to:
- Protect the fetus from mechanical injury.
- Permit movement of the fetus while preventing limb contracture.
- Prevent adhesions between fetus and amnion.
- Permit fetal lung development in which there is two-way movement of fluid into the fetal bronchioles. Absence of AF in the second trimester is associated with pulmonary hypoplasia.

Major alterations in AF volume occur when there is reduced contribution of fluid into the amniotic sac in conditions such as renal agenesis, cystic kidneys or intrauterine growth restriction, all of which cause oligohydramnios. Reduced removal of fluid in conditions such as anencephaly, oesophageal and duodenal atresia is associated with polyhydramnios (see Chapter 14).

References for further reading

Rutter N. The extremely preterm infant. *British Journal Obstetrics and Gynaecology.* 1995; **102:** 682-7.

Hanson MA, Spencer AD, Rodeck CH. *Fetus and Neonate: Physiology and Clinical application. Vol 3: Growth.* Cambridge: Cambridge University Press, 1995.

Gardosi J, Mongelli M, Wilcox M, Chang A. An adjustable fetal weight standard. *Ultrasound Obstetrics and Gynecology* 1995; **6:** 168-74.

Nathanielsz P. *A time to be born. The life of the unborn child.* Oxford: Oxford University Press, 1994.

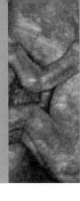

Chapter 7

Antenatal imaging and assessment of fetal wellbeing

OVERVIEW

There is one principal imaging modality in obstetrics, namely diagnostic ultrasound, which is employed in many clinical situations and indeed is used routinely to screen all pregnancies in most developed countries. Ultrasound is used to date and chart antenatal growth of the fetus and to identify congenital abnormalities. Magnetic resonance imaging (MRI) is only occasionally used to provide further information when a fetal structural abnormality is suspected and computerized tomography (CT) scanning has a role in assessing the size of the maternal pelvis; for example, when there is a breech presentation.

Antenatal tests of fetal wellbeing are now principally based on ultrasound techniques and are designed to identify the fetuses that are in the early or late stages of fetal asphyxia. Continuous wave Doppler ultrasound is employed to provide continuous tracings of the fetal heart rate, the patterns of which alter when the fetus is asphyxiated. Colour and spectral Doppler can identify placental and fetal blood vessels and provide information on placental function and the fetal circulatory response to asphyxia.

ANTENATAL IMAGING

Diagnostic ultrasound

This technique employs high frequency (3–7.5 MHz), low-intensity sound waves, which are transmitted through the abdomen or pelvis by an ultrasound transducer. The transducer consists of piezo electric crystals, usually mounted in a curved array. Small groups of crystals are triggered in sequence and each emits a focused ultrasound beam in a series of pulses and then receives the reflected signals from within the uterus between the pulses. These return-ing signals generate small electric charges (piezo electricity), which are transformed into visual signals on a cathode ray tube or video screen. This means that a two-dimensional map of the contents of the uterus is provided in thin slices. Because the complete array is triggered twenty or more times per second, the image is constantly updated in real time and fetal, cardiac and other movements can be studied. Also, as the operator can move the transducer easily across the abdomen, they can build the two-dimensional slices into a three-dimensional mental image of the uterine contents. For imaging in the first trimester, a small array is mounted on a long probe and placed in the vagina (Fig. 7.1a). Transvaginal sonography is also useful for examining the cervix later in pregnancy and for identifying the lower edge of the placenta. In general, however, after 12 weeks an abdominal transducer, which is a flat probe with a much wider array, is used (Fig. 7.1b).

Before we discuss the applications of diagnostic ultrasound, certain aspects of ultrasound imaging should be stressed at this stage.

The obtaining of good images is very dependent on the skill of the operator. The manipulation of the probe and transducer is a key factor in obtaining good diagnostic sections of the fetus and uterine contents.

There is good reason to suppose that ultrasound scanning is safe for both mother and fetus, which is why routine scanning is recommended by many Governments and the Royal College of Obstetricians and Gynaecologists. The safety of ultrasound has been studied epidemiologically by analysing the childhood incidence of childhood cancer, dyslexia, speech development and other variables in women exposed to routine antenatal ultrasound examination, compared to those who had an ultrasound examination on indication. These studies have been reassuring and no woman or baby has ever been shown to have been damaged directly by the use of diagnostic ultrasound in pregnancy. This is all the more striking when one considers that routine ultrasound scanning has been used in most developed countries for many years and many millions of women have been exposed prenatally. However, it is not true to say that ultrasound is a non-invasive method of investigation. Ultrasound can cause bio-effects on cells by inducing heating and other effects. Some of the newer ultrasound equipment uses more focused beams, which result in higher focal intensity than have been hitherto used. Furthermore, the development of spectral Doppler and transvaginal scanning may expose the fetus to higher intensities than those used in the older machines, which were shown to be safe. While there are no restrictions on the use of ultrasound in pregnancy, care should be taken to avoid unnecessarily prolonged exposure or the use of ultrasound for frivolous indications.

Clinical applications of ultrasound

Early pregnancy problems

Transvaginal sonography now plays a pivotal role in the diagnosis of disorders of early pregnancy, such as incomplete or missed abortion and ectopic pregnancy. The early development of the embryo and clinical problems arising in early pregnancy are described in Gynaecology by Ten Teachers.

Fetal measurements

The external dimensions of the fetus can be used to chart the growth rate of the fetus *in utero*. Before 12 weeks' gestation, the crown–rump length (CRL) is

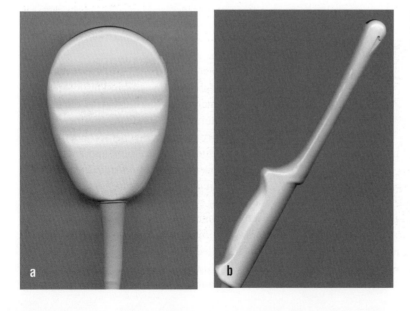

Figure 7.1 (a) Transabdominal ultrasound transducer. (b) transvaginal ultrasound transducer.

measured (Fig. 7.2). After 12 weeks the standard measurements are the biparietal diameter (BPD), head circumference (HC), abdominal circumference (AC) and femur length (FL) (Fig. 7.3). It is customary now to measure all these parameters when assessing fetal size, as it provides information about fetal symmetry. In addition, when combined in an equation, these measurements provide a more accurate estimate of fetal weight (EFW) than any of the parameters taken singly. All measurements can be immediately compared with a normal reference range taken from an unselected population. The following observations can be made about the normal graph. Firstly, that the increase in fetal size is exponential until 12 weeks, linear until 36 weeks and then slows thereafter. Secondly, that the spread of values about the mean increases progressively throughout gestation, but especially after 24 weeks, reflecting an increased variation in fetal growth rate (Fig. 7.4a and b).

Gestational age assessment

Fetal age can be assessed accurately in the first half of pregnancy from any of the fetal measurements described above, for at this stage the range of values around the mean is narrow. In clinical practice, the CRL and biparietal diameter are the most often used, because they are the most reproducible measurements. Essentially the earlier the measurement is made, the better the prediction and measurements made from an early CRL (accuracy of prediction ±5 days) will be preferred to a biparietal diameter at 20 weeks (accuracy of prediction ± 7 days). Predictions of gestational age by ultrasound before 20 weeks have

been shown to be more accurate than predictions from the last menstrual period, even if the woman is certain of her dates. This has led to calls for the ultrasound prediction to be accepted for all pregnancies, but conventionally the ultrasound date is only taken if the discrepancy in the EDD calculated from ultrasound and the date of the last menstrual period is greater than ten days.

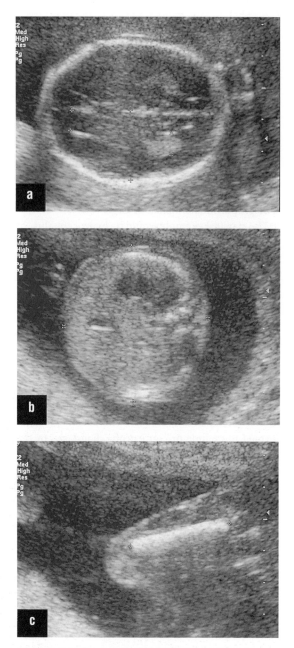

Figure 7.3 Measurements of (a) BPD, HC; (b) AC; and (c) FL taken at 24 weeks' gestation.

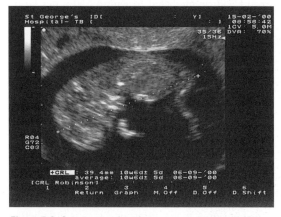

Figure 7.2 Crown–rump length measurement taken at 12 weeks' gestation. This view is also used for measurement of the nuchal translucency.

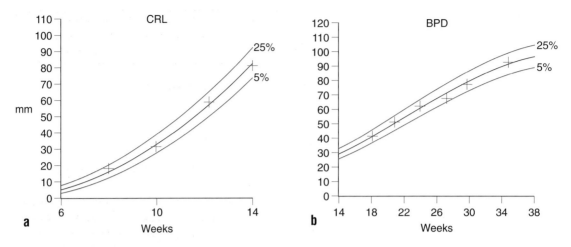

Figure 7.4 (a) Typical crown–rump length chart showing normal growth. (b) Typical biparietal diameter chart demonstrating normal growth.

Fetal symmetry

Not infrequently, when the standard four external fetal measurements are made, one of the dimensions is disproportionately small or large.

The classical example would be hydrocephalus, in which the head circumference is large, although this does not usually occur until late in gestation and the diagnosis is usually based on the identification of enlarged ventricles. A small head circumference would raise the suspicion of microcephaly, a small femur of achondroplasia and a small abdomen of triploidy or trisomy 18. At the time of the mid-pregnancy scan, it is important not to worry parents unnecessarily; for example, a femur just below the normal reference range in most cases merely reflects constitutional short stature. Nevertheless, serial measurements will usually be performed to exclude or confirm the diagnosis. In the third trimester, asymmetry can be caused by intrauterine growth restriction (IUGR) where a brain sparing effect will result in a relatively large head circumference compared with the abdominal circumference. The opposite would occur in a diabetic pregnancy, where the abdomen is disproportionately large due to the effects of insulin on the fetal liver and fat stores.

Fetal growth

In pregnancies at high risk of IUGR, serial measurements are plotted on the normal reference range (see Chapter 11). Growth patterns are helpful in distinguishing between different types of growth restriction (symmetrical and asymmetrical). Cessation of growth is an ominous sign of placental failure. However, the importance of serial measurements has lessened with more dynamic tests of fetal wellbeing, such as umbilical and fetal Doppler and the antenatal cardiotocograph.

Fetal weight

Of all the parameters measured, the abdominal circumference is the most accurate predictor of fetal weight because it is reduced in both symmetric and asymmetric IUGR. However, equations combining several parameters will reduce the random variation in the accuracy of the predictions. For example, by combining biparietal diameter, head circumference, abdominal circumference and femur length, fetal weight will be predicted to within 150 g per kg of true weight. This is especially valuable in predicting the weight of small fetuses, such as growth restricted preterm infants, to provide information as to their potential viability. For example, an estimated birthweight of less than 600 g would generally be considered non-viable. Birthweight assessments, however, are less accurate with larger babies and, above 3 kg, ultrasound assessments are very little better than estimates made by abdominal palpation. This is why routine screening in the third trimester to detect the small-for-gestational age (SGA) infant is not usually performed, because the detection rate of the late SGA fetus on a single ultrasound scan is little better than that obtained by serial measurements of the symphysis–fundal height.

Fetal anatomy

In 3 per cent of all pregnancies, there will be a serious structural abnormality of the fetus, the most common being central nervous system abnormalities and cardiac defects. The detection of these defects is discussed in Chapter 12. The most detailed survey of fetal anatomy is carried out at the mid-pregnancy scan at 20–22 weeks' gestation, but a screen of fetal anatomy will be carried out at any stage if there are risk factors for congenital abnormality. The aim of this scan is to examine every organ and structure in the fetus in the shortest possible time. Fetal measurements and anatomical features that should be visualised are summarised in Table 7.1. The operator will examine each structure in a series of well-rehearsed movements and should complete the examination in 15 minutes. The overall detection rate for abnormalities varies from centre to centre, but most studies report a 70–80 per cent detection rate for disabling or lethal conditions. Fortunately, the false positive rate is low and termination of a normal fetus because of a mistaken diagnosis, is a rare event. However, anxiety is engendered is some parents when waiting for a second opinion on a suspected abnormality. Once a serious abnormality is detected, evidence shows that parents will elect to terminate the pregnancy in 80–90 per cent of cases.

Placental location

Placenta praevia is a cause of life-threatening haemorrhage in pregnancy. Before any major antepartum haemorrhage occurs, there is usually a warning haemorrhage and any woman with a blood-stained vaginal loss should immediately have a scan to determine placental location. If the lower edge of the placenta appears to lie close to the cervix, then a gentle transvaginal scan should be performed to determine whether the placenta covers the internal os, indicating a major placenta praevia (Fig. 7.5). In the third trimester, if the lower edge of the placenta lies within 3 cm of the internal os, then the provisional diagnosis would be type I (minor) placenta praevia. At the mid-pregnancy scan, it is customary to identify women who have a low-lying placenta. At this stage, the lower uterine segment has not yet formed and

Table 7.1 – Fetal measurements and anatomic features visualised on the routine scan between 18 and 22 weeks' gestation

Standard fetal measurments
  Biparietal diameter
  Head circumference
  Abdominal circumference
  Femoral length
Fetal anatomic features and measurements
Brain
  Ventricular section: anterior and posterior horns of the cerebral ventricles; measurement: anterior and posterior ventricle-hemisphere ratio
  Posterior fossa section: cerebellum, vermis, cisterna magna, and nuchal skinfold; measurement: transcerebellar diameter and nuchal skinfold thickness
Skull
  Shape, e.g. lemon-shaped as in spina bifida
Face
  Orbits (and both lenses) measurement: interorbital, external orbital diameters
  Nose, lips, palate, and mandible
Spine
  'Anterior' view of spinous processes down to tip of sacrum; clear view of skin margin throughout length of spine
Chest
  Heart: 4-chamber view, aortic root and arch, pulmonary artery and ductus
  Lungs
Abdomen
  Diaphragm
  Cord insertion
  Liver, stomach, and intestines
  Both kidneys for parenchyma and renal pelvis size
  Bladder
  Genitalia
Limbs
  Femur, tibia, fibula, foot, and toes (both limbs)
  Humerus, radius, ulna, hand, and fingers (both limbs)
Placenta
  Morphology and site
Cord
  Number of vessels
Amniotic fluid
  Volume assessment

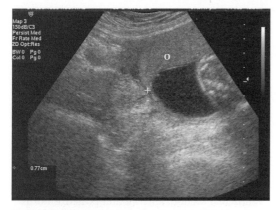

Figure 7.5 Transvaginal scan showing cervix and placenta covering internal os. o = placenta, + = placenta covering internal os

most low-lying placentas will appear to 'migrate' upwards as the lower segment stretches in the late second and third trimesters. About 5 per cent of women will have a low-lying placenta at 20 weeks and only 5 per cent of this group will eventually be shown to have a placenta praevia. Recent studies have shown that a transvaginal scan performed in women with a low-lying placenta will identify cases of true placenta praevia with more precision.

Placental morphology

The appearance of the placenta in the second and early third trimesters is one of a fairly uniform texture (echogenicity). Towards the end of the third trimester, the placenta develops a mature appearance, being distinctly lobular with white echoes demarcating the cotyledons. While there is some evidence that premature maturation of the placenta is associated with impaired function, this is not strong enough to make it a useful test.

Amniotic fluid volume

The amount of amniotic fluid in the uterus is a guide to fetal wellbeing and is affected by fetal abnormalities. A precise evaluation cannot be made by ultrasound, as the fluid gathers in irregular pockets around the fetus, demonstrated on ultrasound as echo-free spaces. Two relatively crude methods are used as indicators of volume. The maximum vertical pool is measured after a general survey of the uterine contents.

Measurements of less than 2 cm suggest oligohydramnios and greater than 7 cm, polyhydramnios. More effective is the amniotic fluid index (AFI), which is the sum of all the maximum vertical pool measurements from the four quadrants of the uterus. The AFI alters throughout gestation, but in the third trimester, it should be between 10 and 25 cm; values below 10 indicate a reduced volume and below 5, oligohydramnios, while values above 25 indicate polyhydramnios.

Umbilical cord

Some abnormalities of the umbilical cord can be identified by ultrasound during the antenatal period and visualization is improved with the use of colour Doppler (*vide infra*). A single umbilical artery is associated with congenital abnormalities of the fetus and intrauterine growth restriction and is looked for at the time of the mid-pregnancy scan. Nuchal displacement is a common event, but occasionally may be associated with fetal distress in labour or intrauterine death. This is more likely if there is more than one loop of cord around the neck. Cord presentation and vasa praevia can also be recognized and both are associated with a low-lying placenta.

Invasive procedures

Ultrasound is used to guide invasive diagnostic procedures, such as amniocentesis, chorion villus sampling and cordocentesis, and therapeutic procedures such as the insertion of fetal bladder shunts or chest drains. If fetoscopy is performed, the endoscope is inserted under ultrasound guidance. This use of ultrasound has greatly reduced the possibility of fetal trauma, as the needle or scope is visualised throughout the procedure and guided with precision to the appropriate place.

Doppler ultrasound

The ability to identify blood vessels in the uterus, placenta and fetus, and measure aspects of blood velocity has led to major advances in the management of pregnancy. Doppler ultrasound makes use of the phenomenon of the Doppler frequency shift, where the reflected wave will be at a different frequency from the transmitted one if it interacts with moving structures, such as red blood cells flowing along a blood vessel. If the red blood cells are moving towards the beam, the reflected signal will be at a higher frequency than the transmitted one and lower if the flow is away from the beam. The original equipment displayed spectral signals with inexpensive continuous wave (CW) Doppler equipment. As the vessels are not visualized, this equipment is only suitable for detailing signals from the umbilical artery, which is easy to isolate from surrounding vessels. In modern equipment, the same transducer has the ability to perform conventional imaging and display Doppler frequency shifts. The Doppler shifted signals can be displayed in two ways. Firstly, they can be shown as a colour map of blood vessels superimposed on top of the grey scale image. This is called colour Doppler imaging (or just colour Doppler). Blood flowing towards the transducer is shown in shades of red, the brighter shades indicating high velocity. Flow away from the transducer is shown is shades of blue. By this means, nearly all the major blood vessels in the placenta and fetus can be displayed (Fig. 7.6). Quantitative information about the velocity or resistance to flow in any of these vessels can be obtained by means of pulsed or spectral Doppler. In this modality, signals from a particular vessel can be isolated (gated) and displayed in graphic form, the velocity being plotted against time. Arterial flow is pulsatile; venous flow is usually constant, but is pulsatile in veins that are close to the heart (central veins). In general, most studies have been carried out on arterial flow, although recently there has been an increasing interest in central veins.

The pulsatile arterial flow velocity waveform has a systolic and diastolic component. If the angle of the ultrasound beam to the long axis of the vessel is known, the absolute blood velocity in centimetres per second can be determined. However, velocity has not been used much in obstetrics, except in assessing the rhesus-affected fetus when high blood velocities are associated with fetal anaemia. Most studies have looked at resistance to flow, which is reflected in the diastolic component. A small amount of diastolic flow implies high resistance downstream to the vessel being studied and implies low perfusion. A high diastolic component indicates low downstream resistance and implies high perfusion (Fig. 7.7). A measure of the amount of diastolic flow relative to systolic is provided by several indices such as the pulsatility index or resistance index, which essentially compare the amount of diastolic flow to systolic. When these indices are high, this indicates high resistance to flow; when the indices are low, resistance to flow is low. Another feature of the waveform is a 'notch' in the waveform in early diastole. This is particularly important in the uterine artery because it indicates that the spiral arteries, which are downstream from the uterine artery, are muscular and compliant and, therefore, that trophoblast invasion of these arteries is incomplete or inadequate.

Clinical applications of Doppler ultrasound

Essentially, Doppler ultrasound is mainly employed to predict and monitor pregnancies at risk of pre-eclampsia and intrauterine growth restriction. This is discussed more fully in Chapter 11 but a brief summary is given here.

Uterine artery (maternal) Doppler

Study of the uterine arteries provides information of the maternal blood supply to the placenta. Both arteries are studied around 20 weeks and provide long-term prediction of the risk of developing pre-eclampsia, intrauterine growth restriction and abruptioplacentae. A high resistance waveform or a waveform with a notch implies inadequate or incomplete trophoblast invasion of the spiral arteries, especially if the findings are bilateral (Fig. 7.8).

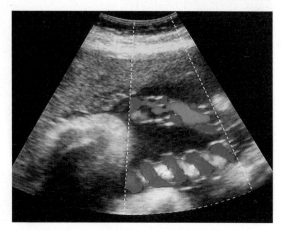

Figure 7.6 Typical colour Doppler image of fetal vessels.

If confirmed at 24 weeks, the pregnancy will require close monitoring of the fetal growth rate and the possible development of maternal hypertension and proteinuria.

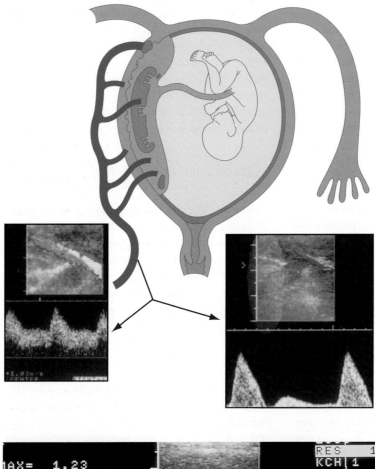

Figure 7.7 Left: a low resistance wave form from the uterine artery; note the abundance of diastolic flow. Right: a high resistance waveform from the uterine artery; note the notches and reduced diastolic flow.

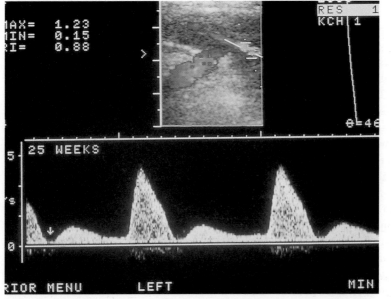

Figure 7.8 The uterine artery is easily identified crossing medial to the external iliac vein. A high resistance waveform is demonstrated.

Umbilical artery and fetal Dopplers

These vessels are studied to provide information on placental function and fetal oxygenation. This is discussed in the next section on assessment of fetal wellbeing.

The routine ultrasound scan

A routine scan between 16 and 22 weeks is practised in most hospitals in Europe. There is now a tendency to delay this to between 20 and 22 weeks, as this improves the opportunity to diagnose cardiac and late developing abnormalities, such as microcephaly. Furthermore, performing the mid-pregnancy scan slightly later will provide improved opportunities to identify women at increased risk of pre-eclampsia and preterm labour by assessment of the uterine artery flow velocity waveforms and measurement of the cervical length.

An increasing number of hospitals are also offering an early scan at about 11 to 14 weeks gestation. A routine two pregnancy scan policy is also recommended by the Royal College of Obstetricians and Gynaecologists.

Early scan (11–14 weeks)

This scan is normally performed transabdominally, but in some countries the transvaginal route is preferred. The principle aim of this scan is:

- To provide an accurate estimation of gestational age by measurement of the fetal CRL.
- To diagnose multiple gestation, and in particular to identify monochorionic twins which are at increased risk of fetal abnormality, and twin–twin transfusion syndrome.
- To identify markers which would indicate a risk of fetal chromosome abnormality, such as Down's syndrome. This is principally achieved by measuring the small pool of fluid underneath the skin at the back of the neck (nuchal translucency). It is important to stress that this test only identifies a high-risk group and is not diagnostic.
- To identify fetuses with gross structural abnormalities, such an anencephaly or encephalocoele.

As experience increases, the early scan will assume an ever increasing importance, but it is unlikely to supplant the mid-pregnancy scan, which affords more detailed information on fetal anatomy and is used to identify women at risk of pre-eclampsia, IUGR and preterm labour.

Mid-pregnancy scan (18–22 weeks)

This scan is performed transabdominally and usually takes about 20 minutes. It provides the most detailed survey of the fetus and uterine contents. Indeed it is the most detailed physical examination the individual will ever receive for the remainder of his or her life. The aim of this scan is to:

- Provide an accurate estimation of gestational age if an early scan has not been performed, through measurement of the BPD, HC, AC and FL.
- Carry out a detailed fetal anatomical survey to detect any fetal structural abnormalities or markers for chromosome abnormality. At the present time, this is probably the principal reason for the mid-pregnancy scan, for the vast majority of fetal abnormalities will not be anticipated and, therefore, would not be detected without this routine scan.
- Establish the presence of multiple gestation if an early scan has not been performed and determine the chorionicity.
- Locate the placenta and identify the 5 per cent of women who will have a low-lying placenta. A small percentage of such women will eventually be shown to have a placenta praevia.
- Estimate the amniotic fluid volume.

Two further tests are now being used in some centres to identify women at high risk of developing pregnancy complications. Uterine artery Doppler employs colour and spectral Doppler to obtain waveforms from both uterine arteries. Waveforms with a high resistance index or a notch indicate poor trophoblast invasion and a significant risk of pre-eclampsia and IUGR or abruptio placentae developing later. At 20 weeks' gestation, 5 per cent of women will have bilateral notches and they have a 60 per cent risk of subsequently developing one or more of these complications. Cervical length measurement requires transvaginal scanning but there is now evidence that

50 per cent of women who deliver before 34 weeks will have a short cervix. The average length of the cervix at 23 weeks in 3.4 cm and if the measurement is less than 1.5 cm, a recent study suggests that there is a 50 per cent chance of spontaneous preterm labour and delivery before 34 weeks' gestation.

The importance of the routine scan

The early and mid-pregnancy routine scans have assumed great importance in the effective management of pregnancy. It allows parental choice if a fetal abnormality is detected. For example, if an abnormality is lethal or will result in serious long-term handicap, most parents will opt for termination of pregnancy. On some occasions, early diagnosis may allow the prenatal treatment of certain conditions, such as an obstructed fetal bladder, which can give rise to renal damage without insertion of a vesico-amniotic shunt. Even if the parents do not want a termination of pregnancy, it will allow arrangements to be made for delivery in a tertiary centre, which will provide optimal care for the baby. A routine scan will also allow triaging of women for hospital care if high-risk factors are found, such as multiple gestation, abnormal uterine artery Doppler or a short cervix.

A routine scan is also the parent's first glimpse of their new baby. Much has been written about the importance of involving the parents in the examination as the scan is performed. This is indeed important, for it has been shown in randomized studies that parents bond with their future baby much better if they can see the ultrasound image on the screen. As a consquence the parents are more likely to comply with health recommendations, such as improving diet or reducing smoking and alcohol consumption.

The scan has now become a family event and it is important the routine scan should be an informative and enjoyable experience. It should not be assumed that the parents wish to know the sex of their child and the information should not be gratuitously given or officiously withheld. If a fetal abnormality is detected, this should be discussed with the parents at the end of the scan. Although parents can recognize anatomical features when they are pointed out, it is extremely rare for them to recognize an abnormality without it being demonstrated to them on the screen. The image of the anomaly should be videotaped and shown to the parents afterwards, for distressed par-

ents can have exaggerated imaginings of fetal abnormalities and they cope much better when they see the apparent lesion on the screen. On many occasions, the operator will need a second opinion and may be uncertain as to whether there is an abnormality. It is always better to explain why a second opinion is required rather than give some reassuring but dishonest explanation, such as 'the baby is in a difficult position'. The doctor–patient relationship and sonographer–patient relationship is based on trust and it is important to tell parents that the recognition of fetal anomalies is not 100 per cent and that false positive and false negative diagnoses are possible.

The impact of the mid-pregnancy routine scan can be shown in the meta-analysis shown in Figure 7.9, where eight studies comparing random allocation of antenatal patients to routine scanning or scanning on indication, are compared. In the routine scan group, there is a significant increase in the number of terminations of pregnancy for fetal abnormalities and a significant reduction in undiagnosed twins. Because ultrasound corrects mistakes in gestational age, assigned from the last menstrual period, there is also a significant reduction in the number of inductions for post-term pregnancy. These are all tangible benefits, but some criticism of the routine scan has been made because there does not appear to be any change in the perinatal mortality rate, the incidence of low birthweight or the neonatal condition as the result of the introduction of the routine scan. This is, in fact, not surprising as there is unlikely to be a change in these outcomes unless routine ultrasound

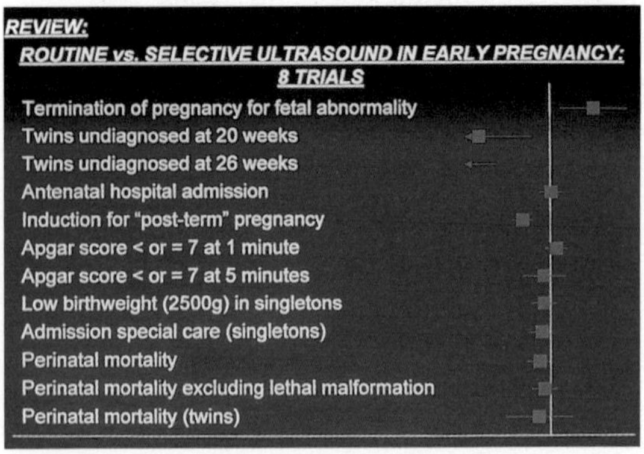

REVIEW:
ROUTINE vs. SELECTIVE ULTRASOUND IN EARLY PREGNANCY:
8 TRIALS
Termination of pregnancy for fetal abnormality
Twins undiagnosed at 20 weeks
Twins undiagnosed at 26 weeks
Antenatal hospital admission
Induction for "post-term" pregnancy
Apgar score < or = 7 at 1 minute
Apgar score < or = 7 at 5 minutes
Low birthweight (2500g) in singletons
Admission special care (singletons)
Perinatal mortality
Perinatal mortality excluding lethal malformation
Perinatal mortality (twins)

Figure 7.9 Meta-analysis of eight studies comparing routine and selective scanning. Routine ultrasound reduces the number of undiagnosed twins, unnecessary inductions of labour and increases number of terminations of pregnancy for fetal anomalies, but as yet does not reduce prenatal mortality or morbidity.

causes a change in management. In future we might anticipate improvements if triaging of care, based on the identification of high-risk pregnancies by uterine artery Doppler or assessment of cervical length, can be made. Successful prophylactic treatment of pre-eclampsia or preterm labour can only be instituted if women at high risk are identified. This must be the future goal of the routine scan.

New developments

3-D Scanning

This technique may transform ultrasound imaging in the future. In conventional scanning, the ultrasound beam is swept electronically in a single plane across a flat transducer. In three-dimensional scanning, the beam is swept in two orthogonal planes to capture a block or volume of echoes which are digitally stored. The aim of the operator is to capture a volume from the region of interest and this is normally completed in 5 to 15 seconds, depending on the required volume for diagnosis. After this, the volume of echoes can be resliced in any plane to provide the appropriate two-dimensional image. Furthermore, by surface or volume rendering, lifelike three-dimensional reconstructions of surface features of the fetus, or particular organs, can be made and surface or volume rendering can remove artefacts or structures that obscure the image. The advantages are that the scanning time can be drastically shortened and volumes can be stored for later analysis. In the future, volumes will be transferred electronically to tertiary centres for expert diagnosis. From the parents' perspective, the images, especially of the fetal face, have a life-like photographic quality (Fig. 7.10) and are likely to improve antenatal parental bonding. The images are at the moment static, but real-time 3-D imaging should be available within a few years. At the moment there is evidence that 3-D imaging improves the diagnosis of certain fetal abnormalities, such as cleft lip and palate.

Magnetic resonance imaging (MRI)

This technique utilizes the effect of powerful magnetic forces on spinning hydrogen protons, which when knocked off their axis by pulsed radio waves, produce radio frequency signals as they return to their basal state. The signals reflect the clinical composition of tissue (i.e. the amount and distribution

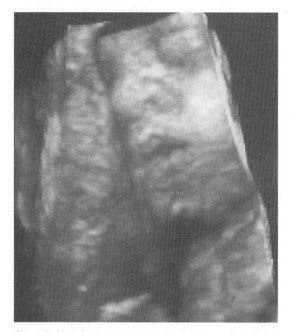

Figure 7.10 3-D ultrasound scan of fetal face.

of hydrogen protons) and thus the images provide significant improvement over ultrasound in tissue characterisation. The technique also has the advantage of providing sectional images in any plane. The main disadvantage is that MRI is many times more expensive than ultrasound and images are more likely to be affected by movement artefacts. Many centres sedate the mother prior to an examination to reduce fetal movement.

MRI does provide superb images of fetal anatomy and is extremely useful when ultrasound images are not diagnostic or when they are suboptimal because of maternal obesity. An example of a fetal MRI scan is given in Figure 7.11.

ASSESSMENT OF FETAL WELLBEING

Obstetricians have searched for tests which could be applied during the antenatal period to identify fetuses at risk of intrauterine hypoxia and death. Although biochemical assessment of placental function (measuring plasma hPL and oestriol) gained popularity in this context in the 1960s and 1970s, these tests have all been abandoned from clinical use, as they are poor predictors of fetal outcome. In Europe and the USA the most widely used tests of

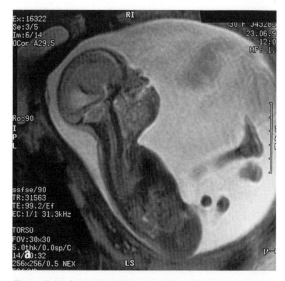 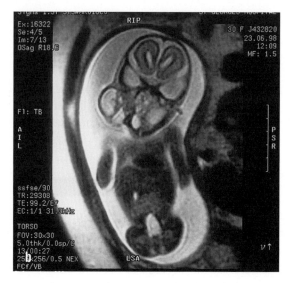

Figure 7.11 (a) and (b) MRI scan of fetus showing thyroid tumour.

fetal wellbeing are now biophysical; namely, Doppler ultrasound and antenatal cardiotocography (CTG). Doppler ultrasound can involve simple assessment of the umbilical artery pulsatility index, which measures placental resistance to blood flow, or detailed assessment of arterial and venous blood flow within the fetus. While these sophisticated fetal Doppler studies provide the most accurate information on fetal oxygenation and cardiac function, antenatal CTG will continue to play an important part in the evaluation of fetal wellbeing. This is because sophisticated fetal Doppler studies are only as yet performed in a few centres due to a lack of expensive colour Doppler equipment and a deficiency of trained personnel in this technique. In contrast, antenatal CTG equipment is less expensive and midwives, or even the patient herself, can make recordings. Secondly, monitoring of the fetal heart rate can sometimes give earlier warning of acute fetal changes in conditions such as abruptio placentae and fetal infection. It must be emphasized that these biophysical tests should always be considered together and be taken in conjunction with the overall clinical picture and the gestational age of the fetus before any management decisions are made.

Cardiotocography

Antenatal CTG uses external (and therefore indirect) methods of monitoring the fetal heart rate. The most widely used method for obtaining this information is ultrasound fetal CTG. This utilizes the physical principle of the Doppler effect to detect fetal heart motion. Signals can also be obtained from antenatal fetal electrocardiography but this is more prone to failure. The interval between successive beats is measured thereby allowing a continuous assessment of fetal heart rate. Most modern transducers have increased numbers of transmitting crystals and detectors so that failure to detect signals from cardiac valve or wall movement is a relatively rare event.

The woman should be comfortable and in a left lateral or semi-recumbent position (avoiding compression of the maternal vena cava). An external ultrasound transducer for monitoring the fetal heart and a tocodynometer (stretch gauge) for recording uterine activity are secured overlying the uterus. Recordings are then made for at least 30 minutes, and the output from the CTG machine is conventionally an ink tracing of fetal heart rate and a second tracing of uterine activity (Fig. 7.12).

Fetal cardiac physiology

Fetal cardiac behaviour is regulated through sympathetic and parasympathetic signals and by vasomotor, chemoceptor and baroreceptor mechanisms. Pathological events such as fetal hypoxia modify these signals and also fetal cardiac response.

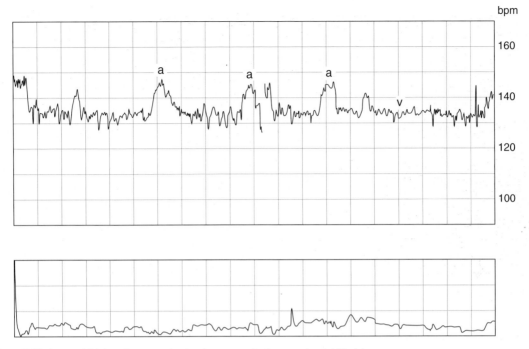

Figure 7.12 A normal fetal cardiotocograph, showing a normal rate, normal variability (v), and the presence of several accelerations (a).

Fetal heart rate variability

Under normal physiological conditions the interval between successive heart beats (beat-to-beat) varies. This is called 'short-term variability' and increases with increasing gestational age. It is not visible on a standard CTG (although this information can be obtained from fetal electrocardiograms, see below). In addition to these beat-to-beat variations in heart rate, there are longer-term fluctuations in heart rate occuring between two to six times per minute. The preferred term for this variation in fetal heart rate is 'baseline variability'. Normal baseline variability reflects a normal fetal autonomic nervous system. As well as gestational age, baseline variability is modified by fetal sleep states and activity, and also by hypoxia, fetal infection, and drugs suppressing the fetal CNS, such as opioids, and hypnotics, all of which reduce baseline variability. Baseline variability is considered abnormal when it is less than 10 beats per minute (Fig. 7.13). As fetuses display deep sleep cycles of 20–30 minutes at a time, baseline variability will be normally reduced for this length of time, but will be preceded and followed by a more normal period of trace if the CTG is continued for a sufficient duration.

Baseline fetal heart rate

Fetal heart rate falls with advancing gestational age as a result of maturing fetal parasympathetic (vagal) tone. It is best determined over a period of 5–10 minutes. The normal fetal heart rate at term is 110–150 beats per minute (bpm), whilst prior to term 160 bpm is taken as the upper limit of normal. A rate lower than 110 bpm is termed a fetal bradycardia. If all other features of the CTG are normal this is unlikely to represent fetal hypoxia unless the rate is less than 100 bpm. Fetal heart rates between 150–170 bpm are again unlikely to represent fetal compromise if the trace is otherwise normal (normal baseline variability in the presence of accelerations and in the absence of decelerations) and there are no antenatal risk factors. Fetal tachycardias (Fig. 7.14) can be due to congenital tachycardias and are also associated with maternal or fetal infection, acute fetal hypoxia, fetal anaemia and drugs such as adrenoceptor agonists (ritodrine).

Fetal heart rate accelerations

These are increases in the baseline fetal heart rate of at least 15 bpm, lasting for at least 15 seconds. The presence of two or more accelerations on a 20–30 minute CTG defines a reactive trace. The importance of

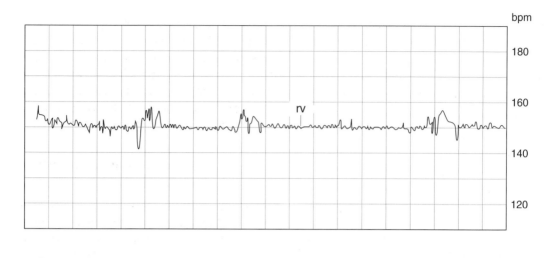

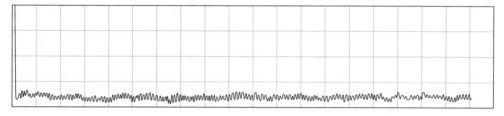

Figure 7.13 A fetal cardiotocograph showing a baseline of 150 beats per minute but with reduced variability (rv).

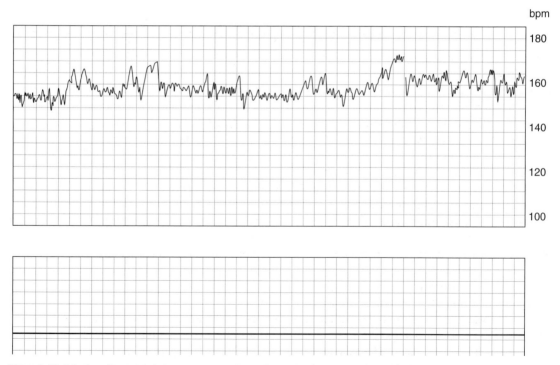

Figure 7.14 A fetal cardiotocograph from a term pregnancy. The true baseline is about 150 beats per minute, as seen at the start of the trace. This baby was very active and the apparent raised baseline rate for the majority of the tracing is due to almost continuous accelerations.

accelerations is that they are only observed very rarely in the presence of fetal hypoxia; i.e. normally they are a good sign of fetal health. Accelerations can be so frequent as to suggest a fetal tachycardia (Fig. 7.14) and this emphasizes the need to interpret CTG tracings carefully in the light of the overall clinical picture.

Fetal heart rate decelerations
These are transient reductions in fetal heart rate of 15 bpm or more, lasting for more than 15 seconds. Occasional decelerations are frequently seen on otherwise normal CTG tracings. When occurring in relation to isolated uterine contractions or fetal movements they do not appear to be associated with a poor fetal outcome. Decelerations that occur in the presence of other abnormal features (Table 7.2), such as reduced variability or baseline tachycardia, are more likely to reflect fetal hypoxia. When baseline variability is reduced, decelerations can be less than 15 bpm from baseline and still be highly significant (Fig. 7.15).

From the above descriptions a normal antepartum fetal CTG can therefore be defined as a baseline of 110–150 bpm, with baseline variability exceeding 10 bpm, and with more than one acceleration being seen in a 20–30 minute tracing. Reduced baseline variability, absence of accelerations and the presence of decelerations are all suspicious features. A suspicious CTG must be interpreted in clinical context. If many antenatal risk factors have already been identified a suspicious CTG may warrant delivery of the baby although where no risk factors exist a repeated investigation later in the day may be more appropriate.

Stress and non-stress cardiotocography

Performing an antenatal CTG with the mother positioned comfortably is called a non-stress test. In this situation the 'stress' of the title refers to what the fetus is experiencing (not the mother). Although not popular in the UK, in the USA fetuses that demonstrate suboptimal non-stress CTG tracings may be subjected to contraction stress tests. These tests are carried out in the same way as non-stress tests except that an oxytocin infusion is administered intravenously to induce uterine contractions. Oxytocin has no direct effect on fetal cardiac activity. A positive test result is fetal cardiac decelerations in response to uterine contractions, and is abnormal. The test has not been adopted in the UK as it is thought to be a poor predictor of fetal

Table 7.2 – Cardiotocography – summary of fetal heart rate patterns and their implications

Normal	Baseline rate 110–150 bpm Variability 10–25 bpm Two accelerations in 20 min No decelerations
Suspicious	Absence of accelerations (important), + Abnormal baseline rate (<110, or >150 bpm) Reduced variability (<10 bpm) Variable decelerations

Abnormal	No accelerations and two or more of the following:
	Abnormal baseline rate
	Abnormal variability
	Repetitive late decelerations
	Variable decelerations with ominous features (duration >60s, late recovery baseline, late deceleration component, poor variability between/during decelerations)
	Others: Sinusoidal pattern
	        Prolonged bradycardia
	        Shallow decelerations with reduced variability in a non-reactive trace

outcome, have unacceptably high false-positive and uterine hyperstimulation rates (5–10 per cent each) and be too time-consuming and invasive. An alternative to oxytocin infusion that can be used for inducing uterine activity is repetitive nipple stimulation. Whilst less invasive, this technique does not overcome the problems of poor prediction of fetal outcome. Fetal provocation using acoustic, light or exercise stimuli have all been documented, but again have not been shown to improve the detection of the at-risk fetus.

The computerized CTG

As the basis of fetal CTG is pattern recognition, which is open to both accurate interpretation and differences in interpretation between different clinicians, computerized CTG interpretation packages have been developed. These packages have been thoroughly field tested in comparison with human experts and have been shown to be equal, or superior, to human interpretation in differentiating normal from abnormal outcome.

One commonly used package relies on the computer's ability to calculate heart rate variability by measuring the variation in frequency of individual heart beats, and assessing increased variability with fetal movements. In this way fetal heart rate accelerations are identified by a reduced interval between beats and decelerations are identified from an increased interval. A sinusoidal trace can be recognized by short-term variation of more than two standard deviations below the mean value expected for a given gestation.

Several potential advantages of a computerized

🔑 Key Points

The computerized CTG
- Introduced by Dawes and Redman, 1987
- Analysis of fetal data performed at 10 minutes and every 2 minutes thereafter
- Dawes and Redman criteria 'MET'/'NOT MET'
- Fits a baseline to the trace
- Measures accelerations and decelerations
- Calculates fetal heart rate range in milliseconds with gestational age
- Calculates high/low variation
- Correlates loss of contact against analysis
- Incorporates fetal movements felt by the mother

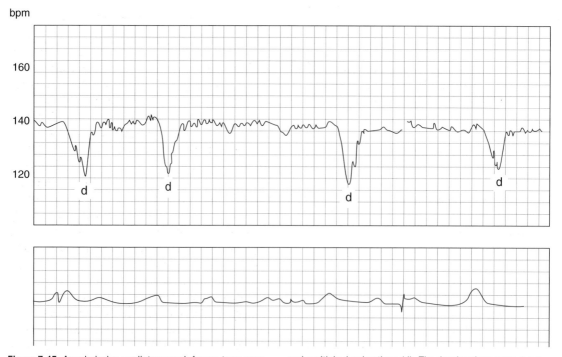

Figure 7.15 An admission cardiotocograph from a term pregnancy. Although the baseline fetal heart rate is normal there is reduced variability, an absence of fetal heart rate accelerations, and multiple decelerations (d). The decelerations were occurring after uterine tightenings and are therefore termed 'late'.

bpm

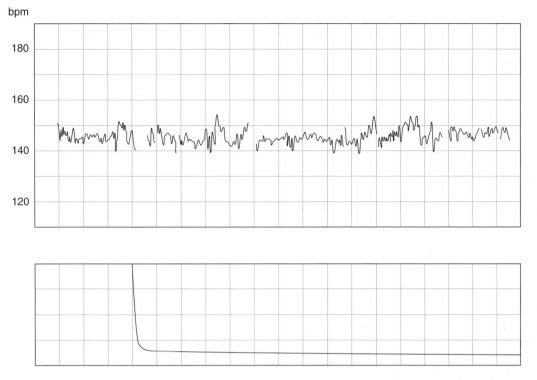

Figure 7.16 A normal 'computerized' CTG.

interpretation seem to exist. The computer is often able to declare a CTG normal after 10 minutes (rather than the more standard 30-minute tracing normally performed manually). Secondly, if signal contact is lost during the tracing the machine alarms, requiring the Doppler transducer to be repositioned. The interactive nature of this monitoring also reduces the total duration of CTG recording and aids interpretation. Examples of computerized CTGs are shown in Figures 7.16 and 7.17.

The CTG Litigation Safeguards
Name of patient
Date and time commenced
Auto clock time check
End of trace recorded
'Abnormalities' noted
'Wait and see' decision noted
Interventions recorded
Pinard record of fetal heart rate
Signatures
Calling appropriate medical aid
Storage for 25 years

Biophysical profile

In an effort to refine the ability of fetal CTG to iden-tify antenatal hypoxia, investigators have looked at additional fetal parameters. In experimental animals, fetal hypoxia can be induced by making the mother breathe hypoxic gas mixtures. Under these conditions fetal biophysical variables, such as fetal breathing movements and forelimb movements, are abolished. This reduction in movement may persist even after the normal fetal oxygenation has been re-established. Similar changes in those active biophysical variables controlled by the central nervous system have been noticed in human fetuses that are acutely hypoxic. These include breathing movements, gross body movements, flexor tone and accelerations in fetal heart rate related to movements. If chronic fetal hypoxia occurs there is an associated reduction in amniotic fluid volume, and fetal growth restriction is seen. By assigning each of the active variables, and also amniotic fluid volume and the CTG scores of either 2 (= normal) or 0 (= suboptimal), it is possible to assign an individual fetus score of between 0 and 10. This is the basis of fetal biophysical profiling (Table 7.3).

The first prospective, blind clinical study using

Table 7.3 – Biophysical profile scoring

Biophysical variable	Normal (score 2)	Abnormal (score 0)
Fetal breathing movements	>1 episode for 30s in 30 minutes	Absent/ <30s in 30 minutes
Gross body movements	>3 body/ limb movements in 30 minutes	<3 body/limb movements in 30 minutes
Fetal tone	>1 episode body/ limb extension followed by return to flexion, open-close cycle of fetal hand	Slow, or absent extension-flexion of or body or limbs
Reactive fetal heart rate	>2 accelerations with fetal movements in 30 minutes	<2 accelerations, or 1+ deceleration in 30 minutes
Qualitative amniotic fluid	>1 pool of fluid, at least 1 cm x 1 cm.	Either no measurable pool, or a pool <1 cm x 1 cm

biophysical profile scores to predict fetal outcome was reported in 1980. Scores were recorded in 216 women but the data were not available to the clinicians managing the pregnancies. The perinatal mortality varied between 600/1000 when all five variables were abnormal, to 0/1000 when all variables were considered to be normal. Intermediate scores were associated with intermediate mortality rates. This study did not allow an assessment of whether performing biophysical profiles was able to reduce perinatal mortality, as clinicians responsible for the care of individual women were unable to act on the results of this new, and at that time, unproven test. Larger studies, where women at high risk for fetal hypoxia were delivered if biophysical scores were abnormal, suggested that delivery at a score of <6 was associated with a lower perinatal mortality than either high-risk pregnancies in which biophysical profiles were not performed, or even low-risk pregnancies. The implication from this latter observation was that even in low-risk antenatal populations some fetuses will be hypoxic with no apparent risk factors. These same large series have suggested that the false-negative rate for the test (a normal score with subsequent death of the fetus within one week of the test) is very low.

These results would appear to argue strongly in favour of the widespread and routine use of biophysical profiling for all pregnancies. However such widespread use has not occurred in many countries, including the UK. There appear to be several reasons for this lack of implementation. Biophysical profiles can be time-consuming. Fetuses spend approximately 30 per cent of their time in non-REM sleep, during which time they are not very active and do not exhibit breathing movements. It is therefore necessary to scan them for long enough to exclude this physiological cause of a poor score. The longer individual ultrasound scans take to perform, the more machines and operators are required to apply the test to the whole antenatal population. This problem is compounded when the

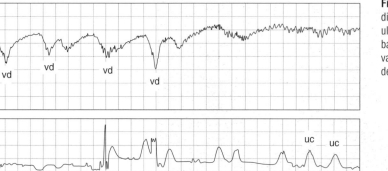

Figure 7.17 An admission cardiotocograph. This CTG shows irregular uterine activity (uc), a rising baseline fetal heart rate with reduced variability and variable heart rate decelerations (vd).

test is performed earlier and more frequently. Another problem with fetal biophysical profiles is that by the time a fetus develops an abnormal score prompting delivery it is already severely hypoxic. Whilst delivery may reduce the perinatal death rate (death *in utero*, or within the first week of life) it may not be increasing long-term survival, and in particular, survival without significant mental and physical impairment.

Doppler investigation

The principles of Doppler have already been discussed. The umbilical artery has been the most extensively studied vessel probably because signals can be obtained with inexpensive continuous wave Doppler equipment. It should be regarded as a placental vessel, however, and only by studying fetal vessels with the more expensive colour Doppler machines can important information on the fetal response to hypoxia be made.

Umbilical artery

Waveforms from these vessels provide information on feto-placental blood flow and should be performed on high-risk mothers, for example with hypertension, or where there is an SGA fetus or an elevated uterine artery resistance index or notch. Normally diastolic flow in the umbilical artery increases (i.e. resistance falls) throughout gestation. If the resistance in the umbilical artery rises above the 95 centile of the normal graph, this implies faulty perfusion of the placenta, which may eventually result in fetal hypoxia. Absent or reversed endiastolic flow in the umbilical artery is a particularly serious development with a strong correlation with fetal distress and intrauterine death (Fig. 7.18). Meta-analysis of several randomized studies shows that umbilical Doppler monitoring will reduce perinatal mortality in high-risk pregnancies.

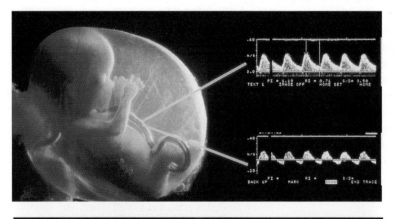

Figure 7.18 Normal (top) and abnormal (bottom) Doppler signals from the umbilical artery. Reversed flow in diastole indicate poor placental function and impending fetal demise.

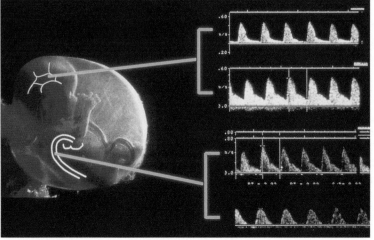

Figure 7.19 Normal and abnormal Doppler signals from the middle cerebral artery and thoracic aorta. Increasing flow in the middle cerebral artery and absence of diastolic flow in the aorta indicates fetal acidaemia.

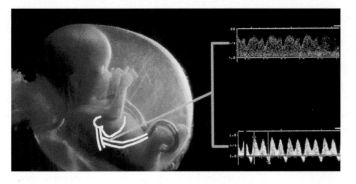

Figure 7.20 Normal and abnormal Doppler signals from the ductus venosus. There is progressive reduction of flow to the heart in late diastole (i.e. with atrial contraction) with increasing fetal acidaemia.

Fetal vessels

Falling oxygen levels in the fetus result in a redistribution of blood flow to protect the brain, heart, adrenals and spleen, and vasoconstriction in all other vessels. Several fetal vessels have been studied, which reflect this 'centralization' of flow. The middle cerebral artery will show increasing diastolic flow (falling PI) as hypoxia increases, while a rising resistance in the fetal aorta reflects compensatory vasoconstriction in the fetal body. When diastolic flow is absent in the fetal aorta, this implies fetal acidaemia (Fig. 7.19). Perhaps the most sensitive index of fetal acidaemia and incipient heart failure is demonstrated by increasing pulsatility in the central veins supplying the heart, such as the ductus venosus and inferior vena cava. When late diastolic flow is absent in the ductus venosus, then delivery should be considered, as fetal death is imminent (Fig. 7.20). The significance of these findings is discussed in Chapter 11.

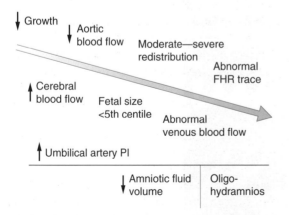

Figure 7.21 Sequential changes in tests of fetal wellbeing in uteroplacental failure.

Key Points

- Abnormalities of fetal well-being are usually the result of impaired transfer of nutrients and oxygen across the placenta leading to the development of intrauterine growth restriction and chronic asphyxia.
- The fetal response to placental insufficiency is
  - A reduction of growth rate in response to impaired transfer of nutrients and to conserve oxygen
  - Redistribution of the circulation to preferentially perfuse the brain, myocardium and adrenal gland with a consequent reduction in blood flow to other organs. This will lead to asymmetrical growth with relative brain sparing and oligohydramnios due to reduced renal perfusion
  - Reduction of fetal activity to conserve oxygen and reduce anaerobic metabolism. This will result in a reduction of general body and breathing movements
  - Modification of the autonomic control of the fetal heart with a reduction in baseline variability
- Ultimately as fetal acidaemia develops as a result of anaerobic glycolysis there will be abnormal Doppler waveforms in the ductus venosus as a result of right heart failure and decelerations in the fetal heart trace as a result of increased vagal tone
- Most of these changes can now be documented by means of Doppler ultrasound and antenatal cardiotocograph. A brief summary of the sequence of events in given in Figure 7.21
- The decision when to deliver the baby will be taken by the Obstetrician on the basis of an evaluation of several of these antenatal tests together with the maternal condition such as the presence of pre-eclampsia or diabetes mellitus. For example, after 32 weeks, the decision to deliver might be based on an SGA infant with oligohydramnios and evidence of circulatory redistribution. Before 32 weeks, delivery may be delayed in order to achieve greater fetal maturity, so tests of fetal cardiac function (ductus venosus and cardiotocography) become critical

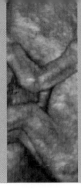

Chapter 8

Antenatal care

OVERVIEW

Antenatal care is the clinical assessment of mother and fetus during pregnancy, for the purpose of obtaining the best possible outcome for both the mother and the child.

To achieve this objective, history and examination are complemented by screening and assessment using a combination of methods, including biochemical, haematological and ultrasound. Efforts are made to maintain maternal physical and mental wellbeing, prevent preterm delivery, anticipate difficulties and complications at delivery, ensure the birth of a live healthy infant and assist the couple in preparation for parenting. The main aims of antenatal care are listed below.

The aims of antenatal care

- Assessment and management of maternal risk and symptoms.
- Assessment and management of fetal risk.
- Prenatal diagnosis and management of fetal abnormality.
- Diagnosis and management of perinatal complications.
- Decision regarding timing and mode of delivery.
- Parental education regarding pregnancy and childbirth.
- Parental education regarding child-rearing.

Antenatal care traditionally involves a number of 'routine' visits for assessment to a variety of healthcare professionals, on a regular basis throughout the pregnancy. This approach to antenatal care evolved in an era that preceded the current, evidence-based approach to medicine.

Early monitoring and on-going care during pregnancy is associated with more favourable birth outcomes. Compared with no antenatal surveillance, some antenatal healthcare has a beneficial effect on adverse factors such as preterm delivery, low birth weight, maternal and perinatal mortality. While some traditional practices, such as strict weight-gain restriction, the use of diuretics and the liberal use of X-rays, have been discontinued, many of our current clinical practices fail to stand up to scientific scrutiny. Despite this, antenatal care continues to be centred around clinical assessment, with an emphasis on the regularity of visits, rather than a focus on what can be achieved at key visits during the antenatal period.

Maternity care remains a mixture of both art and

science, with advances in medical technology now allowing us to focus more on the specific requirements of the mother and fetus, with an increasing drive towards the re-appraisal of current practices. A number of the more specialized aspects of antenatal care are covered in detail elsewhere in this book. This chapter will therefore concentrate on routine antenatal care as it is currently practised, referring to the relevant chapters where greater detail is required.

Achieving the aims of antenatal care

In order to achieve the aims of antenatal care, an efficiently organized and implemented programme is necessary. This should be based on the individual requirements of both mother and fetus, as judged by the initial assessment, and within a cost-effective framework.

Previously, the schedule of hospital antenatal visits was not ordered by a set of clearly defined maternal or fetal requirements, but by a routine established in the 1920s. The current emphasis is on increasing maternal and primary healthcare team involvement, with as much provision in the community as possible. However, the groups most likely to be satisfied with traditional or reduced antenatal visit schedules cannot be easily identified. Ideally, each woman should have their care tailored to their particular needs or preferences, but this must be contained within a reasonable framework of cost versus benefit.

Providers of antenatal care

Antenatal care is provided within a team framework, which includes the general practitioner, midwives, obstetricians, neonatologists, other medical specialists, clinical geneticists, health visitors, social workers, counsellors and health advocates. Although each may have a specific role to play in each individual case, who provides care is dictated by the needs specific to each pregnancy. There are usually three schemes of care:
1. Community care, supervised predominantly by the midwife.
2. Shared care between the woman's general practitioner, midwife and obstetrician, with the visits interspersed between all the health professionals concerned.

3. Hospital-only care in cases where there is increased risk to either the mother, the fetus, or both.

Schedule of visits during pregnancy

The pregnant woman is seen by her general practitioner as soon as possible following the first missed period and after an initial assessment is referred to the hospital for her first (booking) hospital visit between 8–14 weeks. Hospital referrals are increasingly instituted earlier nowadays, especially among the more health conscious, older, educated women, who may request screening tests for the early detection of fetal abnormality. Previously, the antenatal visits were: monthly until 32 weeks' gestation; then fortnightly until 36 weeks; and weekly thereafter until delivery, resulting in up to 14 hospital visits during pregnancy. Although antenatal care improves the outcome in terms of maternal and perinatal morbidity and morality, there appears to be little difference in outcome between a four-visit schedule and a twelve-visit schedule. Currently the trend is towards reducing the number of visits, while at the same time establishing clearly defined objectives to be achieved at each visit. The schedule of key visits is listed below.

Schedule of key antenatal visits

Preconception clinic visit
8–14 week visit
20–24 week visit
36–38 week visit
41–42 week visit

The preconception visit
The ideal first antenatal visit is at a preconception clinic where health education and risk assessment can be directed towards the planned pregnancy. At that time the patient's general health and wellbeing can be fully assessed, rubella, hepatitis and HIV status can be established and appropriate action taken where indicated. General advice regarding nutrition and lifestyle can be given at this time. Even a single antenatal nutritional education session during pregnancy has a significant effect on birth weight.

Advice can be given regarding the avoidance of teratogens, including those linked with dietary excesses such as vitamin A, cigarette smoking and alcohol, while ensuring an optimal dietary intake of folic acid. It has been demonstrated that folate supplementation reduces the risk of a subsequent neural tube defect by 72 per cent in those considered at high-risk by virtue of a previous affected pregnancy. It is recommended that at least 0.4 mg folic acid is taken daily during the periconceptional period. For a woman with diabetes mellitus, abnormal blood glucose control during the periconceptional period is associated with an increased incidence of fetal abnormalities. This is also an ideal time to ensure that such factors have been taken care of by sound dietary education and, where necessary, adjustment of insulin dosage.

The first trimester

The first trimester remains a critical period in determining the outcome of a pregnancy, with miscarriage the single most common complication of pregnancy. A dedicated early pregnancy unit, set up to deal with complications that present with symptoms of vaginal bleeding and abdominal pain, is invaluable in modern day practice. Following carefully established guidelines, and with dedicated medical and nursing staff, women can be investigated using history, examination, biochemical testing and transvaginal ultrasound. Women with non-viable pregnancies may be cared for in a supportive environment, with the help of trained counselling staff, while those with progressing pregnancies may be reassured and special needs, such as administering anti-D immunoglobulin, attended to.

Booking visit (8–14 weeks)

The main purpose of the booking visit is to obtain a comprehensive history (see Chapter 1), establish the gestational age and identify maternal and fetal risk factors. Baseline investigations are performed (see below). Where there is asymptomatic bacteriuria, or evidence of anaemia or infection, the patient can be contacted and the problem resolved as early as possible in the pregnancy. In most centres, women are offered a first trimester ultrasound scan for pregnancy dating, the exclusion of structural fetal abnormalities and measurement of the fetal nuchal translucency (see Chapter 12).

Typical schedule of antenatal investigations

Booking (8–14 weeks)

Blood tests

Haemoglobin and full blood count, atypical antibodies (if severe anaemia <8.5g/dL, send blood for a film and transferrin, ferritin, RBC folate and B12 assays)

Haemoglobin electrophoresis (sickle and thalassaemia status) or women at particular risk (Mediterranean, Afro-Caribbean and Asian)

Microbiological: rubella, hepatitis B and syphilis status (VDRL); HIV (different screening policies exist); toxoplasma (depending on history)

Urine tests

Dip for glucose, ketones, protein; certain reagent strips test for bacterial activity. If proteinuria or suspicion of UTI, send for microscopy, culture and sensitivities

Vaginal speculum examination

Perform only if indicated, for instance, if a cervical smear has not been performed recently, or the last smear test was abnormal. If there is vaginal discharge, a high vaginal swab (HVS) should be sent for microbiology studies

Ultrasound

As for 'early scan' (see Chapter 7, page 75)

Mid-trimester visit (20–24 weeks)

Blood tests

Haemoglobin and atypical antibodies

Blood glucose measurement (for gestational diabetes screening)

Urine tests

Dip for glucose, ketones and protein

Ultrasound

As for 'mid-pregnancy scan' (see Chapter 7, page 75)

36–38 week visit

Blood tests

Haemoglobin and atypical antibodies

Urine tests

Dip for glucose, ketones and protein

Ultrasound

Not performed routinely unless an indication (see Chapter 7)

A management plan is then drawn up for the pregnancy, based upon the risk assessment. It is by no means inflexible and is subject to alteration at subsequent visits. If the patient has a known medical problem, e.g. diabetes, the patient is referred to a dedicated combined clinic. If there is a history of genetic or familial problems, referral to a feto-maternal specialist is arranged. A typical risk assessment chart is presented in Figure 8.1. This is a checklist of the most common problems that can be identified at the time of the booking visit. Fortunately the risk of serious complications in pregnancy, particularly in the antenatal period, are low and there is a low recurrence rate for most pregnancy complications. The majority of 'risk' factors identified at the booking visit carry very little actual increase in risk for the current pregnancy, with the odds of a complication typically not even being double that of the general obstetric population. Investigations, such as biochemical placental protein assay, ultrasound and uteroplacental Doppler ultrasound are more likely to provide us with groups of women that have significantly increased risk of complications in pregnancy (see Chapters 7 and 11).

There are several sources of psychosocial stress during pregnancy because it is a period of considerable change in life events. There is an association between maternal psychosocial factors and low birth weight and preterm delivery. Negative mood states such as anxiety, depression, and/or hostility, and rejection of the pregnancy are all associated with low birth weight. Often women have insufficient knowledge of what to expect in pregnancy and at delivery, and worries about personal health and the outcome of the pregnancy, are common concerns. It is important that women are given the opportunity to discuss such problems at an early stage in the pregnancy, and that remedial action is initiated. Acceptance of the pregnancy, emotional support, strengthening of the woman's social network and other efforts to improve self-esteem, help to promote the health of the mother and prospective baby.

The mid-trimester risk assessment visit (20–24 weeks)

The results of tests performed at the first trimester visit and at 16 weeks are reviewed with the mother. The results of the ultrasound scan for fetal abnormality are also reviewed (see Chapters 7 and 12). In some centres, Doppler ultrasound screening of the uterine arteries, which is used to identify women at high risk of subsequent pre-eclampsia and intrauterine growth restriction, is offered at this stage. Further care is then planned in line with the risk assessment based on the ultrasound scan and other findings.

Antenatal visits in the second half of pregnancy

Assessment of maternal health and fetal growth and wellbeing are pursued through these visits, which can take place in the community setting. Any incidental maternal symptoms are dealt with. This period is also important in ensuring the education of the woman regarding the rest of pregnancy and her delivery. Plans for the birth and postpregnancy contraception should also be discussed from an early stage especially with regards to sterilization or other permanent contraception.

Antenatal classes and the familiarization hospital visit

During the antenatal visits informal education is provided for the pregnant woman and those supporting her through pregnancy. There are formal parenting (or parent craft) classes organized in most units where the prospective parents are encouraged to discuss the pregnancy and delivery, and any apprehensions they may have. There are also usually sessions with others involved in their care to discuss topics such as breastfeeding, pain management during the delivery, etc. The common objectives of these formal educational sessions include:

- the promotion of good health habits;
- allaying anxiety;
- increasing the mother's feelings of control and satisfaction with the pregnancy and delivery;
- preparation for the postnatal period;
- infant feeding;
- subsequent contraception.

Antenatal visit with hospital team (usually around 36–38 weeks)

The primary objective of this visit is to anticipate any problems regarding the prospective delivery. Several factors are considered, including the past obstetric history, e.g. a previous caesarean delivery for lack of progress in labour. Fetal malpresentation or

Name	LMP	Team
Number	EDD	

AT BOOKING	YES	NO
Problems arising during pregnancy		
MATERNAL FACTORS		
Age <18 / age > 40		
Grandmultip		
Booked after 20 weeks		
IUCD in situ		
Infertility >2 years		
Fibroid/ovarian cyst at booking		
Unsupported mother / social problem		
Smoking > 5 per day		
Drinking > 10 units per week		
Drug use (including partner)		
Not fluent in English		
RELEVANT MEDICAL CONDITION		
Hypertension		
Diabetes		
Heart disease		
Haemoglobinopathy		
Other		
PREVIOUS OBSTETRIC HISTORY		
Stillbirth/nnd		
Congenital abnormality		
Baby <2.5 kg / > 4.5 kg		
Diabetic pregnancy		
Hypertension in pregnancy		
Aph/pph		
Late pregnancy loss (14-24 weeks)		
Pre-term delivery		
Cervical suture		
Labour <2 hours		
Caesarean/hysterotomy/myomectomy		
Manual removal		
3rd degree tear		
Postnatal depression		
Top ‡ 2		
BOOKING EXAMINATION		
Weight < 45 kg / weight > 90 kg		
Height <5' (1.5m)		
BP ‡ 140/90		
Proteinuria		
Uterus inconsistent with dates		

ACTION PLAN (please sign)

Figure 8.1 A typical risk assessment sheet used at the booking antenatal visit.

malposition is sought because these may also indicate a high likelihood of operative delivery. With the increasing number of planned home births, the final place of choice for the delivery is also decided. This is also a good time to finalize the discussions on planned contraception after delivery, especially if sterilization is being considered.

Postdates visit (41–42 weeks)

With accurate pregnancy dating, true postdates pregnancies are identified. At this visit a joint decision is taken as to whether an induction of labour is appropriate. This is current practice because of the reported association between postdates pregnancies and poor pregnancy outcome. Induction of labour is used to prevent stillbirths due to the lack of an accurate, reliable test of fetoplacental reserve during those final few weeks of pregnancy. Induction of labour is usually performed by the 42nd week. There are two main methods of induction:

1. amniotomy or surgical induction;
2. medical methods using prostaglandin or oxytocin.

When appropriately selected, there is a high probability of a safe, uneventful vaginal delivery. If vaginal delivery does not ensue by the 43rd week the likelihood of a caesarean delivery is high, irrespective of the mode of onset of labour. As the perinatal morbidity and mortality continue to rise at this stage, intervention is recommended. Factors that are unfavourable for a vaginal delivery are shown in Table 8.1.

History and physical examination

Obstetric history

A good obstetric history is invaluable for the initial and on-going assessment of the mother and fetus during antenatal care. Enquiry about maternal age is one of the oldest screening tests in the history of antenatal care. The mother's age is particularly important because of the increased risk of chromosomal disorders with increasing maternal age, while the incidence of spontaneous miscarriage is also higher among older women. An accurate menstrual history is equally important.

The assessment of gestational age depends on the estimated date of delivery calculated according to

Naegele's rule (280 days from the LMP) and its correlation with the gestational age as estimated by ultrasound measurements of the crown–rump length (CRL), biparietal diameter, fetal abdominal circumference and femur length. Longitudinal data pose problems in analysis, and the numbers in this study are relatively small.

A reassessment is necessary where a disparity of more than ten days occurs between the two calculations. A dating ultrasound scan should be performed by mid-pregnancy to be reliable. A history of prior menstrual irregularity or oral contraceptive pill use around the period of conception may indicate incorrect menstrual dating. If the menstrual cycle is regular, and the dates accurate, then the finding of a small fetus should arouse suspicion of fetal growth complications.

The previous obstetric and gynaecological history, and past medical and surgical history are relevant to antenatal care, as a number of obstetric, gynaecological, and medical factors affect pregnancy outcome. The parity and gravidity of the mother is important. Gravidity records the number of pregnancies, while parity records the number of pregnancies that have reached viability. It is important to note that, using this classification, the outcome of pregnancies that reached viability is unknown. It is therefore important to be tactful in enquiring about the fate of these pregnancies, as they may have resulted in a perinatal death, or other

Table 8.1 – Factors unfavourable for a vaginal delivery at the 41–42 week visit

• High head	Occipito-posterior position
	Large baby/small pelvis
	Deflexed head (face/brow)
	Placenta praevia
	Pelvic tumour (e.g. fibroid, ovarian cyst)
	Full maternal bladder
	High pelvic inclination (common in Afro-Caribbean women)
• Suspicious CTG	Reduced variability (<10 bpm)
	Variable decelerations
• Reduced amniotic fluid	
• Low Bishop score of the cervix	

complication. Certain conditions, such as pre-eclampsia are more likely to occur in a first pregnancy, while there are also potential complications such an antepartum and postpartum haemorrhage at the other extreme of high parity. The presence of large pelvic masses, previous pelvic surgery, and medical conditions like diabetes mellitus could all affect the pregnancy adversely.

Physical examination

The woman's height and weight are recorded at the first visit, and a respiratory and cardiovascular examination performed to exclude any complications in these systems. The use of centile charts of maternal weight gain during pregnancy is not effective in predicting those likely to give birth to small for gestational age (SGA) infants but there is an increased risk of perinatal complications in association with a maternal weight of <45 kg or >100 kg. Maternal weight loss or a failure to gain weight over a two-week period has also been reported in up to 46 per cent of pregnant women with normal outcomes at term. Maternal weight needs be recorded only at booking, with the exception of patients in whom nutrition is of concern.

Whereas the history can provide a wealth of information that is useful for the carer, much of the physical examination carries little real weight in terms of predicting adverse events later in pregnancy. Where the level of maternal morbidity is high, a thorough physical examination remains an essential part of the booking visit. In areas where morbidity is low, a more specific examination, based on history and symptoms, is often favoured. A more detailed appraisal of history and examination is presented in Chapter 1.

A typical examination at each antenatal visit

- Blood pressure
- Check for oedema: fingers, pretibial
- Symphysis–fundal height
- Presentation
- Lie
- Engagement
- Fetal heart auscultation

Investigations

Urine

Urine is examined for the presence of abnormal constituents, such as protein and glucose. If proteins are present, urine is sent for microscopy and culture, so that the 5–9 per cent of women with asymptomatic bacteriuria can be identified and treated. In some centres, urine analysis is now done only at booking, and only at later visits if there are urinary complaints or if the maternal blood pressure is elevated. As with much of current antenatal practice, the scientific evidence does not support the use of routine urinalysis, or indeed routine visits for their own sake. If glucose is persistently present, a random blood sugar test should be sent to the laboratory.

Blood

Blood investigations include a full blood count and haemoglobin estimation, as well as haemoglobin electrophoresis in populations where there is a risk of haemoglobinopathy, and blood group and rhesus antibody testing. Serum glucose screening for diabetes mellitus is also performed as this aids the early detection of gestational diabetes. Serum screening for Rubella antibody is performed routinely because of the grave risks to the fetus if an infection is contracted during the pregnancy. The timing is less than ideal; Rubella status should be known prior to conception to enable immunization before a pregnancy begins. Screening for treponemal infection is still performed routinely in most centres, although the prevalence and pick-up rates do not justify this procedure. This serves as a good example of the need for a regular review and modernization of antenatal care procedures.

It is estimated that by the millennium up to 10 million children will be infected with the human immuno-deficiency virus (HIV). It is unfortunate that even in places where antenatal testing is available, up to 80 per cent of infected mothers go through pregnancy unaware of their HIV status. The previously poor fetal outlook is now significantly improved, with a reported reduction in vertical transmission from 25–30 per cent to <5 per cent following treatment of the mother during the antenatal period. Anonymous testing of a sample antenatal population (combined with screening of high-risk patients) has been advocated for monitoring the prevalence of HIV infection and estimating any future need for generalized screening. In some centres, HIV screening is already offered universally to all women booking for pregnancy because of high positive rates in the community, and the fact that knowledge of maternal status helps to improve the fetal outcome. In some London hospitals, up to 1 per cent of booking mothers are HIV positive, therefore counselling and screening such women forms an important part of their antenatal care.

Seroprevalence rates for hepatitis B are generally higher than for HIV. Antenatal maternal serum screening for hepatitis B carriers is advocated in most centres because of the evident benefits in preventing the occurrence of hepatoma and chronic liver disease in their offspring in later life. Other infections, such as varicella zoster, toxoplasma gondii and cytomegalovirus (CMV), which may affect the fetus adversely, are not routinely screened for by laboratory testing, but action is taken in cases where there is a history of exposure. There have recently been calls for preconception varicella screening since the introduction of a new vaccine in 1994. The routine tests performed during pregnancy are listed on page 89.

Screening

Patients and doctors alike are used to associating an investigation with the confirmation or exclusion of a diagnosis. It is not surprising, therefore, to find that an enormous amount of anxiety can be created by the use of screening tests, particularly in pregnancy. Screening tests simply alter an individual's risk of having or developing a condition. This in turn allows us to place populations into low- and high-risk groups, for the purpose of planning the next level of care for the particular issue or diagnosis. Screening tests can be useful in a variety of situations in pregnancy. It is essential that a patient understands the nature of a screening test before agreeing to the investigation, so that true informed consent is obtained, to minimize the anxiety of a false positive result, and to appreciate the possibility of a false

negative result. The situation is made more confusing by the fact that many diagnostic tests applied to the whole population are described as 'screening the population', using the lay, rather than scientific meaning of the word.

At this visit, a biochemical screening test for chromosomal abnormality is also discussed, especially if booking at a later gestation, i.e. if the first trimester ultrasound screen was missed. Various biochemistry screening programmes exist, with a range of two to four biochemical markers. These include: serum oestriol, alpha fetoprotein, human chorionic gonadotrophin (total or free-beta subunit), and more recently, inhibin. The only way to diagnose a chromosomal anomaly is to perform an invasive test, e.g. amniocentesis, chorion villus sampling, or cordocentesis. As these procedures have an associated 1 per cent risk of miscarriage, many women contemplating a diagnostic test will elect to have a screening test prior to making a final decision.

The influence of one screening test on the other is uncertain. It may turn out to be complementary in some cases, e.g. biochemical screening and nuchal translucency. In other situations, appropriate prior screening practically eliminates the possibility of a further screen positive being of any use. For instance, nuchal translucence screening identifies between 60–80 per cent of chromosomal anomalies by 14 weeks' gestation. Soft markers, e.g. hydronephrosis, have a weak link to chromosomal anomaly. If over two-thirds of chromosomal anomalies are already identified and excluded, it renders the finding of hydronephrosis as a marker of chromosomal anomaly meaningless. However, it may still require follow-up as a renal lesion.

Ultrasound

The ultrasound scan has now been integrated into antenatal care, so that in many hospitals it is routinely offered to women at 11–14 weeks and 20–22 weeks for accurate dating, the diagnosis of multiple gestation and chorionicity. It is also used in the diagnosis of structural and chromosomal abnormalities (see Chapter 12) and for the identification of pregnancies at high risk of pre-eclampsia, intrauterine growth restriction and placenta praevia.

Ultrasound scanning will also be performed when

there are clinical indications, such as antepartum haemorrhage, suspected PPROM, low symphysis–fundal height, reduced fetal movements or suspected malpresentation. These are further discussed in Chapter 12.

Key symptoms in pregnancy

There are some major symptoms that require immediate attention during pregnancy. While the occurrence of these symptoms does not assume an adverse outcome for the pregnancy, they signal the possibility of serious perinatal complications.

Vaginal bleeding, or antepartum haemorrhage (if it occurs after the 24th week of pregnancy up to delivery), should always be investigated promptly, particularly to exclude the possibility of a placental abruption (usually associated with pain) or placenta praevia. If the mother is Rhesus negative, Anti–D should be administered, to minimize the risk of Rhesus iso-immunization. New evidence suggests that universal prophylaxis against Rhesus iso-immunization for all women can further reduce the risks of iso-immunization.

In pregnancy, abdominal pain is a common presenting symptom of a urinary tract infection. Constipation, musculoskeletal strain, uterine contractions or indeed labour and placental abruption are but some of the possible causes. In most cases, a comprehensive history and examination will identify the probable source of the pain, allowing appropriate action to be taken.

Premature rupture of the membranes, presenting as leakage of fluid from the genital tract, is another key symptom in pregnancy. If this occurs before 20 weeks' gestation, the risk of premature delivery, lung hypoplasia and limb deformity, are very high. Later in pregnancy the risk of an associated or concurrent infection (chorioamnionitis) is a constant concern, because of the poor outcome for both mother and child in these circumstances.

While the vast majority of headaches are related to tension, this can be the first symptom of impending pre-eclampsia. A headache is particularly worrying if it is accompanied by visual disturbances, alteration in consciousness, or epigastric pain. An assessment of blood pressure is always recommended with the first symptoms, and again if circumstances change.

As the pregnancy progresses, the pattern of fetal movements changes in two ways. The length of time between cycles of activity increases and the number of fetal 'kicks' decreases, but fetal trunk movement continues at the same rate. If the patient is not made aware of these changes, she can naturally become anxious as the pattern of the movements change. In this situation an ultrasound scan can help reassure the mother that the fetus is active, while the operator can spot the very small number of complications associated with this complaint. Abrupt cessation of fetal movements, however, is an ominous finding, with studies quoting perinatal mortality as high as 50 per cent in this group. The patient should be encouraged to visit the labour ward as soon as possible for assessment.

Collapse and convulsions are clearly ominous, and require urgent attention. Eclampsia, haemorrhagic shock, and pulmonary embolus may present in this way.

Acute leg pain and swelling should always arouse suspicion of a deep venous thrombosis in pregnancy. Although the risk of thromboembolism increases in pregnancy, the greatest risk is postpartum. Generalized itch is commonly a symptom associated with skin disorders of pregnancy. Women with persistent itch should have their liver function checked, as this symptom also occurs with obstetric cholestasis, which in turn can have an adverse effect on the fetus. The most common obstetric complications associated with these symptoms are dealt with in Chapter 14, while the medical conditions that affect pregnant women are discussed in Chapter 16.

Minor disorders of pregnancy are discussed in detail in Chapter 14.

S Symptoms

Major symptoms requiring urgent investigation
- Vaginal bleeding – antepartum haemorrhage
- Abdominal pain, including contractions
- Premature rupture of membranes
- Headache, unwell
- Cessation of fetal movements
- Collapse, including convulsions

Special problems

Obstetric problems among teenagers

Teenage mothers deserve special mention because they constitute a high-risk group. The pregnancy is often unplanned therefore there is usually no pre-pregnancy preparation. The mothers are more likely to be single and unsupported and on occasion, the pregnancy may be concealed until a late stage. There is a greater risk of pre-eclampsia, premature labour and low birth weight. Special teenager clinics with specialist midwife practitioner involvement can improve outcome for this group of women.

Obstetric problems among ethnic minority groups

An example of this is the ethnic minority population in Britain. In the Asian community there have been consistent reports of higher perinatal mortality and morbidity rates, irrespective of social class. Low birth weights are also more common among this population. The implicated factors include: poor education; different attitudes to health care; unplanned pregnancies, often at the extremes of maternal age; poor birth spacing; poor housing; chronic ill-health; poor nutrition.

There have been reports of variation in biochemical screening programmes for fetal chromosomal abnormality due to ethnicity. For example, the sensitivity of biochemical screening for chromosomal anomaly is different for Afro-Caribbean and Asian populations, when compared with Caucasians. A higher rate of caesarean deliveries has been reported for Afro-Caribbean women, although the reasons for this remain controversial. Various medical complications of pregnancy are also more prevalent, while other diseases are specific to certain ethnic minority groups, such as, sickle cell disease in Afro-Caribbean women, thalassaemia in Mediterranean populations, and glycogen storage disorders in the Jewish population. Appropriate testing for these conditions is therefore desirable.

Social problems including drug abuse

The majority of antenatal outpatient services do not specifically address the needs of women with social problems, who often fail to attend, as they are hostile to the 'establishment' services provided. Special services, such as help with drug problems, HIV counselling or screening, may be rejected from a fear of prejudice and consequent repercussions. Antenatal care for women with these social problems should be considered in the context of their families and social interaction, and should be provided by a small number of familiar staff forming part of an integrated multidisciplinary team in close and regular contact.

Antenatal admission, if it is the woman's wish, should be viewed as justified in the management of such social problems; conversely, women should not be pressurized into hospital admission or rehabilitation programmes, or made to feel guilty if they are unable to comply. Outpatient antenatal services should be conveniently sited in the community close to other relevant services and should be flexible, not only in terms of organization and format, but also in the roles of the participants. They should be comprehensive but with special services in addition to, not instead of, routine care, provided by a team of appropriately trained staff. In the provision of antenatal care for women with social needs, no single format can be universally applicable or desirable, and the design and content of the service should be varied according to local requirements, taking into account the women's wishes as well as their needs. Ultimately, if the women identify the service as being in their best interests and as meeting their needs, they will use it, thereby giving it a chance of success.

Factors affecting the success of antenatal care

It is unfortunate that rates of under-utilization of antenatal care are greatest among high-risk groups, such as single unsupported mothers and particularly those with unplanned and unwanted pregnancies. Special efforts should therefore be directed towards helping such groups of women.

CASE HISTORY

Mrs J Goldberg, aged 42, journalist, vegetarian

First pregnancy: early ultrasound at 8 weeks shows viable IVF twins; requests vaginal delivery and a labour 'as natural as possible'; no relevant medical and surgical history; on examination, overweight at 106 kg

Mrs Goldberg attends the antenatal booking clinic to see the Consultant. What are the major issues that must be addressed?

Risk assessment

The booking visit is crucial to identify aspects arising from history or examination that may have adverse repercussions on Mrs Goldberg's pregnancy. These include:

Occupation: It is useful to note whether Mrs Goldberg is working at present, and what she does for a living. This is important in general terms, particularly if she performs manual jobs or needs to keep working to support herself.

Age: At 42, Mrs Goldberg is approaching the end of her reproductive lifespan, and represents what is somewhat unfortunately known as 'an elderly primigravida'. This is important from the maternal point of view because all medical conditions are commoner in older mothers (particularly hypertension, diabetes, auto-immune conditions and renal disease). From the fetal aspect, age is a strong risk factor for chromosomal conditions such as Down's syndrome. Finally, obstetricians instinctively regard age over 40 as an independent risk factor for obstetric adverse outcome.

Twins: This was diagnosed on scan at 8 weeks, after successful IVF. A twin pregnancy is a 'high-risk' pregnancy with an increased risk of preterm delivery, pre-eclampsia and perinatal mortality. The definite diagnosis of twins should not be made until at least 11 weeks, however, as it is not uncommon for one to 'disappear'. (This is known as vanishing twins; one is non-viable and becomes resorbed, often leaving little trace at later scans.) The crucial point about twins is whether they are monochorionic (identical) or dichorionic (non-identical)? Monochorionic twins are associated with specific problems that can make their management challenging (see Chapter 13, Multiple Gestation).

Diet: Mrs Goldberg is a vegetarian. She does, however, eat fish, eggs and dairy products so she would not be at high risk of becoming deficient in iron, calcium and folic acid.

Request for a 'natural pregnancy': Mrs Goldberg is at relatively high risk of adverse obstetric outcome as we have discovered. This does not mean, however, that her care must be totally medicalized. If reasons why decisions are taken are explained and agreed with the patients, then normally women and their partners agree to a sensible

course of action. Fortunately, she has decided against her earlier wishes to have a home birth and avoid all ultrasound scans! Mrs Goldberg is keen to avoid syntocinon/ ergometrine injection following the delivery of the babies, and does not wish them to have vitamin K (see Neonatology, Chapter 22): clearly these issues are important and must be tackled at later antenatal visits.

Weight: Being overweight is a further risk factor. Not only does it increase the likelihood of 'minor' complications of pregnancy, but it predisposes her to hypertension, pre-eclampsia and diabetes. It makes obstetric palpation difficult, increasing the reliance of obstetricians and midwives on ultrasound. Any instrumentation or operation (for example, caesarean section) will be more hazardous and increases the likelihood of wound infection, postpartum haemorrhage and deep venous thrombosis.

In addition to normal booking investigations:

- 11-14 week early ultrasound scan to define chorionicity and risk of Down's syndrome from individual twin nuchal measurements (luckily, this showed non-identical twins with low risks for Down's).
- Specific advice on dietary means to reduce weight, and encouragement for sensible exercise (e.g. swimming).
- Iron and folic acid supplements from booking throughout pregnancy.
- Consultant-led care with visits at 14, 20, 24, 28, 32, 34 and 36 weeks; weekly thereafter, with ultrasound growth scans at 24, 28, 32 and 36 weeks. Senior obstetricians must be involved at every step with her care.
- A plan for delivery to be formulated at 34 weeks: her insistence on a vaginal delivery might be accommodated as long as all factors are favourable (cephalic/cephaphic presentation, normal fetal sizes). In view of her size, one might argue that a vaginal delivery would be preferable to the operative risks of a Caesarean Section. However, a vaginal delivery might be associated with a higher risk of birth trauma to the babies. Attempting a vaginal delivery might also be hazardous in view of her size; this makes fetal monitoring and external manipulation difficult, thus increasing the risk of caesarean for the second twin. As long as she is aware of the risks involved, and discussions with senior staff have taken place and are documented clearly in the notes, she may proceed with the delivery of her choice.

Cost

Cost-effectiveness is an issue that applies to all aspects of health care. Conventional antenatal care is not cost-effective. The majority of women in an antenatal population are at low risk of pregnancy-related complications, and traditional antenatal care schedules are notoriously poor at identifying relatively common obstetric problems such as pre-eclampsia in low-risk populations. Improving cost-efficiency involves an estimation of the resources used nationally, particularly in relation to the type of populations served. More appropriate allocation of funds could be arranged, or even allocated to more efficient alternatives. The management of labour and delivery remain by far the most expensive part of maternity care. A pertinent observation is the fact that around 70 per cent of babies are delivered by midwives and at present home births account for less than 5 per cent. An increase in home deliveries may reduce costs. If costs were all, however, the most cost-effective option would be for all women to be delivered by elective Caesarean Section, eliminating most potential intrapartum complications, and reducing delivery room costs significantly. While this may be an absurd notion in everyday clinical practice, it serves to highlight the importance of evaluating cost versus care in a practical and realistic manner.

Concept of risk and women's rights and responsibility of care

In the past, women were often excluded from the process of medical decision making during pregnancy, even though medical decisions that are made by healthcare professionals affect them personally and affect the future wellbeing of their unborn children. There are increasing numbers of new genetic tests and technologies, designed to predict and even treat certain genetic problems during pregnancy, through prenatal diagnosis, fetal surgery and fetal gene therapy. The impact of such developments is that the number of choices being given to pregnant women regarding prenatal diagnosis continues to increase and with it the uncertainty in the minds of many women as to the next step to take. It is imperative that a great deal more time and effort be paid to the education and counselling of pregnant women in the future.

A good example of the increasing accountability of pregnant women for their pregnancies is seen in the fact that in many centres the mothers now carry their own case notes and 'cooperative cards' are no longer used. The disadvantage of this concept however, is that the assessment and management of risk is not standardized or consistently applied. However, to the lay public, healthcare providers and the legal system it may seem as if 'risk' is synonymous with indisputable 'fact'. Inequality in social status is the most important factor linked with women's compliance with prescribed health needs. In some countries, to improve compliance, certain payments, e.g. antenatal allowances, or maternity benefits, are linked with improved antenatal attendance and compliance. Obstacles to care may include the pregnant woman's personal beliefs, knowledge, attitudes, fears and lifestyles. The mother's socio-economic status and level of education are important factors.

Clinical risk management and antenatal care

Clinical risk management is a natural development of the 'best practice' approach to antenatal care. It is emerging as an integral aspect of care, especially in obstetrics. The main objectives of clinical risk management are: to reduce the likelihood of causing harm to women and their babies in the process of obstetric care; to minimize the damage (and costs) to those who are affected, despite the care taken; and to limit the possibility of subsequent litigation. There has been increased pressure for alternative methods of antenatal care and childbirth. In 1994, the government in the UK accepted the 'Changing Childbirth' report, which strongly recommends an increased choice for women in their pregnancy. The diversity of people interested or involved in maternity services has resulted in an ever-increasing amount of conflicting information and advice being offered to women.

Reduction of risk requires the identification and breakdown of the patterns of maternal and fetal risk, and improvements in clinical practice affected by concentrating on problem areas. The more common complications in this category include:

- antepartum, intrapartum and neonatal deaths;
- neurological complications and handicap;
- congenital abnormalities.

This also introduces ethical and financial considerations. Stillbirths, neonatal death and neurological damage are now less linked to birth injury; the result is an increased scrutiny of antenatal care, and a search for contributory deficiencies in such care. The vast majority of current litigation concerns incidents that occur during delivery, but the focus may well change with time.

The important factors in risk reduction include improvements in communication among the carers, and between staff and patients, more appropriate staffing in units, and relevant education and updating training. The regular maintenance and upgrading of infrastructure and equipment is also important. The standardization of practice using protocols is helpful but should only be used as guidelines because of the wide individual differences in pregnancy complications in different areas.

The book 'Effective care in Pregnancy and Childbirth' sought to review all the known trials of obstetric management, in order to ascertain the usefulness of these practices. It has since emerged as an electronic publication, which is updated regularly. Science and statistics however, have their own limitations and failings. Many of the analytical processes used in producing evidence-based medicine are themselves flawed. The good clinician must keep this in mind when contemplating a change in practice and use his or her judgement to good effect. Good practice remains the best form of defence.

New developments in antenatal care

Abandoning outdated practices: the slavish following of routines established over the last 40 or so years is giving way to a less formal approach for 'low-risk' antenatal women. Routine weight measurement is now rarely performed, and vaginal examination should only be performed if there is a clinical indication or prior to induction of labour.

Antenatal HIV testing: there is now good evidence that HIV vertical transmission can be reduced to considerably below 10 per cent with careful antenatal, delivery and

postnatal management. This provides a strong rationale for antenatal testing. The current policy of offering HIV tests to those considered to be at high risk is giving way to more widespread 'opt out' screening programmes, such as those now offered in the UK.

Nuchal translucency measurement for risk of Down's syndrome (11–14 weeks) and uterine artery Doppler screening for pre-eclampsia and small babies (20–24 weeks). Rather than basing a decision on invasive prenatal diagnosis purely on age, a risk assessment of pre-eclampsia and delivering a small baby on past obstetric history, parents-to-be can be given accurate and targetted risk levels that will allow rational decisions on obstetric management.

The concept of the 'lead professional': The Changing Childbirth report (HMSO, 1993) suggested that women should be able to choose the professional most closely involved with their antenatal care. The thrust of this concept is that antenatal care could be devolved from hospitals into the community, and the role of the obstetrician redefined as someone who looks after women with risk factors or an actual problem. This means that low-risk multiparas might be predominantly looked after by a community midwife, low-risk primigravidae might choose their GP and those with risk factors or medical/obstetric problems are under the care of an obstetrician. There is no data yet to assess how popular or effective this pattern of care is.

Key Points

- Antenatal care improves pregnancy outcome. A variety of models of antenatal care exist, each providing similar benefits
- There are key visits during the pregnancy when essential investigations or decisions are taken regarding antenatal care and delivery
- The integration of care and education is necessary and the two should not be separated. It is important that the patient is aware of the key symptoms that may occur in pregnancy which require prompt assessment
- The service provided requires continual reappraisal in the light of new scientific information, accepting the limitations of such data
- We must continue to find ways of ensuring that those in most need are included in the process of antenatal care

Conclusion

Antenatal care is an essential aspect of health care delivery for improving pregnancy outcome, although the methods may vary. It should always remain a combination of art and science, with the clinician integrating scientific developments when the need arises. Antenatal care and education should be integrated not separated. The increasing focus on prenatal diagnosis and seeking the 'perfect child' should not detract from the joys of pregnancy. There is a need to continually update and improve our current mould of antenatal care. The move towards a more educational approach to antenatal care, based on sound scientific evidence, is to be encouraged.

Reference for further reading

Effective care in pregnancy and childbirth. Series; Oxford Medical Publications. Edited by Iain Chalmers, Murray Enkin and Marc J.N.C. Keirse, Oxford University Press, 1989.

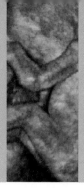

Labour

OVERVIEW

Labour is defined as the onset of painful, regular contractions, more than one every ten minutes, with progressive cervical effacement and dilatation accompanied by descent of the presenting part. A more utilitarian definition is 'the process by which the fetus is expelled from the uterus'. These mechanical definitions do not do justice to the complex interplay of medical, social and ethical aspects that combine to make the obstetric management of labour such a challenge. A doctor or midwife who manages labour must be aware of the normal anatomy and physiology of the mother and fetus, what marks out an abnormal from a normal labour, when to adopt a 'hands off' approach and when, and how, to intervene. This chapter contains the basic information that you must know before embarking on the complex but rewarding process of care of a woman in labour.

Introduction

Labour and delivery is the focus and climax of the reproductive process. It is both a physical and emotional challenge for the mother. It is also a hazardous journey for the fetus. There is an interplay between the powers of the uterus, the passages of the birth canal and the passenger, single or multiple. Each contraction necessary to promote dilatation of the uterine cervix and descent of the fetus transiently deprives the placenta of blood flow and consequently the fetus of oxygen. Our duty is to ensure this process achieves completion with all parties healthy and satisfied.

As well as bringing great joy and happiness to the majority of families, labour has brought death and catastrophe to others. In historical documents and literature there is ample reference to the death of the mother in childbirth. Sadly, maternal death, often associated with emergencies in labour, remains frequent in many countries that have less developed health care systems. This is not natural childbirth: it is medically unattended childbirth. In developed countries a significant minority of women seek natural childbirth but this implies childbirth with minimal technology and natural methods of pain relief. In the modern environment of changing childbirth this is an option. Women seeking this are sometimes responding to a perception that birth has been 'hijacked' by modern medicine and modern doctors. Conversely, there is now a small but significant minority of women who have responded in the opposite direction. They have opted to avoid labour altogether and elect for planned Caesarean Section. They have reasons for doing this and as long as they are making an informed choice and are aware of the risks of either option, then this is also part of the modern menu. About 5 per cent of women have elective Caesarean Section and another 10 per cent have emergency Caesarean Section after a period of labour. In most centres the Caesarean Section rate is higher or lower than this. This could be due to differing case mix or to differing obstetric and midwifery practices.

Labour begins when uterine contractions become painful and progressive, more then one in every ten minutes, with or without a show or rupture of the membranes leading to progressive changes in the cervix. A show is the release from the cervix of a bloodstained mucus plug, which is then expelled from the vagina. Rupture of the membranes is when the chorioamniotic membrane breaks and releases amniotic fluid. A show and rupture of the membranes can both occur without labour being in progress and vice versa. However when they occur with painful contractions present it is highly suggestive that the process of labour has begun.

Any definition of labour that includes pain must be partly subjective. Women are in varying frames of mind in late pregnancy. Anxious, poorly supported women may present several times with painful Braxton Hicks contractions in late pregnancy and not be in labour. This has been called false or spurious labour. A better expression is painful prelabour. Contractions, whether of prelabour or labour itself, present a stress to the fetus. Studies of the length of labour have been hampered by incorrectly establishing the time at which it started. There has been an essential misunderstanding of this: labour does not begin at a point; it is a transition from the physiology of late pregnancy to labour. We can only establish a time of the start of 'observed' labour whether at home or in hospital. This will coincide with a confirmatory vaginal examination showing progressive dilatation and/or effacement. Obsession with the diagnosis of the onset of labour has been part of the medicalization of labour as a medical condition rather than a biological event.

The majority of women experience normal labour and normal delivery. They often do so with minimal pain relief in the form of good support from a friend, husband or partner, family member, midwife and sometimes a medical student! Good preparation for labour is essential to reduce the fear of the unknown. Pain relief in labour starts in the antenatal preparation classes. Staffing aims at one-to-one care in labour. If nature is doing a good job it is important to let it take its course and not interfere unnecessarily. Careful assessment of fetal condition on admission, mobilization in early labour and midwifery skills are all that is required. The record of labour is kept on a partogram (Fig. 9.1). This is indispensable, containing all the important information at a glance. It is from this that any deviation may become apparent.

Anatomy of the female pelvis and fetus relevant to labour

Knowledge of the anatomy of the normal female pelvis, the fetal skull and the soft tissues is essential to the understanding of the mechanism of labour.

The pelvis

The pelvic brim or inlet

The pelvis is sometimes divided into the true and false pelvis, which are separated by the pelvic brim or inlet. The plane of the pelvic brim is bounded in front by the symphysis pubis (the joint separating the two pubic bones), on each side by the upper margin of the pubic bone, the ileopectineal line and the ala of the sacrum, and posteriorly by the promontory of the sacrum (Fig. 9.2). The normal transverse diameter in this plane is 13.5 cm and is wider than the anterior–posterior diameter, which is normally 11 cm (Fig. 9.3). The angle of the brim or inlet is normally 60° to the horizontal in the erect position but in Afro-Caribbean women this angle may be 90° (Fig. 9.4). This increased angle may delay the head entering the pelvis in labour.

The pelvic mid-cavity

This pelvic mid-cavity can be described as an area bounded in front by the middle of the symphysis pubis, on each side by the pubic bone, the obturator fascia and the inner aspect of the ischial bone and spines, and posteriorly by the junction of the second and third pieces of the sacrum. The cavity is almost round as the transverse and anterior diameters are similar at 12 cm. The ischial spines are palpable vaginally and are used as landmarks to assess the descent of the head on vaginal examination (station). They are also used as landmarks for providing an anaesthetic block to the pudendal nerve. The pudendal

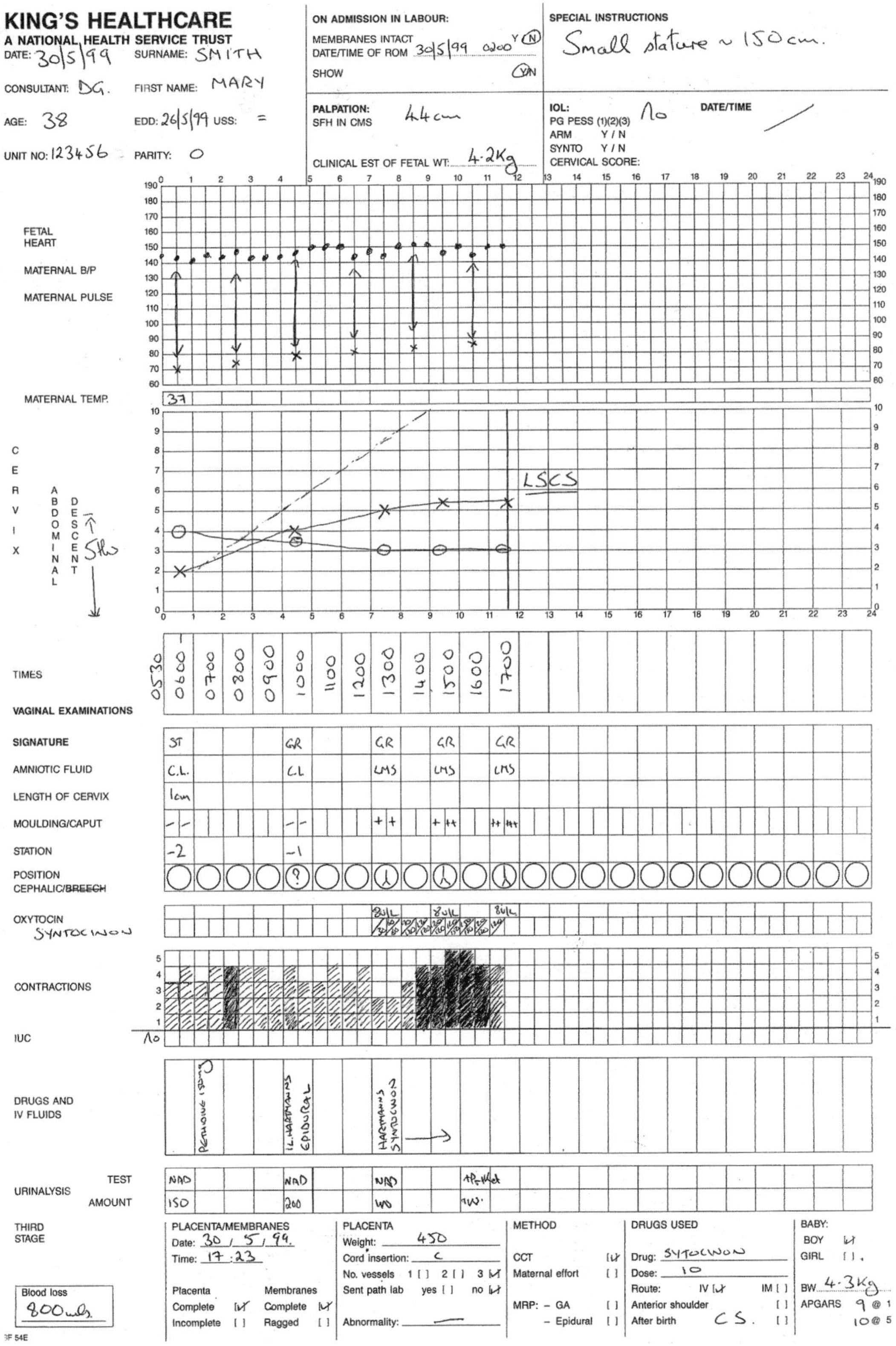

KING'S HEALTHCARE
A NATIONAL HEALTH SERVICE TRUST
DATE: 30/5/99   SURNAME: SMITH

CONSULTANT: DG.   FIRST NAME: MARY

AGE: 38   EDD: 26/5/99 USS: =

UNIT NO: 123456   PARITY: O

ON ADMISSION IN LABOUR:
MEMBRANES INTACT
DATE/TIME OF ROM 30/5/99 0200 Y (N)
SHOW   (Y) N

PALPATION:
SFH IN CMS   44 cm

CLINICAL EST OF FETAL WT: 4.2 Kg

IOL:
PG PESS (1)(2)(3)   No   DATE/TIME
ARM   Y / N
SYNTO   Y / N
CERVICAL SCORE:

SPECIAL INSTRUCTIONS
Small stature ~ 150 cm.

FETAL HEART
MATERNAL B/P
MATERNAL PULSE
MATERNAL TEMP.   37

CERVIX
ABDOMINAL DESCENT   SHO

LSCS

TIMES: 0530 0600 0700 0800 0900 1000 1100 1200 1300 1400 1500 1600 1700

VAGINAL EXAMINATIONS

SIGNATURE	ST		GR	GR	GR	GR			
AMNIOTIC FLUID	C.L.		CL	LMS	LMS	LMS			
LENGTH OF CERVIX	1cm								
MOULDING/CAPUT	- -		- -	+ +	+ ++	++ +++			
STATION	-2		-1						

POSITION CEPHALIC/~~BREECH~~

OXYTOCIN SYNTOCINON   8u/L   8u/L   8u/L

CONTRACTIONS

IUC   No

DRUGS AND IV FLUIDS   PETHIDINE 100mg   IL HARTMANS EPIDURAL   HARTMANS SYNTOCINON

URINALYSIS
TEST: NAD   NAD   NAD   +Prot/Ket
AMOUNT: 150   200   50   50

THIRD STAGE

PLACENTA/MEMBRANES
Date: 30 / 5 / 94.
Time: 17 : 23

Placenta   Membranes
Complete [✓]   Complete [✓]
Incomplete [ ]   Ragged [ ]

PLACENTA
Weight: 450
Cord insertion: C
No. vessels 1 [ ] 2 [ ] 3 [✓]
Sent path lab   yes [ ]   no [✓]
Abnormality: —

METHOD
CCT [✓]
Maternal effort [ ]
MRP: – GA [ ]
– Epidural [ ]

DRUGS USED
Drug: SYNTOCINON
Dose: 10
Route: IV [✓]   IM [ ]
Anterior shoulder [ ]
After birth   CS. [ ]

BABY:
BOY [✓]
GIRL [ ].
BW 4.3 Kg
APGARS 9 @ 1
10 @ 5

Blood loss   800 mls

Figure 9.1 A typical partogram. This is a partogram of a nulliparous woman of short stature with a big baby and an augmented labour. The labour culminates in an emergency caesarean section for cephalo pelvic disproportion.

nerve passes behind and below the spine. The pelvic axis describes an imaginary curved line, which shows the path that the centre of the fetal head takes during its passage through the pelvis.

The pelvic outlet

The pelvic outlet is bounded in front by the lower margin of the symphysis pubis, on each side by the descending ramus of the pubic bone, the ischial tuberosity and the sacrotuberous ligament, and posteriorly by the last piece of the sacrum. The anterior–posterior diameter of the pelvic outlet is 13.5 cm and the transverse diameter is 11 cm (Fig. 9.5).

The pelvic floor

This is formed by the two levator ani muscles, which with their fascia form a musculofascial gutter during the second stage of labour (Fig. 9.6).

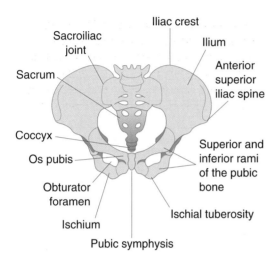

Figure 9.2 The bony pelvis.

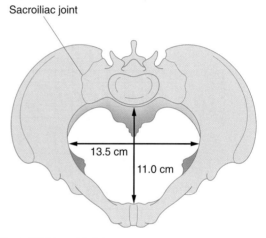

Figure 9.3 The pelvic brim.

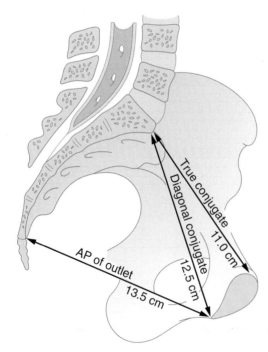

Figure 9.4 Sagittal section of the pelvis with conjugate diameters and AP diameter of the outlet shown.

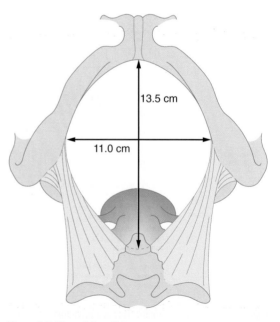

Figure 9.5 The pelvic outlet.

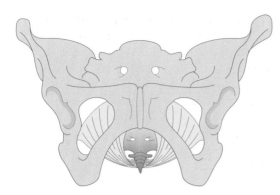

Figure 9.6 The musculofascial gutter of the levator sling.

🔑 **Key Points**

- A variety of pelvic shapes described may explain difficulties in labour. The gynaecoid pelvis is the most favourable for labour, and the most common (Fig. 9.7a–c). Other shapes of pelvis predispose to the following clinical scenarios
  Android: deep transverse arrest (Fig. 9.8a–c)
  Anthropoid: persistent occiputo-posterior (OP) position (Fig. 9.9a–c)
  Platypelloid pelvis: obstructed labour (Fig. 9.10a–c)
- Previous pelvis fracture may be relevant in labour
- All pelvic measurements relate to bony points. As the pelvic ligaments loosen in pregnancy, the pelvis is often more flexible than the measurements would suggest, which is why pelvic measurements may not be helpful clinically

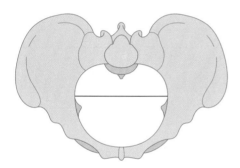
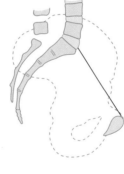
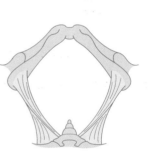

a Brim   b Lateral view   c Outlet

Figure 9.7 The gynaecoid pelvis. (a) Brim, (b) lateral view, (c) outlet.

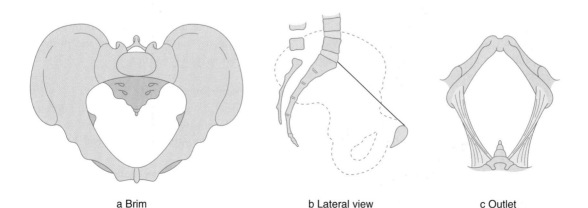

a Brim   b Lateral view   c Outlet

Figure 9.8 The android pelvis. (a) Brim, (b) lateral view, (c) outlet.

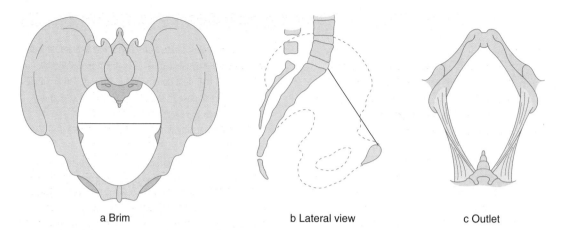

a Brim   b Lateral view   c Outlet

Figure 9.9 The anthropoid pelvis. (a) Brim, (b) lateral view, (c) outlet.

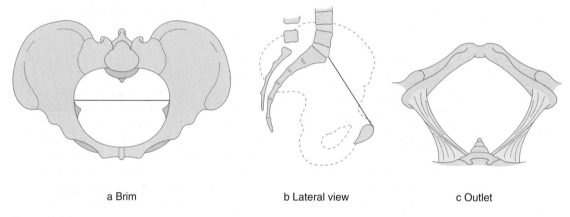

a Brim   b Lateral view   c Outlet

Figure 9.10 The platypelloid pelvis. (a) Brim, (b) lateral view, (c) outlet.

The fetal skull

The bones, sutures and fontanelles

The fetal skull is made up of the vault, face and the base. At the time of labour only unossified membranes at the sutures join the bones of the vault, unlike the face and the base which are all firmly united (Fig. 9.11).

The bones that form the vault, are the parietal bones and parts of the occipital, frontal and temporal bones. Between these bones there are four membranous sutures: the sagittal, frontal, coronal and lambdoidal sutures.

Fontanelles are the junction of the various sutures. The anterior fontanelle or bregma (diamond shaped) is at the junction of the sagittal, frontal and coronal sutures. The posterior fontanelle (triangular shaped) lies at the junction of the sagittal suture and the lamdoidal sutures between the two parietal bones and the occipital bone.

The area of the fetal skull bounded by the two parietal eminences and the anterior and posterior fontanelles is termed the vertex.

The diameters of the skull

The fetal head is ovoid in shape. There are different longitudinal diameters that may present in labour depending on the attitude of the fetal head (Fig. 9.12).

The longitudinal diameter that presents in a well-flexed fetal head (vertex presentation) is the suboccipito-bregmatic diameter. This is usually 9.5 cm, and is measured from the suboccipital region to the centre of the anterior fontanelle (bregma). The longitudinal diameter that presents in a less well-flexed

P   Understanding the physiology

The physiology of labour

The mechanism responsible for initiating human parturition is still unknown. There are certain things that seem to be important. Firstly, the duration of the pregnancy seems to be influenced by the fetal genotype. Secondly, prostaglandins are involved in some way.

The onset of human parturition does not fit into many of the animal models used. It is thought that the mechanism may depend on an interaction between the contiguous tissues of the fetus and the mother, namely the chorion (both membranous and placental) and the decidua. The action of prostaglandins in initiating labour is partly by stimulating contractions, but probably mainly by ripening and increasing the sensitivity of the cervix to oxytocin. The exact mechanism by which this happens is unknown, but it is likely to involve the synthesis of proteins that link smooth muscle cells electrically into a functional syncytium permitting coordinated activity. At the same time cervical ripening occurs, resulting in structural changes to the collagen and connective tissue matrix. The softening of the cervix occurs by the destruction of collagen fibres, a decrease in dermatin sulphate, which has a strong affinity for collagen, and an increase in hyaluronic acid.

Steroid hormones, oxytocin, cytokines, platelet-activating factor, and endothelin-1 may stimulate prostaglandin synthesis. Progesterone and phospholipase A2 inhibitors may inhibit prostaglandin synthesis. Corticotrophin-releasing factor fulfils many of the requirements of an agent initiating labour, but evidence regarding its role remains circumstantial.

Myometrial cells contain filaments of actin and myosin, which are the two key proteins for contraction. The interaction of myosin and actin brings about contraction, while their separation brings about relaxation under the important influence of intracellular free calcium. An increase in intracellular free calcium ions results in the formation of the contractile entity of actin-phosphorylated myosin. Beta-adrenergic compounds and calcium channel blockers decrease intracellular calcium. Prostaglandins and oxytocin increase intracellular free calcium ions.

Individual myometrial cells are laid down in a mesh of collagen. There is a cell-to-cell communication system by means of gap junctions which facilitates the passage of various products of metabolism and electrical current between cells and are actual bridging connections between the cells that form at various times. Of interest is that these gap junctions are absent for most of the pregnancy but appear in significant numbers at term. It also appears that the gap junctions increase in size and number with the actual labour process and tend to disappear afterwards. Prostaglandins stimulate their formation, while beta-adrenergic compounds possibly inhibit them being formed. The probability of a uterine pacemaker is likely but histologically has not been proven.

Retraction is a major feature of uterine contractility during labour. This is the progressive shortening of the uterine smooth muscle cells in the upper portion of the uterus as labour progresses. After the cells contract they relax but they do not return to their original length. The result of this retraction process is the development of the thicker, active, contracting segment in the upper portion of the uterus. At the same time the lower segment of the uterus becomes thinner and more stretched. Eventually this results in the cervix being taken up into the lower segment of the uterus and forming a continuum with the lower uterine segment (Fig. 9.13).

Uterine contractions are involuntary in nature. There appears to be relatively minimal extrauterine neuronal control. The frequency of contractions may vary during labour and with parity. Throughout the majority of labour they occur at intervals of 2 to 4 minutes. Their duration also varies during labour from 30 to 60 seconds, or occasionally longer. The intensity or amplitude of the intrauterine pressure generated with each contraction averages between 30 and 60 mmHg.

---

head, such as is found in occipito-posterior (OP) position, is the suboccipito-frontal diameter, and is measured from the suboccipital region to the prominence of the forehead. It measures 10 cm.

With further extension of the head the occipito-frontal diameter presents. This is measured from the root of the nose to the posterior fontanelle and is 11.5 cm.

The greatest longitudinal diameter that may present is the mento-vertical, which is taken from the

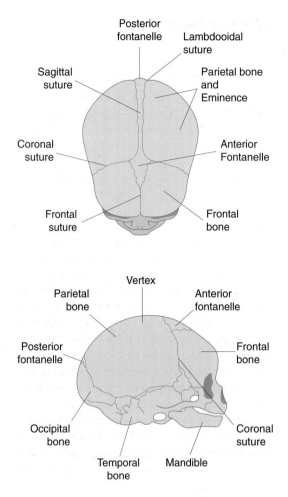

Figure 9.11 The fetal skull from posterior and lateral views.

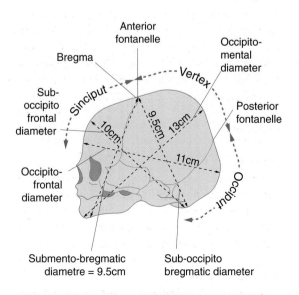

Figure 9.12 The diameters of the fetal skull.

chin to the furthest point of the vertex and measures 13 cm. This is known as a brow presentation and it is usually too large to pass through the normal pelvis.

Extension of the fetal head beyond this point results in a smaller diameter presenting. The submento-bregmatic diameter is measured from below the chin to the anterior fontanelle and measures 9.5 cm. This is clinically a face presentation.

The stages of labour

Labour is divided into three stages, as described below. The definitions of the stages rely predominantly on anatomical criteria and in certain situations this may be a disadvantage as labour is essentially a physiological process. In normal labour, the divisions into three stages are of little clinical significance. The important events in normal labour are the diagnosis of labour and the maternal urge to push, which usually corresponds with full dilatation of the cervix and the baby's head resting on the perineum. The importance of defining the three stages of labour becomes more relevant if the labour does

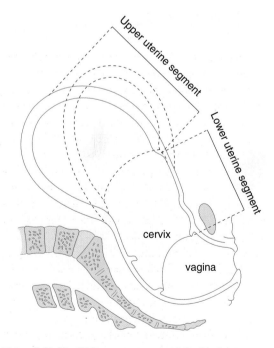

Figure 9.13 The thick upper segment and the thin lower segment of the uterus at the end of the first stage of labour. The dotted lines indicate the position assumed by the uterus during contraction.

not progress normally. Because the definition of a normal labour can only be made retrospectively, there is difficulty in defining exactly when a normal labour becomes abnormal. Indeed this definition will be different depending on the gestation, the category, the previous obstetric record and the onset of labour. It will also depend on what the initial dilatation of the cervix was on the diagnosis of labour.

The stages of labour are as follows.

- 1st Stage. From the diagnosis of labour to full dilatation of the cervix.
- 2nd Stage. From full dilatation of the cervix to delivery of the fetus or fetuses. The second stage of labour may be subdivided into two phases. Phase one is where there is no maternal urge to push and the fetal head is high and the sagittal suture is in the transverse position. Phase two is when there is a maternal urge to push, the head is low and the sagittal suture is in the anterior–posterior position. Epidural anaesthesia affects the length of the stages of labour and their management.
- 3rd Stage. From delivery of the fetus or fetuses until delivery of the placenta(s).

The duration of labour

More than any other objective measurement, the duration of labour determines the impact of childbirth, particularly on mothers but also on babies, and also on those who care for both of them. A prolonged labour has an effect on the efficient running of the delivery ward and therefore indirectly an effect on every aspect of a woman's care.

The morale of most women starts to deteriorate after six hours in labour, and after 12 hours the rate of deterioration significantly accelerates. There is a greater incidence of fetal hypoxia after a long labour and often a greater incidence of vaginal operative deliveries. Shorter labours will also mean that personal attention for each woman in labour is a realistic possibility. An early artificially ruptured membrane (ARM) does shorten the length of labour, but does not necessarily alter the outcome.

It is difficult to define prolonged labour, but it would be reasonable to suggest that labour lasting longer than 12 hours in nulliparous women and eight hours in multiparous women should be regarded as prolonged.

The mechanism of labour

This refers to the series of changes in position and attitude that the fetus undergoes during its passage through the birth canal. It is described here for the vertex presentation and the gynaecoid pelvis. The relation of the fetal head and body to the maternal pelvis changes as the fetus descends through the pelvis. This is essential so that the optimal diameters of the fetal skull are present at each stage of the descent.

Engagement
The head normally enters the pelvis in the transverse position or some minor variant of that position. The anterior parietal bone slides past the symphysis followed by the posterior parietal bone, so that the sagittal suture stays synclitic, or evenly orientated between the sacrum and the symphysis. Engagement is said to have occurred when the widest part of the presenting part has passed successfully through the inlet. Engagement has occurred in the vast majority of nulliparous women prior to labour, but not in the majority of multiparous women.

The number of fifths of the fetal head palpable abdominally is often used to describe whether engagement has taken place. If more than two-fifths of the fetal head is palpable abdominally then the head is not said to be engaged.

Descent
Descent of the fetal head is needed before the further series of changes of flexion, internal rotation and extension (Fig. 9.14). During the first stage and first phase of the second stage of labour, descent of the fetus is secondary to uterine action. In the second phase of the second stage of labour, descent of the fetus is helped by voluntary use of abdominal musculature.

Flexion
The fetal head may not always be completely flexed when it enters the pelvis. As the head descends into the narrower midcavity, flexion should occur (Fig. 9.15). This is probably as a passive movement in part due to the surrounding structures.

Internal rotation
The anatomy of the lower pelvis and the resistance of the pelvic floor predispose the head to arrive at the

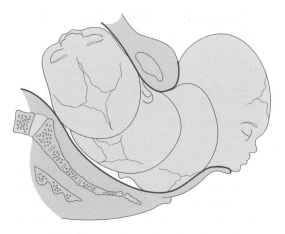

Figure 9.14 Descent and flexion of the head followed by internal rotation and ending in birth of the head by extension.

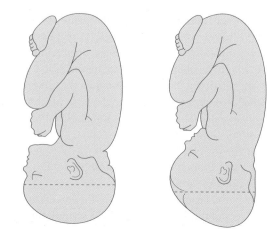

Figure 9.15 Flexion of the head during labour. The dotted line indicates the reduction in diameter of the head when it flexes.

pelvic outlet in the anterior–posterior position, and usually occipito-anterior rather than occipito-posterior. This internal rotation occurs because with a well-flexed head the occiput is leading and meets the sloping gutter of the levator ani muscles, which by their shape direct it anteriorly. If the fetus has engaged in the occipito-posterior position, internal rotation can occur from an occipito-posterior position to an occipito-anterior position. This long internal rotation may explain the increased duration and dystocia associated with this malposition. Alternatively, an occipito-posterior position may persist resulting in a 'face to pubes' delivery.

Extension
Following completion of internal rotation the occiput is underneath the symphysis pubis and the bregma is near the lower border of the sacrum. The soft tissues of the perineum still offer resistance, and may be traumatized in the process (see Chapter 10). The well-flexed head now extends, with the occiput escaping from underneath the symphysis pubis and starting to distend the vulva. This is known as the crowning of the head. The head extends further and the occiput underneath the symphysis pubis almost acts as a fulcrum point as the bregma, face and the chin appear in succession over the posterior vaginal opening and perineal body. This extension and movement minimize soft tissue trauma by utilizing the smallest diameters of the head for the birth.

Restitution
When the head is delivering, the occiput is directly anterior. As soon as it escapes from the vulva, the head aligns itself with the shoulders, which have entered the pelvis in the oblique position. The slight rotation of the occiput through one-eighth of a circle is called restitution.

External rotation
In order to be delivered, the shoulders have to rotate into the direct anterior–posterior plane. When this occurs, the occiput rotates through a further one-eighth of a circle to the transverse position. This is called external rotation (Fig. 9.16).

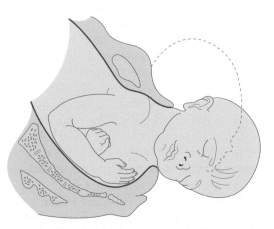

Figure 9.16 External rotation of the head after delivery as the anterior shoulder rotates forward to pass under the subpubic arch.

Shoulder rotation

When restitution and external rotation have occurred, the shoulders will be in the anterior–posterior position. The anterior shoulder is under the symphysis pubis and delivers first, and the posterior shoulder delivers subsequently.

Delivery of the fetal body

Normally the rest the fetal body is delivered easily occasionally aided by lateral movements.

A typical normal labour

A midwife usually looks after a woman who is admitted in normal labour. Medical involvement is not necessary unless labour deviates from its expected progress, there is a fetal problem or a maternal medical condition.

On admission, a midwife will normally take a brief history and look through the mother's notes in order to be re-acquainted with any important details of the antenatal course of the pregnancy. The midwife will then perform a vaginal examination and auscultate the fetal heart. In most units a 30-minute cardiotocograph (CTG) is the norm; an 'admission CTG'. If the woman is in labour, analgesia would be discussed and the membranes might be ruptured depending on how advanced labour was.

The mother-to-be may eat a light diet (heavy foods are not recommended in view of the commonness of nausea and vomiting), and her partner may be with her throughout.

On admission the midwife will normally perform blood pressure and pulse rate measurements and analysis. If these are normal, then BP and pulse rate are recorded every 2–4 hours, or more frequently if an epidural is sited. The midwife normally performs vaginal examinations every 4 hours.

In early labour, providing the admission CTG is normal and there is no meconium in the amniotic fluid (meconium is the intestinal content of the fetus), the mother would be encouraged to mobilize and intermittent CTG might be performed. As delivery becomes imminent, she would normally return to the delivery bed and lie semi-inclined, tilted slightly to the left (to avoid aorta-caval compression). Occasionally, delivery in other positions, such as on all fours or standing is requested. These requests can usually be accommodated providing the midwife feels sufficiently experienced to deal with the situation and if fetal and maternal condition remain satisfactory.

Admission assessment

History

The history of previous births and the size of previous babies are crucial. The uneventful birth of normal or large babies previously is encouraging. Nulliparity provides no such proof of delivery ability. A previous Caesarean Section is an adverse feature especially if it was performed because of a mechanical problem. Enquiry should be made about:
- fetal movements;
- abnormal vaginal discharge or bleeding;
- whether the membranes are ruptured and if so, the colour and amount of amniotic fluid lost.

General examination

An observation of maternal height and weight is important. The midwife will already have recorded the temperature, pulse and blood pressure.

Abdominal examination

After the initial inspection for scars indicating previous surgery, it is important to determine the position of the fetus and presenting part. An attempt to estimate the size of the fetus should be made. A vertex presentation is optimal for successful delivery as it indicates a well-flexed head but this may be difficult to determine especially if the mother is obese. It is crucially important however to determine whether it is a cephalic or breech presentation. If it is cephalic the degree of engagement must be determined in fifths palpable. A head that remains high and unengaged is a poor prognostic sign for successful delivery. If there is any doubt as to the presentation or if the head is high (five-fifths palpable), an ultrasound scan will determine the presenting part or the reason for the high head (e.g. OP position, deflexed head, placenta praevia, fibroid, etc.) Abdominal examination includes an assessment of the contractions: this takes time (at least 10 minutes) and is done by the midwife or the medical student.

Vaginal examination

A full explanation of the purpose and technique of vaginal examination is given to the woman and her consent is obtained. The vaginal introitus is initially examined and the consistency of the soft tissues assessed. The index and middle fingers are then passed to the top of the vagina and the cervix. The cervix is examined for dilatation, effacement and application to the presenting part. The dilatation is estimated digitally in centimetres. When no cervix can be felt this means the cervix is fully dilated (10 cm) and the presenting part can descend for delivery to occur. Effacement of the cervix is the shortening of cervical length. The cervix at 36 weeks is about 3 cm long. It then gradually shortens but in early labour may still be uneffaced. At about 3 cm of dilatation the cervix should be fully effaced and then thinning. The mechanism of this and subsequent dilatation may depend on tight application of the presenting part to the cervix with a contraction. This should be observed on examination. Providing the cervix is at least 3 cm dilated, the position and station of the presenting part can now be determined. In a normal labour, the vertex will be presenting and the position can be determined by locating the occiput. The occiput is identified by feeling for the triangular posterior fontanelle with three sutures running into it. Failure to feel the posterior fontanelle may be because the head is deflexed, the occiput is posterior or because there is so much caput that the suture cannot be felt. All of these indicate the possibility of a prolonged labour. Normally the occiput will be transverse (OT position) or anterior (OA). Relating the lowest part of the head to the ischial spines will give an estimation of the station. If the station is 1 cm above the spines or higher, then the head is probably not engaged although this should always be taken together with assessment of fifths palpable by abdominal palpation. If the head is at or below the ischial spines (0 to +1 or more) and the occiput is anterior (OA), the outlook is favourable for vaginal delivery. The condition of the membranes should also be noted. If they have ruptured, the colour and amount of fluid draining should be noted. Copious amounts of clear fluid is a good prognostic feature; scanty, heavily blood- or meconium-stained fluid may herald fetal distress.

Admission management

A simple system for triaging further care of the woman following admission to either midwife or medical supervision is shown as a flow chart (Fig. 9.17).

Fetal assessment in labour

After a woman is admitted to the labour ward a review of her history and examination should be made for risk factors. There are many conditions such as diabetes, hypertension, intrauterine growth restriction, previous poor outcome, bleeding during pregnancy, etc., which are markers of risk. Examination may reveal factors that indicate risk, in particular: breech presentation, small for dates, large baby, twins, etc. A review of the clinical scenario is essential.

In many hospitals an admission CTG will be recommended. When the history, examination and the admission CTG are found to be reassuring then the woman can mobilize for the next few hours. In this time intermittent auscultation of the fetal heart is undertaken with a fetal stethoscope. This can be at intervals of 15–30 minutes. Should any abnormality be heard then further electronic monitoring is undertaken to elucidate the situation. The appearance of meconium staining of the amniotic fluid is an important sign. In most cases it is old dilute meconium passed physiologically because of maturity but in other occasions it can indicate the fetus becoming compromised. The appearance of meconium is an indication for electronic fetal monitoring.

Information about fetal condition comes from clinical and electronic assessment. The evolution of the process is important. The healthy human fetus is well able to withstand the stresses of labour: head compression, umbilical cord compression and reduced placental blood flow. It responds to stress but on occasion may become distressed. Fetal distress should not be the description of a CTG but a more comprehensive analysis of the overall situation. The use of electronic fetal monitors, only introduced in the 1970s, has been controversial and the reader is referred to further reading for more detail. Education and training is crucial in the proper use of all

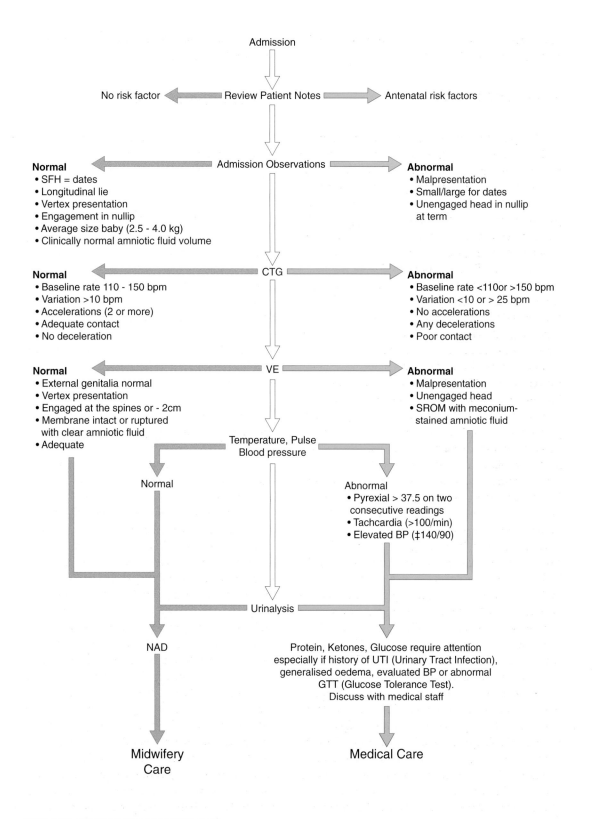

Figure 9.17 Admission management flow chart.

equipment. Unfortunately these devices were introduced before their understanding was fully developed. They can be used with adjunctive tests such as fetal scalp pH measurement. There is little doubt that babies' lives have been saved by the use of electronic fetal monitors but they have contributed to the rise in the Caesarean Section rate. This remains a challenge.

The fetus is assessed in labour for any evidence of growth restriction. The colour, consistency and amount of amniotic fluid are also used to assess the fetus. This is the most important reason why some would advise an early ARM in labour. All high-risk fetuses are monitored electronically using external monitoring providing the quality of recording is adequate. Intrapartum risk factors include oligohydramnios, meconium, labour of more than eight hours, the use of epidurals and oxytocin, and induced labours.

The CTG records the fetal heart rate on a paper strip. This is carried out either by an external abdominal transducer or a fetal scalp attachment inserted through the vagina. The uterine contractions are also recorded on the same strip of paper by either external or internal monitoring. Interpretation requires training. The normal and common abnormal features are described below.

There are four components to interpreting any CTG (Fig. 9.18).

1. Baseline rate: this is the average fetal heart rate in-between accelerations and decelerations. The normal value is 110–150 bpm.
2. Baseline variability: this is the variation in the baseline rate over one minute, excluding accelerations and decelerations. The normal value is 10–25 bpm.
3. Accelerations (reactivity): the presence or absence of accelerations. These are increases in the fetal heart rate from the baseline. Accelerations must have an amplitude of >15 bpm (be greater than baseline variability) for at least 15 seconds to be counted as such. The normal value is at least two accelerations per 15 minutes.
4. Decelerations: these are slowing of the fetal heart rate from the baseline. They are significant when they are at least 15 bpm less than the baseline for at least 15 seconds. Each deceleration should be described in terms of the amplitude (the difference between the baseline rate and the lowest fetal heart rate in beats per minute), duration (the length of the deceleration in seconds), shape

(whether the deceleration is v- or u-shaped) and lag time of the deceleration in relation to the peak of the contraction. Decelerations which are u-shaped and whose lag time is relatively long (late deceleration) are more significant. Decelerations occurring with a contraction and with a short lag time (early decelerations), and v-shaped are less significant and occasionally indicate quick progress.

The partogram

The introduction of a graphic record of labour in the form of a partogram has been an important development. This record allows an instant visual assessment of the rate of cervical dilatation against an expected norm, according to the parity of the woman, so that active management can be speedily instituted if progress is slow. Other key observations are entered onto the chart including the frequency and strength of contractions, the descent of the head in fifths palpable, the amount and colour of the amniotic fluid

Ultrasound scan on the labour ward

Most labour wards will now have an inexpensive portable ultrasound machine for bedside diagnosis. The principal use will be:

- confirmation of fetal viability if the fetal heart is difficult to auscultate;
- estimation of fetal size if the fetus is thought to be large or small for gestational age;
- determination of presenting part when palpation is difficult (for example of the second twin);
- position of fetal head when high in early labour;
- location of placental edge if there is brisk bleeding in early labour to exclude placenta praevia;
- investigation of sudden abdominal pain and/or bleeding to exclude intraperitoneal bleeding;
- determination of the amount of amniotic fluid, i.e. AFI, if there is suspected rupture of membranes;
- measurement of the length of the cervix when there are preterm contractions (if the cervix is >3 cm, labour rarely progresses);
- to confirm position of curettes/sponge forceps and retained tissue when performing surgical removal of products of conception or manual removal of placenta

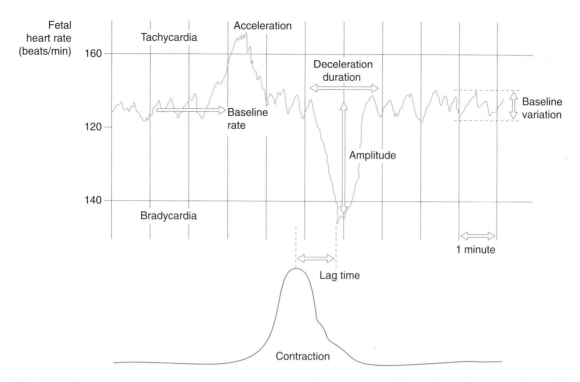

Figure 9.18 The components of a typical CTG.

The management of normal labour

The first stage

The first stage of labour is timed from the diagnosis of onset of labour to full dilatation of the cervix. The key principles of management are as follows.
1. Provision of continuity of care and emotional support to the mother.
2. Observation of the progress of labour with timely intervention if it becomes abnormal.
3. Monitoring of fetal wellbeing.
4. Adequate and appropriate pain relief consistent with the woman's wishes.
5. Adequate hydration to prevent ketosis.

Dilatation of the cervix occurs in two phases. The latent phase begins with the onset of labour and ends when the cervix is 3 cm dilated. This phase is variable

draining and basic observations of maternal wellbeing, such as blood pressure, pulse rate and temperature (Fig. 9.1).

in duration depending on the effacement of the cervix at the onset of labour and could be the longest phase if the Bishop score is initially low. The active phase occurs from 3 cm to full dilatation and the rate of cervical dilatation occurs normally at approximately 1 cm per hour in a primigravida and 2 cm per hour in a multigravida.

During the first stage, the membranes may be intact, have been ruptured artificially (ARM) or ruptured spontaneously. Generally speaking, if the membranes are intact, it is not necessary to rupture them if the progress of labour is satisfactory.

A woman in the first stage of labour should undergo intermittent monitoring of both her condition (BP, pulse rate, temperature) and that of her fetus by CTG. This is as long as labour is progressing normally. If labour is abnormal (see later) continuous CTG monitoring, antacid administration to the mother, epidural and urinary catheter insertion may be required.

In a normal first stage of labour, the woman should be encouraged to mobilize and may eat a light diet. The midwife would normally perform vaginal examinations every four hours, and the progress of the labour is plotted on a partogram. If an epidural is sited, an indwelling catheter should be positioned or the bladder emptied every few hours by an 'in and out' catheter.

Second stage

If the labour has been normal, the first sign of the second phase of the second stage is an urge to push by the mother. Full dilatation of the cervix should be confirmed by a vaginal examination if the head is not visible. The woman will get an expulsive reflex with each contraction, and will generally take a deep breath, hold it, and strain down. The pushing needs to be organized so that it is effective. Early in the second stage it does not matter what position the woman adopts, but if she is well propped up with her head upright and her hands behind her knees she will be in a comfortable position to push effectively with some assistance from gravity. Alternatively pushing can be quite effective in the left lateral position, which has the advantage of removing the weight of the uterus from the inferior vena cava and aorta. There may be requests by women to deliver in different positions, or in water. There are differences of opinion about this. In general, as long as mother and baby are well, and there is good progress in labour, then the outcome will be good, but the possible risks or disadvantages should be explained to the mother.

Descent and delivery of the head
The progress of the descent of the head can be judged by watching the perineum. At first there is a slight general bulge as the woman strains. When the head stretches the perineum, the anus will begin to open, and soon after this the baby's head will be seen at the vulva at the height of each contraction. Between contractions the elastic tone of the perineal muscles will push the head back into the pelvic cavity. The perineal body and vulval outlet will become more and more stretched until eventually the head is low enough to pass forwards under the subpubic arch. When the head no longer recedes between contractions (crowning) this indicates that it has passed through the pelvic floor, and delivery is imminent. If delivery of the baby is left entirely to nature, laceration of the perineum often occurs during the birth. Therefore, at this stage the midwife must control the head to prevent its being born suddenly, and it must be flexed until the largest diameter has passed the vulval outlet. Once the head has crowned, the woman should be discouraged from bearing down by telling her to take rapid shallow breaths. The head may now be delivered carefully by pressure through the perineum onto the forehead by means of a finger and thumb placed one each side of the anus, pushing the head forward slowly before it is allowed to extend and complete its delivery, and controlling the rate of escape with the other hand.

If extension of the head begins before the biparietal diameter has passed through the vulval orifice, a larger diameter than the suboccipital-frontal diameter will distend the vulva and a tear may result, unless an episiotomy is performed. Even if the head has crowned gradually, perineal rupture may occur if the head is allowed to expel suddenly and rapidly.

Delivery of the shoulders and rest of the body
Once the fetal head is born, a check is made to see whether the cord is wound tightly around the neck, thereby making delivery of the body difficult. If this is the case, the cord may need to be clamped and divided before delivery of the rest of the body. If there is any meconium staining of the amniotic fluid, naso-pharyngeal suction should be performed to prevent meconium aspiration. With the next contraction, there is external rotation of the head and the shoulders can be delivered. To aid delivery of the shoulders, the head should be pulled gently downwards and forwards until the anterior shoulder appears beneath the pubis. The head is then lifted gradually until the posterior shoulder appears over the perineum and the baby is then swept upwards to deliver the body and legs. If the infant is large and traction is necessary to deliver the body, it should be applied to the shoulders only, and not to the head. Shoulder dystocia (difficulty in delivering the shoulders) is discussed in Chapter 19.

Immediate care of the neonate

After the infant is born, it lies between the mother's legs and usually takes its first breath within seconds. There is no need for immediate clamping of the cord, as about 80 mL of blood will be transferred from the placenta to the baby before cord pulsations cease. The baby's head should be kept dependent to allow mucus in the respiratory tract to drain and oropharyngeal suction should be applied if necessary. After clamping the cord, the baby should have a one-minute APGAR (see Chapter 22) score assessed and then be placed on the mother's abdomen for cuddling and suckling. This will help bonding and the release of oxytocin will encourage uterine contractions. Before being taken from the delivery room, the first dose of vitamin K should be given (see Chapter 22) and the infant should have a general examination for abnormalities and a wrist label attached for identification.

Third stage

This is timed from the delivery of the baby to the expulsion of the placenta and membranes. This normally takes between 5 and 10 minutes. If longer than 30 minutes, it should be regarded as prolonged.

Separation of the placenta occurs because of the reduction of volume of the uterus due to uterine contraction and the retraction (shortening) of the lattice-like arrangement of the myometrial muscle fibres (see Chapter 5). A cleavage plane develops within the decidua basalis and the separated placenta lies free in the lower segment of the uterine cavity. Signs of separation are:
- lengthening of the cord protruding from the vulva;
- a small gush of blood from the placental bed which normally stops quickly due to a retraction of the myometrial fibres;
- a rising of the uterine fundus to above the umbilicus (Fig. 9.19). The fundus becomes hard and globular compared to the broad, softer fundus prior to separation.

Traditionally, it was considered prudent to await signs of placental separation before expelling it by pressing down on the fundus. This process could, however, last for as long as 20 minutes and was associated with a 5 per cent risk of postpartum haemorrhage.

The modern management of the third stage is active and involves a procedure called controlled cord traction (Fig. 9.20). This technique is as follows:
1. Synthetic oxytocin 10iu or syntometrine (5iu oxytocin, 0.5 mg ergometrine) is given by intramuscular injection following delivery of the anterior shoulder. Syntometrine gives a more sustained contraction due to the ergometrine but should not be given if the woman is hypertensive. This injection will cause the uterus to contract soon after delivery of the baby.

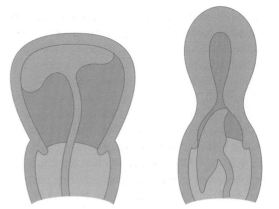

Figure 9.19 Signs of separation and descent of the placenta. After separation, the uterine upper segment rises up and feels more rounded.

2. After delivery of the baby, the attendant should place the left hand on the uterus to identify when a contraction has occurred. During this time, the vulva should be observed for any haemorrhage. The cord should be double clamped approximately 1–2 minutes after delivery of the baby. It is wise to place a clamp close to the vulva so that lengthening of the cord can be better identified.
3. When a contraction is felt, the left hand should be moved suprapubically and the fundus elevated with the palm facing towards the mother. At the same time, the right hand should grasp the cord and exert steady traction so that the placenta separates and is delivered gently, care being taken to peel off all the membranes, usually with a twisting motion.

In a small percentage of cases (approximately 2 per cent), the placenta will not be expelled by this

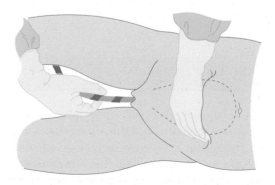

Figure 9.20 Delivering the placenta by controlled cord traction.

method. If no bleeding occurs, a further attempt at controlled cord traction should be made after 10 minutes. If this fails, then the placenta is 'retained' and will require manual removal under general or regional anaesthesia in the operating theatre.

Controlled cord traction is the favoured way of managing the third stage in most hospitals as it shortens the third stage and is associated with a significant reduction in postpartum haemorrhage. It is of crucial importance that controlled cord traction is not performed in the absence of a uterine contraction, otherwise uterine inversion may occur (see Chapter 19).

After completion of the third stage, the placenta should be inspected for missing cotyledons or a succenturiate lobe. If these are suspected, then manual removal of the placenta (possibly under ultrasound guidance) should be arranged, for in this situation the risk of postpartum haemorrhage is high.

Finally, the vulva of the mother should be inspected for any tears or lacerations. Minor tears do not require suturing, but tears extending into the perineal muscles (or, indeed, an episiotomy) will require careful repair (see Chapter 19).

🔧 Key Points

The key features of normal labour are:
- Spontaneous onset
- Single cephalic presentation
- 37–42 weeks gestation
- No artificial interventions
- Unassisted spontaneous vaginal delivery
- Less than 12 hours in nulliparous women, and less than eight hours in multiparous women
- Healthy mother and baby
- Retrospective diagnosis

ABNORMAL LABOUR

Labour becomes abnormal when there is poor progress (as evidenced by a delay in cervical dilatation), and/or the fetus shows signs of compromise. Similarly, by definition, if there is a malpresentation, a uterine scar or labour is induced then labour is not normal.

Poor progress in the first stage

Progress in labour is dependent on three variables.
1. The powers, i.e. uterine efficiency.
2. The passenger, i.e. the fetus with particular respect to its size, presentation and position.
3. The passages, i.e. the uterus, cervix and bony pelvis.

Abnormalities in one or more of these factors can slow the normal progress of labour.

Poor progress in the first stage is diagnosed when there is slow dilatation of the cervix. If the cervical dilatation in centimetres is two hours to the right of the partogram action line, then labour should be considered abnormal. If more than four hours, then action should be considered by the senior obstetrician. The slowing of cervical dilatation can occur in any of the two phases of the first stage (see types of partogram abnormalities). A prolonged latent phase is generally associated with a failure of cervical effacement, primary dysfunctional labour with inefficient uterine action and secondary arrest with cephalo-pelvic disproportion but these are only guidelines and a careful clinical assessment is required to more accurately determine the cause for delay.

1. Inefficient uterine action

This is the most common cause of poor progress in labour. It is more common at the extremes of reproductive age, in primigravidae and in women who are unusually anxious. It is also associated with uterine overdistension (e.g. twins) and minor degrees of cephalo-pelvic disproportion or malposition of the fetal head. Traditionally, inefficient uterine action was divided into hypotonic and hypertonic inertia, although it is only the latter that is of clinical concern. Hypotonic inertia implies that contractions are weak and infrequent and there is normal uterine tone between contractions. Treatment is by rupture of the membranes, and intravenous oxytocin if this is not effective. Hypertonic inertia implies that the contractions are irregular and that there is a high resting basal tone between contractions. In this circumstance, the uterine circulation does not return to normal between contractions and consequently fetal distress is more

Types of partogram abnormalities

Prolonged latent phase, primary dysfunctional labour and secondary arrest.

These terms are used by some obstetricians and all relate to poor progress in labour. They all share the problem of being difficult to define and therefore as a reason for poor progress their use is more of theoretical than practical benefit:

- Prolonged latent phase implies a failure of thinning of the lower segment, effacement and dilatation of the cervix despite several hours of painful contractions.
- Primary dysfunctional labour is most common in a first labour, and implies a slow progress during the active phase of labour. Usually associated with inefficient uterine contractions.
- Secondary arrest implies appropriate progress of labour in the initial phase, but arrest of cervical dilatation typically after 7 cm. Commonly associated with malposition and cephalo-pelvic disproportion.

likely. At one time, it was considered that oxytocin infusion would exacerbate the situation but it is now shown that epidural analgesia, together with intravenous oxytocin, helps to make uterine activity more coordinated and efficient.

2. Cephalo-pelvic disproportion (CPD)

This implies anatomical disproportion between the fetal head and maternal pelvis. This can be due to a large head, small pelvis or a combination of the two. Women of small stature (<1.60 m) with a large baby in their first pregnancy are likely candidates to develop this problem. Relative cephalo-pelvic disproportion can also occur with malposition of the fetal head together with deflexion such as occurs in the occipito-posterior position (this is categorized as either direct OP, right OP or left OP, Fig. 9.21). CPD is suspected in labour if:

- progress is slow or arrested despite efficient uterine contractions;
- the fetal head is not engaged;
- vaginal examination shows severe moulding and caput formation;
- the head is poorly applied to the cervix.

Oxytocin can be given carefully to a primigravida with mild-moderate cephalo-pelvic disproportion as long as fetal distress is not present.

3. Abnormalities of the passages

Both the bony pelvis and maternal soft tissues may cause delay in progress in labour. Severe pelvic contracture, sufficient to obstruct labour, is now rare in developed countries, although it can occur in women of very small stature or in association with previous fracture of the pelvis. Relative cephalo-pelvic disproportion described above is a more common cause of first stage delay. Abnormalities of the uterus and cervix can also delay labour. Unsuspected fibroids of the lower uterine segment can prevent descent of the fetal head. More commonly, delay can be caused by cervical dystocia. This is caused by severe scarring of the cervix from previous operations, such as cervical cautery, cone biopsy or loop excision. The scar tissue does not dilate like the collagen matrix found in the normal cervix. If scarring is severe, Caesarean Section should be performed, otherwise annular detachment of the cervix will occur. However, if the cervix becomes effaced, the tight fibrous ring of the external os can usually easily be stretched by the examining fingers and normal delivery achieved.

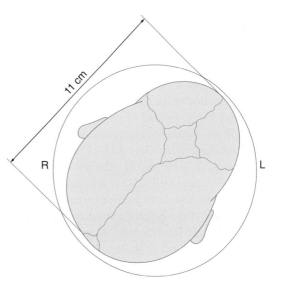

Figure 9.21 Vaginal palpation of the head in the right occipito-posterior position. The circle represents the pelvic cavity with a diameter of 12 cm. The head is poorly flexed, so that the anterior fontanelle is easily felt.

Delay in the second stage

The second stage of labour is the time of descent of the presenting part and lasts from full dilatation to delivery of the baby. It is important to be certain that the woman is fully dilated before delay in the second stage is diagnosed. In the first phase of the second stage, the woman has no urge to push, so vaginal examination is the only means of determining that she is fully dilated. Even when she has the urge to push, it is not certain that full dilatation has occurred, for in many labours where the fetus is in the persistent occipito-posterior position, the woman will have the urge to bear down before full dilatation.

The causes of second stage delay can again be classified as abnormalities of the powers, the passenger and the passages. Secondary uterine inertia is a common cause of second stage delay, and may be exacerbated by epidural analgesia. Having achieved full dilatation, the uterine contractions become weak and ineffectual and this is sometimes associated with maternal dehydration and ketosis. If no mechanical problem is anticipated, the treatment is with rehydration and intravenous oxytocin. Delay can also occur because of a persistent occipito-posterior position of the fetal head. In this situation, the head will either have to undergo a long rotation to occiput-anterior or be delivered in the occiputo-posterior position, i.e. face to pubes. Either way, the second stage is usually prolonged and if the contractions are not strong, oxytocin infusion may help to speed up the process. Delay in the second stage can also occur because of a narrow mid-pelvis (android pelvis), which prevents internal rotation of the fetal head. This results in the fetal head being arrested at the level of the ischial spines in the transverse position, a condition called deep transverse arrest (Fig. 9.22). Under these circumstances, delivery may be achieved by means of rotational forceps (Kjelland's) or ventouse extraction, but frequently Caesarean Section is required. When there is doubt as to whether vaginal delivery is achievable, the obstetrician may decide to perform a trial of forceps in the operating theatre. If any difficulty is encountered, then Caesarean Section is performed.

In the past, obstetricians regarded delivery of a baby, in an obstructed second stage, as a test of their prowess in the art of instrumental delivery. Nowadays, it is regarded as prudent not to attempt to

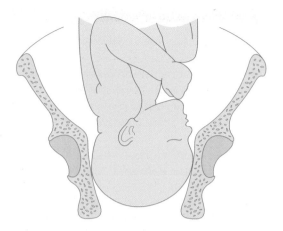

Figure 9.22 Deep transverse arrest of the head.

Risk factors for abnormal labour

- Small woman
- Big baby
- Malpresentation
- Malposition
- Early membrane rupture
- Soft tissue/pelvic malformation

deliver the baby if there is any chance of a difficult delivery, which may cause trauma to the baby's skull and brain, for example intracranial haemorrhage, torn falx cerebri or skull fractures.

The management of poor progress in labour

The active management of labour should lead to shorter labours and more unassisted deliveries. Historically this was introduced in the 1970s because of concerns about very long labours that resulted in damage to mother and baby, as still happens in less developed countries. The sun should never set twice on a woman in labour. It did set the style for a more proactive approach to anticipating problems in labour rather than obstetricians appearing as 'fire fighters' when the fire was already burning. On the other hand some women saw it as unwarranted medical interference. A balance between intervention and

Active management of labour

- One-to-one care
- Early detection of abnormal labour
- Pain relief
- Oxytocin augmentation of abnormal labour

allowing a normal physiological process to proceed has to be achieved.

In nulliparous women, the treatment of poor progress in the absence of any fetal problems is early ARM. If there continues to be poor progress in nulliparous women, an oxytocin infusion to augment labour is started.

The treatment of poor progress in labour with oxytocin should never be carried out if there is any suspicion of fetal distress. The nulliparous uterus should be considered immune to rupture; but the multiparous uterus prone to rupture. Oxytocin should therefore only be given to augment the multiparous uterus with care. Rupture of the multiparous uterus can take place in the absence of oxytocin if prolonged, obstructed labour is not treated appropriately by Caesarean Section

The assessment of uterine contractions is most commonly carried out by clinical examination and by using external uterine tocography. Intrauterine pressure catheters are rarely used, as they offer little advantage over external uterine contraction monitoring, providing the frequency and duration of contractions can be properly ascertained. Starting oxytocin may not always make the contractions more frequent, but instead more efficient. In multiparous women the assessment of contractions is more critical as the likelihood of inefficient uterine action is rare and therefore the requirement for oxytocin is much less. In addition, the risks of oxytocin in multiparous women (uterine rupture) are much greater.

When pain has been relieved then augmentation of the contractions with an oxytocin infusion (Syntocinon) is used. This intravenous infusion is started at a rate of 2 milli-units per minute and increased at intervals. It is important that the fetal heart is electronically monitored during this time because oxytocin increases the strength and frequency of contractions thereby also reducing oxygenation. This process is called augmentation of labour. The Syntocinon is then titrated to generate four to five contractions in 10 minutes. After two hours vaginal examination is undertaken to assess any change in the cervix. As well as dilatation and effacement, the degree of caput and moulding is assessed. A major degree of caput and moulding suggests that there is a mechanical obstruction to the labour process. If there have been strong contractions but little progress then the situation developing is suggestive of CPD. It may be appropriate to perform a Caesarean Section for CPD or to continue for a maximum of two more hours to see whether there is any improvement. To permit this there must be a normal fetal heart pattern. The other common pathology is that there is an occipito-posterior position with consequent deflexion of the fetal head and arrest of labour. If the second stage of labour has been reached then a skilled attempt at assisted vaginal delivery may be undertaken.

CPD exists when a well-conducted trial of labour fails to bring about rotation and descent of the baby in a woman with a suspect fetopelvic relationship. It is important that the doctor performing the Caesarean Section should document the position of the occiput, the head level and the presence of caput or moulding at the time of the delivery. This will assist an analysis to advise how a future pregnancy should be managed.

🔍 Key Points

- The use of oxytocin is relatively safe in nulliparous women. It is less safe in the multiparous woman because of the risk of uterine hyperstimulation in the face of obstruction, fetal distress and uterine rupture. Its use must always be carefully supervised
- Women with breech presentation or previous caesarean section require careful consideration. Oxytocin treatment can be appropriate but should be used with great caution

Women with a uterine scar

Some women will have a pre-existing uterine scar, usually because of a previous Caesarean Section. Nowadays, Caesarean Section scars are made on the lower segment because this part of the uterus is less active in the puerperium and, therefore, healing is better. Nevertheless, it is estimated that rupture occurs in approximately 1 in 200 women who labour with a pre-existing uterine scar. As about 20 per cent of all deliveries in developed countries are by Caesarean Section, the care of these women in a subsequent pregnancy has become a significant problem.

Rupture of the uterus is particularly likely to occur:
- late in the first stage of labour;
- with induced or accelerated labour;
- in association with a large baby.

Early signs of uterine rupture are severe lower abdominal pain, cessation of contractions, signs of fetal distress and maternal tachycardia. Late risks of uterine rupture are profound maternal shock and intrapartum death of the fetus.

In general it is not advisable for a woman to labour if she:
- has two or more previous Caesarean Section scars;
- has a high head at term;
- requires induction of labour.

When the agreed policy is for a woman to labour with a Caesarean Section scar, intense surveillance is required to identify early signs of uterine rupture. Some obstetricians believe it is not advisable for a woman to have epidural analgesia, in case this masks local signs of tenderness indicative of uterine rupture.

Some women will have scars on the uterus as a result of a previous myomectomy operation. In general, there is minimal danger of rupture of a myomectomy scar unless the uterine cavity has been extensively opened during the procedure. Normally, women will labour satisfactorily with a previous myomectomy scar, but many of these women are older, with perhaps a history of infertility, and Caesarean Section may be advisable for these reasons.

Fetal distress

Definition

The term fetal distress is poorly defined and is often a clinical assessment. In labour it should be thought of as hypoxia which if allowed to persist may result in fetal death or permanent fetal damage. About 10 per cent of cerebral palsy cases are associated with possible intrapartum causes.

Aetiology

The most common risks to the fetus during labour are hypoxia and trauma. Infection, meconium aspiration, and fetal blood loss are the other risks that may result in fetal death or permanent damage and may be associated with both hypoxia and trauma. Fetuses may already be compromised before labour, and when the uterine contractions start they reduce the placental blood flow resulting in hypoxia. Long labours and prolonged pushing in the second stage may all increase the chance of fetal distress.

Diagnosis of fetal distress

A normal CTG is reassuring (Fig. 9.23), but abnormal patterns are not confirmation of fetal distress. Whenever there is any CTG abnormality, especially decelerations, it is important to carry out an immediate vaginal examination. This is to exclude malpresentation, malposition, a cord prolapse and to assess whether the cervix is not fully dilated and the baby ready to be delivered.

Abnormal antenatal CTG patterns are described in greater detail in Chapter 7.

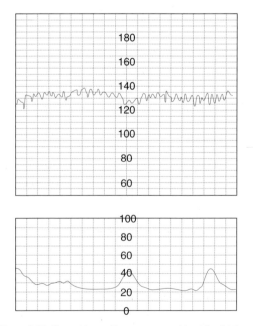

Figure 9.23 Normal trace. The upper record is of the fetal heart reat; the lower record shows uterine activity.

Ominous CTG signs suggestive of distress

- late or variable decelerations (Figs 9.24 and 9.25)
- baseline tachycardia (>150 bpm) with reduced baseline variability (Figs 9.26 and 9.27)
- loss of variability with a 'wandering' baseline
- fetal bradycardia <100 bpm for more than 3–6 minutes

Fetal distress may be confirmed by fetal scalp blood sampling. The indications when to carry out a fetal scalp sample are not specific; it should be thought of as a means of assessing the fetal condition not necessarily to confirm fetal distress. A normal fetal scalp sample result is often more helpful than an abnormal result. A normal fetal scalp sample will

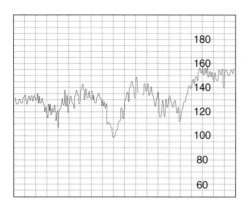
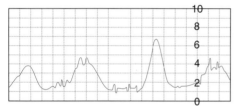

Figure 9.24 Fetal heart rate; late decelerations.

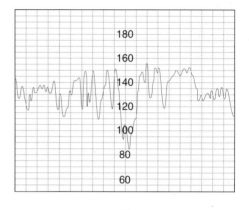
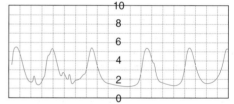

Figure 9.25 Fetal heart rate; variable decelerations.

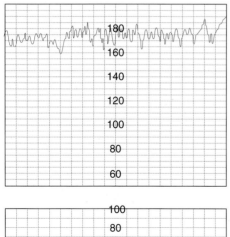
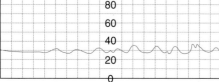

Figure 9.26 Fetal tachycardia.

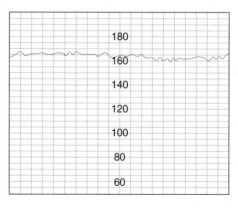
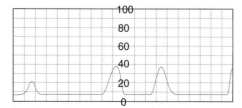

Figure 9.27 Loss of baseline variability in fetal heart rate.

allow you to carry on with the labour, or deliver by Caesarean Section, but with slightly less urgency and therefore hopefully more safely. It may mean the difference between a Caesarean Section using a spinal anaesthetic as opposed to a general anaesthetic.

While an abnormal CTG is the main indication for a fetal scalp sample other factors such as meconium, oligohydramnios, 42 weeks' gestation and suspected intrauterine growth restriction may often reduce the threshold for carrying out a fetal scalp sample for any particular CTG.

Fetal scalp blood sampling

- An amnioscope is inserted into the vagina and its distal end is placed at right angles on to the fetal head. The scalp is cleaned and a small cut is made using a blade with a guard. The resulting blood is collected into a microtube. The amount of blood required is approximately 25 microlitres.
- The normal pH would be above 7.25. A pH below 7.20 would be considered as confirmation of fetal distress. The base deficit can be useful in interpretation of the fetal scalp pH. One fetal scalp pH in labour is not as useful as several. A downward

trend in the fetal scalp pH values is significant and should be assessed together with how the labour is progressing.
- If an abnormal CTG persists in labour, then despite normal values, fetal scalp sampling should be repeated every 30–60 minutes.
- In cases of abruption, infection and fetal blood loss the value of fetal blood sampling is questionable and probably has little, if any, place.

Sequence of events in asphyxia

Fetal distress occurs when there is fetal hypoxaemia leading on to acidaemia. This occurs because the accumulation of acids, such as lactic acid (as a result of anaerobic glycolysis), overwhelms the buffering mechanism of fetal blood. Normally, aerobic glycolysis proceeds through the Krebs Cycle to provide 38 molecules of adenosine triphosphate (ATP) per molecule of glucose. Anaerobic glycolysis is less efficient, producing only 8 molecules of ATP. The net result of inefficient energy production and accumulating acidaemia will affect cardiac contractility and all organ

---

CASE HISTORY

Mrs T S

30 years old, married, Scandinavian

Gravida 3 Para 2: 2 SVDs 3.2 kg and 3.5 kg

Both born in good condition, second with forceps for prolonged second stage.

Height 153 cm

Spontaneous labour

At term

Fundo-symphysis height 43 cm

Arrest of cervical dilatation at 4 cm

Cephalic, left occipito transverse, 3/5 palpable

Poor contractions

Meconium-stained amniotic fluid

What risks do Mrs S and her baby face?

On account of the meconium-stained amniotic fluid the fetus faces the hazard of asphyxia.

She is only 153 cm tall, her last baby was born by forceps for a prolonged second stage and this baby is likely to be bigger than the last one: this is a biological fact. There is a risk of obstruction of labour, failure to progress in labour and a Caesarean Section.

What care should Mrs S receive?

She should receive reassurance and pain relief. Meconium is present and steps should be taken to ensure the fetus is not compromised. This is done by using an electronic fetal monitor. Normal baseline rate, normal baseline variability and accelerations are reassuring.

An experienced obstetric registrar should examine her to verify that there is a vertex presentation and ensure that there is no mechanical obstruction to delivery. The registrar should perform a clinical pelvimetry and be satisfied that no obstruction to delivery is present. Cautious augmentation of labour should be undertaken.

What subsequent assessment should be undertaken?

The situation should be reassessed two hours later by the obstetric registrar. If adequate contractions have been stimulated then a further vaginal assessment should be made. If good progress in labour has not been made in the presence of good contractions, especially with the appearance of caput and moulding, then serious consideration should be given to Caesarean Section.

Fetal distress: emergency management

- Place in left lateral position
- Stop oxytocin
- Give oxygen
- Give IV fluids

systems, eventually leading to fetal demise. Low glycogen levels at the onset of labour, such as occurs in intrauterine growth restriction, leads to rapid deterioration in fetal condition.

Management of fetal distress

The diagnosis of suspected fetal distress in labour occurs most commonly because of CTG abnormalities. A vaginal examination should be performed to exclude cord prolapse or rapid progress to full dilatation. Resuscitative measures should take place at the same time, especially if the CTG abnormalities follow the insertion, or top up, of an epidural. This would include ensuring that there is no aortocaval obstruction by placing the woman in the left lateral position and the administration of intravenous fluids.

Once the diagnosis of fetal distress has been confirmed one of two things must take place. Either the removal of the exacerbating factors which are causing the hypoxia and delivery within a short period of time or the removal of the exacerbating factors and, if the CTG improves, then repeating the fetal scalp sample. The progress in labour and the individual circumstances of the case will determine this. In cases where there are CTG abnormalities associated with antepartum haemorrhage in labour or infection, then the decision to deliver should be taken on clinical grounds.

Malpresentations

Breech presentation

The incidence of breech presentation falls as pregnancy advances, but about 3 per cent of all fetuses present by the breech at term. At least 30 per cent of babies presenting by the breech are now delivered by elective Caesarean Section, because of possible long-term damage, which can result from a vaginal birth. The antenatal management of breech presentation, and the factors that affect the decision on mode of delivery, is discussed in Chapter 14. The delivery of a baby presenting by the breech should be conducted under medical supervision. Principle complications of breech delivery are:

- Prolapse of the cord. This is common with a footling presentation and to a lesser extent with a flexed breech presentation.
- Difficulty in delivering the shoulders. This complication usually arises because the fetus is larger than expected. Damage can be caused to the brachial plexus of the fetus or to the liver.
- Difficulty in delivering the head. The main dangers here are of sudden uncontrolled delivery of the head, which can result in intracranial bleeding due to a tear of the tentorium or a delay in delivery of the head, resulting in prolonged compression of the umbilical cord and asphyxia. In the first circumstance, the fetus is frequently small and in the second, the fetus is probably larger than expected.

With these potential complications in mind, it is vitally important that a mother with a breech presentation should not be encouraged to labour if:

- the baby is a footling presentation;
- the predicted weight is less than 1.5 kg or greater than 3.5 kg, or if the pelvis is narrow in any dimension.

Management of a breech delivery

The conduct of labour is similar to that of a vertex presentation. In general, epidural analgesia is advised, because of the manipulations, which may be necessary to deliver the baby. Poor progress in labour may occur if the sacrum is posterior (in a similar way to occipito-posterior position in a vertex presentation) or if there is poor fit between a flexed breech and the lower segment. This also may result in early rupture of the membranes and if this occurs, a careful vaginal examination should be performed to detect cord prolapse. Poor progress may also be due to a bigger baby than is expected, so oxytocin in fusion is usually not advisable if cervical dilatation is slow. Caesarean section is the wisest course under these circumstances.

The second stage should always be confirmed by vaginal examination because the woman frequently has a desire to bear down before the cervix is fully dilated. When the breech is seen to be distending the perineum, the mother should be placed in a lithotomy position and urged to bear down with contractions. When the buttocks protrude from the vulva, an episiotomy should be performed to provide easy delivery of the body and give greater access to the obstetrician if any manipulations are necessary. Normally the legs are delivered easily, but occasionally extended legs will need to be flexed by pressure in the popliteal fossa before bringing them down.

With delivery of the umbilicus, a small loop of cord may be pulled down and cardiac pulsations felt. It there are no pulsations, delivery is expedited. The rest of the trunk is born by further descent together with the arms, which normally remain flexed in front of the body. The arms and shoulders are delivered by

hooking first the anterior and then the posterior arm from under the symphysis pubis. The operator should avoid interfering if at all possible, but occasionally the arms are extended and will require delivery by Loveset's manoeuvre (Fig. 9.28). This relies on the fact that the posterior shoulder will lie below the level of the pelvic brim when the anterior shoulder lies behind the symphysis pubis. When the baby's body is rotated through 180° (with the back facing upwards) with moderate downwards traction, the arm that was previously posterior is now anterior and either delivers spontaneously or can easily be hooked out by a finger. With delivery of the shoulders, the breech is allowed to hang for at least one minute, so that the weight of the baby will allow the head to flex as it enters the pelvis. When the head has entered the pelvis, it is generally accepted that the

Figure 9.28 Loveset's manoeuvre.

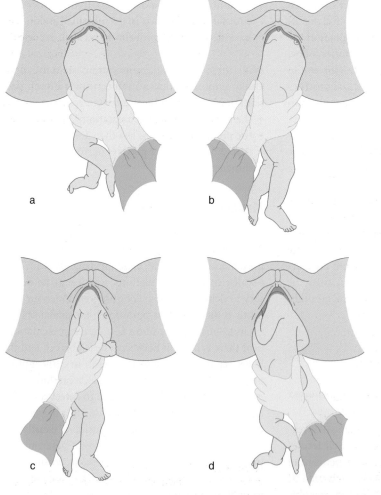

a

b

c

d

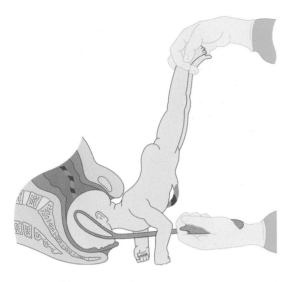

Figure 9.29 Delivery of the aftercoming head with forceps.

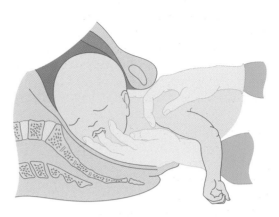

Figure 9.30 Jaw and shoulder traction applied to a fetus with the head at the level of the pelvic brim. Forceps could not be applied at this level.

application of short curved forceps to the head will allow it to be delivered in a steady controlled manner to avoid the complications outlined above (Fig. 9.29). Obstetricians should also learn to deliver the head by the Mauriceau–Smellie–Veit manoeuvre (Fig. 9.30), as occasionally, with rapid delivery of the body, obstetric forceps may not be available.

Face presentation

This malpresentation occurs in about 1:500 labours and is due to complete extension of the fetal head (mento-anterior, Fig. 9.31). In the majority of cases, the cause for the extension is unknown although it is frequently attributed to excessive tone of the extensor muscles of the fetal neck. Certainly, during the antenatal period, full extension of the fetal neck can frequently be identified by ultrasound, which may last for a few hours. Rarely, extension may be due to a fetal anomaly such as a thyroid tumour. The presenting diameter in a face presentation is a sub-mento-bregmatic, which measures 9.5cm, i.e. approximately the same as the suboccipito-bregmatic (vertex) presentation. Despite this, engagement of the fetal head is late and progress in labour is frequently slow, possibly because the facial bones do not mould. It is diagnosed in labour by palpating the nose, mouth and eyes on vaginal examination. If progress in labour is excellent, and the chin remains

mento-anterior then vaginal delivery is possible, the head being delivered by flexion (Fig. 9.32). If the chin is posterior (mento-posterior position) then delivery is impossible, as extension over the perineum cannot occur. In this circumstance, Caesarean Section is performed. Oxytocin should not be used, and if there is any concern over fetal condition, then Caesarean Section should be performed.

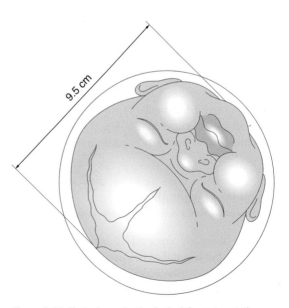

9.5 cm

Figure 9.31 Vaginal examination in the left mento-anterior position. The circle represents the pelvic cavity with a diameter of 12 cm.

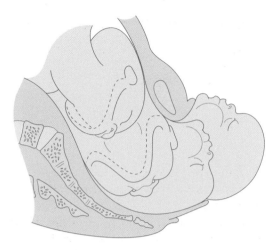

Figure 9.32 The mechanism of labour with a face presentation. The head descends with increasing extension. The chin reaches the pelvic floor and undergoes forward rotation. The head is born by flexion.

Brow presentation

This arises when there is less extreme extension of the fetal neck than is seen with a face presentation (Fig. 9.33). It can be considered a mid-way position between vertex and face. It is the rarest malpresentation, occurring in 1:2000 labours. The causes of this are similar to face presentation although some brow presentations will arise as a result of exaggerated extension associated with occipito-posterior position. The presenting diameter is mento-vertical (measuring 13.5 cm). This is incompatible with a vaginal delivery. It is diagnosed in labour by palpating the anterior fontanelle, supra-orbital ridges and nose on vaginal examination (Fig. 9.34). If this presentation persists, delivery must be achieved by Caesarean Section.

Shoulder presentation

This is frequently reported as occurring in 1:300 deliveries, but few of these women will go into labour. Shoulder presentation occurs as the result of a transverse or oblique lie of the fetus and the causes of this abnormality are discussed in Chapter 14. When the cause is placenta praevia, pelvic tumour or subseptate

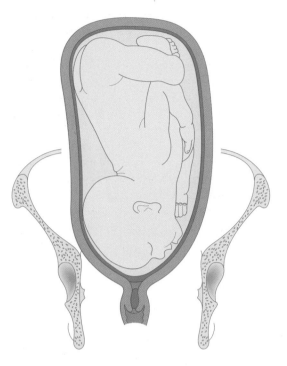

Figure 9.33 Brow presentation. The head is above the brim and not engaged. The mento-vertical diameter of the head is trying to engage in the transverse diameter at the brim.

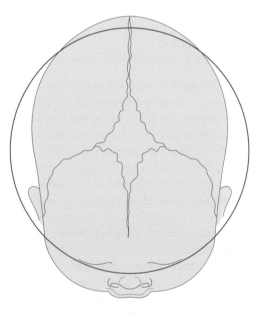

Figure 9.34 Vaginal examination with brow presentation. The circle represents the pelvic cavity with a diameter of 12 cm. The mento-vertical diameter of 13 cm is too large to permit engagement of the head.

uterus, then delivery is by Caesarean Section. Occasionally a woman will present in labour with a shoulder presentation as a result of an uncorrected unstable lie due to uterine laxity, which usually occurs in women of high parity. Normally, the antenatal problem of unstable lie will have been recognized and the woman admitted for observation (see Chapter 14). However, if the woman presents in labour with a shoulder presentation, no attempt should be made to perform external version even if the membranes are intact as the uterine tone may be high and the fetus could be damaged or the uterus ruptured by attempts at vaginal delivery. Early membrane rupture is common with shoulder presentation. If this occurs, vaginal examination should be immediately performed to exclude prolapse of the cord.

Multiple gestations

About 1:80 pregnancies at term are multifetal. High-order multiples such as triplets and quadruplets are now invariably delivered by Caesarean Section, because of the risks to the last fetus if vaginal delivery is attempted. Even in twin gestation, elective (i.e. planned) Caesarean Section is frequently performed in the fetal interest in the following circumstances:

- malpresentation of the first twin;
- second twin larger than the first;
- evidence of IUGR in one or both twins;
- monochorionic twins;
- history of fertility treatment.

There are four principal combinations of presentation (Fig. 9.35):

Cephalic/cephalic	60%
Cephalic/breech	20%
Breech/cephalic	10%
Breech/breech	10%

Essentially, the presentation or even the lie of the second twin is not of crucial importance but planned caeasarean section will usually be performed if the first twin presents by the breech and certainly if it is transverse.

The management of a twin gestation in labour where the first twin presents by the vertex is little different to that of a single fetus.

There is sometimes poor progress in labour, but this is usually of the hypotonic variety and responds well

to oxytocin. Epidural analgesia is an advantage in twin gestation so that delivery of the second twin can be assisted if necessary, or an emergency Caesarean Section can be performed speedily. Monitoring of two fetal heart rates is required; the first usually by means of a scalp electrode and the second by a Doppler transducer. Abnormalities in the heart rate of the second twin usually indicate the need for caearean section as fetal scalp blood sampling cannot be performed.

The management of the second stage in twins must be organized. The delivery should take place in theatre so that delivery of the second twin by Caesarean Section can take place if necessary. There should be adequate staff present including midwives, obstetricians, anaesthetists and neonatal paediatricians. After delivery of the first twin, it is essential not to give syntometrine as this will cause entrapment and asphyxia of the second twin. The cord is clamped in the usual

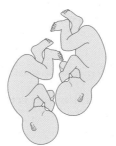

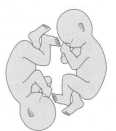

Cephalic/Cephalic (60%)   Cephalic/Breech (20%)

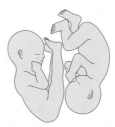

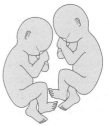

Breech/Cephalic (10%)   Breech/Breech (10%)

Figure 9.35 The four major representations of twin pregnancy.

way, but the contractions will cease after delivery of the first twin and the cervix to some extent reforms. The obstetrician should palpate the abdomen to determine the lie of the second twin; if transverse then external cephalic version (if desired, under ultrasound guidance) is easily performed. There is no need to turn the fetus if the baby is breech as the baby is usually not large, and the delivery is usually uncomplicated. If there is a delay of more than 15 minutes before contractions recommence, and providing the fetus is longitudinal, the membranes can be ruptured and if this does not kick start contractions, then oxytocin infusion may be commenced.

The risks to the second twin are significant in a twin birth due to increased incidence of prolapsed cord, abruption and constriction ring. Delay in delivery of the second twin of more than 30 minutes constitutes a significant risk and in these circumstances, the threshold for performing Caesarean Section should be low.

Additional points specific to the management of twin gestation in labour are found in Chapter 13.

Operative delivery

Operative delivery has been discussed in more detail (see Chapter 19).

New developments

These fall into two groups. Those that follow technological developments and those that revert to a more natural approach. In either event audit and guidelines are important so as to be aware of the outcomes. There is concern about a rising Caesarean Section rate and its consequences.

- Technological developments suggest that the use of an intrauterine probe to assess uterine contractions and head-to-cervix force directly may be of some value. More studies are required. This is, however, physically invasive.

- A return to a more natural approach with less intervention in early labour has been recommended by those that believe that a cascade of intervention may occur after an ill-considered action.
- Better methods are being sought for induction of labour. New prostaglandin analogues such as Misoprostol would ideally recreate a natural labour environment in terms of the right contractions: not too many or too strong to cause fetal asphyxia but enough to make labour progress to a normal birth.

Key Points

- Most labour is natural and uncomplicated
- Obstetricians and midwives must provide full emotional support and relieve pain
- Labour can be a hazardous journey for the baby
- Use oxytocics with care
- At least do no harm

Induction of labour

The incidence of induction varies, but in the UK it is of the order of 15–25 per cent. The reason why the incidence varies is because different definitions are used, the definitions are incorrectly applied or the data is simply poorly collected. In addition a small proportion of single cephalic pregnancies at greater than 37 weeks are delivered by Caesarean Section before either spontaneous labour or induction of labour. An induction of labour is performed when prolongation of hesitation is considered inadvisable for fetal and/or maternal wellbeing. Furthermore, it must be established that vaginal delivery should be achievable, or elective Caesarean Section should be performed. In the past 'social' induction was considered acceptable; this is no longer the case.

All women undergoing induction should be assessed vaginally for the degree of favourability by using the Bishop's score (Table 9.1). The greater the score the easier it should be to initiate labour. Of all the parameters in the Bishop's score the dilatation of the cervix and the station of the presenting part are the most important.

The methods of induction of labour after 37 weeks

most commonly include prostaglandin gel or pessaries and ARM with or without oxytocin. The methods used depend upon the Bishop's score and the indication for induction.

There is a continual search for better agents and methods to induce labour. At the present time, the antiprogestogens such as mifepristone perhaps combined with the prostaglandin misoprostol show promise.

There are circumstances where doctors believe that there is an indication to conclude a pregnancy in the maternal or fetal interest. Essentially this means that there are risk factors present that suggest it is more hazardous for the pregnancy to continue than it is for it to reach a conclusion. Emphasis on some of these factors varies from unit to unit. Hypertension is relatively common in late pregnancy and generally improves after delivery. However, there are varying degrees of hypertension. When it is severe, proteinuric and symptomatic then an indication for delivery is clear. This is only infrequently the case. There are, therefore, varying degrees of concern from place to place. Prolonged pregnancy generates varying degrees of anxiety. The definition of post-dates pregnancy is one that continues beyond 42 weeks' gestation. In general the risks to the fetus increase at this time; it may seem wise to deliver the baby. Social induction of labour is controversial. This is not induction done for maternal discomfort or pain but it is done for social, organizational reasons of the family. If an indication for delivery is 'soft' then the woman and her partner should be given full advice about the risks of the induction. These are determined essentially by the parity and the cervical condition. If the situation is favourable for vaginal birth, with higher parity and

Common indications for induction
• Post dates
• Small for gestational age/IUGR baby
• Pre-eclampsia
• Spontaneous or premature rupture of membranes
• Antepartum haemorrhage
• Intrauterine death
• Diabetes mellitus
• Congenital fetal abnormality requiring optimal timing for surgery

a favourable cervix, then 'soft' indications are more acceptable. In any circumstances induction of labour is abnormal labour and should be carefully supervised by doctors.

History

This depends entirely on the existing condition as an indication for induction of labour. It is useful to know if the woman is experiencing prelabour contractions and pressure on account of the head being in the pelvis. Has she already had a show? A history of normal fetal movements is reassuring.

Examination

General and abdominal examination should be as already outlined. Particular attention should be paid to the size of the baby and the degree of engagement of the head.

Table 9.1 – Modified Bishop score

Score	0	1	2	3
Dilatation of cervix (cm)	0	1 or 2	3 or 4	5 or more
Consistency of cervix	Firm	Medium	Soft	–
Length of cervical canal (cm)	>2	2–1	1–0.5	<0.5
Position of cervix	Posterior	Central	Anterior	–
Station of presenting part (cm above ischial spines)	3	2	1 or 0	Below

Vaginal examination

This is essentially to determine the favourability of the cervix. Bishop (1967) observed that as the time of spontaneous labour approached, the cervix changed. It became softer, shortened, came forward and started to dilate. This reflects the natural preparation for labour. If labour is induced before this process is nearly complete then the induction process must be correspondingly longer.

Treatment

Induction of labour was traditionally done by a surgical method, termed 'surgical induction of labour'. This involved performing an ARM. In the mid-1950s synthetic oxytocin became available and was then used as an intravenous adjunct after rupture of the membranes. In favourable cases this would succeed in inducing labour and often in effecting vaginal delivery. However in unfavourable cases it was not so successful and sometimes it was impossible to rupture the membranes. In the late 1960s prostaglandin by gel or tablet became available. Various routes have used various preparations but the optimal method seems to be Prostaglandin Gel, PGE 1 mg per vaginam. A slow-release prostaglandin preparation is currently under investigation.

The majority of inductions are now performed with prostaglandin gel. A CTG should be performed at the start of every induction. It should then be remembered that, in general, induction of labour is being performed because there is a perceived risk. The stimulation of contractions should be gentle and done with appropriate surveillance of the fetal heart using an electronic fetal monitor when the contractions become established. Prostaglandin gel is re-administered after six hours and an ARM performed when the cervix starts to open. This should not be done too soon after the prostaglandin administration because of the cumulative effect. Intravenous oxytocin can then be used as a further adjunct to maintain contractions until delivery, once the membranes have been ruptured.

Complications

Induction of labour may fail and result in Caesarean Section. Hyperstimulation of the uterus may result in

---

C A S E   H I S T O R Y

Mrs P W
33 years old
First pregnancy
42 weeks pregnancy
156 cm tall
Fundo-symphysis height 43 cm
Oligohydramnios
Cervix unfavourable

What risks do Mrs W and her baby face?
If the pregnancy continues then the combination of being 42 weeks pregnant and having reduced amniotic fluid places the fetus at risk of asphyxia. This may be due to umbilical cord compression or it may be due to an 'ageing' placenta. Tests of fetal wellbeing are not reassuring in these circumstances.

If labour is induced she faces a long labour, an increased chance of an assisted delivery and an increased chance of a Caesarean Section. She faces the associated physical and emotional complications of this.

What care should Mrs W receive?
She should be given full psychological support from the midwifery and medical team. She should have Prostaglandin Gel administered per vaginam up to three times at six-hourly intervals. Electronic fetal heart rate monitoring should be done when significant contractions supervene. ARM should be performed and an oxytocin infusion used when labour has become established but is not progressive. Pain relief should be offered usually in the form of epidural anaesthesia in these circumstances.

What ongoing care should she receive?
Attention should be paid to the need for continuity of care in spite of staff shift changes. A senior doctor should be involved and review the situation at intervals to determine if it is safe to continue or whether emergency Caesarean Section should be performed. If labour is prolonged and difficult then an H2-blocker and an anti-emetic should be given orally to reduce gastric acid secretion to reduce the risks in the event of an anaesthetic becoming necessary.

fetal asphyxia and Caesarean Section. Induction of labour in very adverse circumstances may lead to uterine rupture. After induction of labour there are more long labours and assisted vaginal deliveries. There are also more cases of postpartum haemorrhage due to the uterus failing to contract after delivery of the placenta.

Women and their partners should be advised of these risks before embarking on the procedure.

Pain relief in labour

The provision of analgesia in childbirth varies in different cultures. Some women and their carers believe that there is an advantage in avoiding analgesia at all cost. Likewise some women do not want to feel any pain at all in labour. Professionals who are knowledgeable about labour and are sympathetic to the labouring woman should give advice regarding pain relief in labour. Pain relief is to some extent dependent on the previous obstetric record of the woman, the course of labour and also the estimated length of labour. Just as one woman's labour can be made into an unhappy experience by unsolicited and unnecessary analgesia, pain relief that is inadequate, or offered too late can ruin another's experience. It should be remembered that after advice from professionals regarding analgesia, the final decision rests with the woman.

Non-pharmacological methods

Relaxation and breathing exercises may not relieve pain, but may perhaps make it easier for the woman to manage her pain. Prolonged hyperventilation can make the woman dizzy and alkalotic. Homeopathy, acupuncture and hypnosis are sometimes used, but their use has not been associated with a significant reduction in pain score or in the need for conventional methods of analgesia, and they are probably not widely applicable.

Transcutaneous electrical nerve stimulation (TENS) is more frequently used. It works on the principle of blocking pain fibres in the posterior ganglia by stimulation of small afferent fibres. It has not been shown to reduce pain scores or the need for other forms of analgesia. It does not have any adverse effects, but is often disappointing. It can be of use early in labour.

Relaxation in warm water during the first stage of labour often leads to a sense of wellbeing and allows women to cope with pain much better. Clearly, a woman in labour cannot use an opiate or have an epidural *in situ* whilst in water.

Pharmacological methods

Opiates such as pethidine are still used in most obstetric units. Generally women do not regard it as any better than TENS. It often does not reduce the level of pain, but women are less concerned about it. In conventional doses it may produce severe sedation as well as nausea and vomiting. Pethidine is unsuitable for use in severe pregnancy hypertension since its primary metabolite norpethidine has convulsant properties. It does have a prolonged effect on the newborn by occasionally causing respiratory depression, which may affect bonding and breastfeeding. Giving naloxone to the newborn can counteract any effects. Possibly the most serious adverse effect of pethidine and all the opiate agonists is delayed maternal gastric emptying. This represents a danger to mothers if they require general anaesthesia. In the presence of a full stomach, under general anaesthesia, regurgitation and pulmonary aspiration can occur unless skilled cricoid pressure is applied. Therefore ranitidine should be given to women in labour who opt for pethidine, and to all other women who are at risk of needing a Caesarean Section.

Diamorphine is a better analgesic than pethidine, but has potentially a greater respiratory depressant effect on the newborn. All opiates may be given by subcutaneous or intravenous infusion by PCA (patient-controlled analgesia). This allows the woman, by pressing a dispenser button, to determine the level of analgesia that she requires. This is the preferred method of administering systemic opiates.

Inhalational analgesia

Nitrous oxide (NO) in the form of Entonox (an equal mixture of NO and oxygen) is used on most labour wards. It has a quick onset, a short duration of effect, and is more effective than TENS or pethidine. Its adverse effects are light-headedness and nausea. It is not suitable for prolonged use from early labour because hyperventilation may result in hypocapnoea, dizziness, and ultimately tetany and fetal hypoxia. Its most suitable use is late in labour or while awaiting epidural analgesia.

Epidural analgesia

Epidural (extradural) analgesia is the most reliable means of providing effective analgesia in labour. Failure to provide an epidural is one of the most frequent causes of anxiety and disappointment among labouring women. The epidural service must be well organized to be effective, but unfortunately the resources are not always available at the present time to provide an efficient and universal epidural service.

Indications
The decision to advise women whether or not to use epidural analgesia in labour is a joint midwifery, obstetric and anaesthetic decision. The final decision in most cases rests with the woman unless there is a definite contraindication. The main contraindications are:

- coagulation disorders;
- local or systemic sepsis;
- hypovolaemia;
- a lack of trained staff.

The main indication is for effective pain relief. There are other maternal and fetal conditions where epidural analgesia would be advantageous in labour. These are, in particular:

- prolonged labour;
- multiple gestation;
- certain maternal medical conditions;
- where there is a high risk of operative intervention being necessary.

Advanced cervical dilatation on its own is not a contraindication to an epidural. It is more important to assess the rate of progress, the anticipated length of time to delivery and the type of delivery expected. Conversely a spontaneous multiparous labour at an early cervical dilatation may be expected to deliver within 30–60 minutes and therefore would not benefit from the epidural, but would still be at risk of all the complications of epidural. This should be explained to the mother and professional advice given. It is important, also, to warn the woman that she may lose sensation and movement in her legs.

Technique
An intravenous infusion needs to be set up prior to insertion of the epidural. This is to give intravenous access in case of a problem, and may also be used to give a preload of 500–1000 ml crystalloid in order to prevent hypotension.

The epidural catheter is normally inserted at the L2–L3, L3–L4 or L4–L5 interspace (Fig. 9.36). The catheter is aspirated to check for position and if no blood or cerebrospinal fluid is obtained a test dose is given to confirm the catheter position (Fig. 9.37). The epidural space contains blood vessels, nerve roots and fat. These spaces lie posterior to the dural sac and communicate with one another and with the

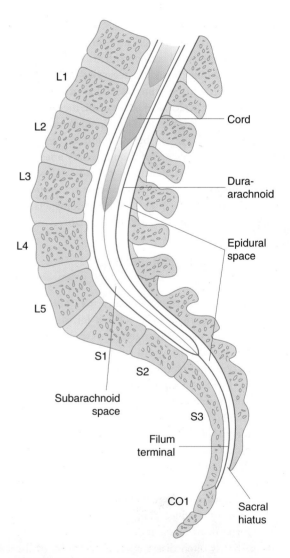

Figure 9.36 Sagittal section of the lumbo-sacral spinal cord.

intervertebral foramina via potential spaces between the dura and surrounding bones and ligaments. The injection of 2 ml of 0.5 per cent bupivacaine has little effect if injected into the epidural space, but a sub-arachnoid injection usually results in a sensory block, leg weakness and peripheral vasodilatation. If none of these signs are observed five minutes after injection of the test dose, then a loading dose can be administered.

After the loading dose is given, the mother should be kept in one or other lateral position, and her blood pressure should be measured every five minutes for 30 minutes. A fall in blood pressure should be treated with intravenous fluids and a change to the other lateral position. Vasoconstrictors such as ephedrine can be used if necessary. The mother should never lie supine, as aortocaval compression can reduce maternal cardiac output and so compromise placental perfusion. Opioids such as fentanyl may be used to supplement the epidural block.

Regional analgesia can be maintained throughout labour with either intermittent boluses or continuous infusions, or occasionally, a combination.

Spinal analgesia

A fine-gauge atraumatic spinal needle is passed through the epidural space, through the dura and into the subarachnoid space which contains the cerebrospinal fluid. A small volume of local anaesthetic is injected, after which the spinal needle is withdrawn. This may be used as the anaesthetic for Caesarean Sections.

Combined spinal–epidural analgesia

Combined spinal–epidural analgesia has gained in popularity recently. This technique has the advantage of producing a rapid onset of analgesia and, provided low-dose local anaesthetic is used, preserving motor function so that labouring women can be more mobile. It remains to be proven whether there are any advantages to this technique.

Complications of regional analgesia

Hypotension is the most common complication and is usually easily treated.

Accidental dural puncture during the search for the epidural space should occur in less than 1 per cent of cases.

Accidental total spinal anaesthesia causes severe hypotension, respiratory failure, unconsciousness and death if not recognized and treated immediately. The mother requires intubation, ventilation and circulatory support. Hypotension must be treated with intravenous fluids, vasopressors and left uterine displacement, though urgent delivery of the baby may be required to overcome aortocaval compression and so permit resuscitation.

Postdural puncture headache can occur in some women. The symptoms are treated initially by bedrest in a horizontal position. If the headache is severe or persistent, autologous epidural patching by an experienced anaesthetist is the treatment of choice. Neurological complications are rare, and are usually associated with other factors. Drug toxicity can occur with accidental placement of a catheter within a blood vessel. This is normally revealed by aspiration prior to injection.

Bladder dysfunction can occur if the bladder is allowed to overfill causing damage to the muscle. To avoid this, catheterization of the bladder should be carried out early or prophylactically if the woman has difficulty in passing urine.

Backache during and after pregnancy is not uncommon. The evidence whether epidural analgesia in

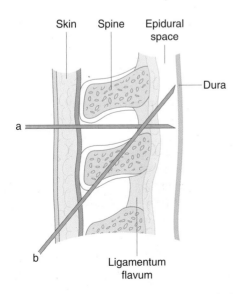

Figure 9.37 Needle positioning for an epidural anaesthetic. Midline (a) and paramedium (b) approaches.

labour causes backache is not clear, but if it does it may be related to poor postural positions during labour.

The effect of epidural analgesia on labour and the operative delivery rate is the most controversial question of all. The evidence is not clear, but it does seem that epidural analgesia can increase the operative delivery rate and the length of labour. However, this seems to be related to the way labour is managed, as there are institutions where a dramatic increase in the incidence of epidural analgesia has not affected either the length of labour or the operative delivery rate. It may, however, result in an increase in the need for oxytocin, especially in the second stage.

In certain clinical situations an epidural in the second stage of labour may assist a vaginal delivery by relaxing the woman and allowing time for the head to descend and rotate.

Labour ward audit

The continual audit of labour is important for quality assurance. Labour ward audit and the labour ward audit cycle are the processes involved in achieving quality assurance (Fig. 9.38).

The organization of labour ward audit needs involvement by all the different professionals on the labour ward. The labour events and outcomes to be measured need to be defined. They then need to be collected, distributed and eventually discussed by multidisciplinary meetings. Standards need to be set and continually assessed. Decisions regarding possible changes need to be made and, finally, these changes need to be implemented and audit continued. The audit of physical outcome needs to be complimented by the audit of women's satisfaction.

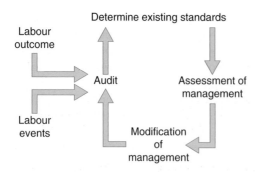

Figure 9.38 The Labour Ward Audit Cycle.

DEFINITIONS AND TERMS USED

Amniotic fluid

This is released from the amniotic sac around the baby when the membranes rupture spontaneously or when they are ruptured artificially. The amniotic fluid is measured in quantity, colour and consistency. There are six common situations.

It may be normal in quantity and clear in colour. There are three grades of meconium (Fig. 9.39).

- Grade 1 meconium is diluted by a large volume of amniotic fluid, which is lightly stained by the meconium.
- Grade 2 meconium is a reasonable amount of amniotic fluid with a heavy suspension of meconium.
- Grade 3 meconium is thick meconium, undiluted with amniotic fluid. If no amniotic fluid is obtained, then this is considered the same risk as Grade 3 meconium.

Lastly the amniotic fluid may be bloodstained.

Amniotomy

This is the artificial rupture of the membranes (ARM). It may be after spontaneous labour has been diagnosed (augmentation) or be part of the process of induction of labour.

Attitude

This refers to the relation of the different parts of the fetus to one another in terms of extension and flexion.

Caput

Caput succedaneum is oedema over the presenting part of the head, crossing the suture lines and is

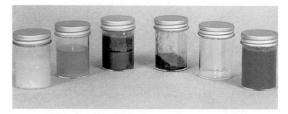

Figure 9.39 Samples of amniotic fluid: from left to right: clear/whitish amniotic fluid; slight meconium staining (grade 1); moderate meconium staining (grade 2); thick meconium (grade 3); no fluid obtained; bloodstained amniotic fluid.

quite common after delivery. It is associated with long labours.

Deep transverse arrest

A condition where normal internal rotation of the fetal head is arrested at the level of the ischial spines in the transverse position. It is usually associated with an android pelvis and is a cause of second stage delay.

Definition of labour

Labour is the onset of regular, painful uterine contractions associated with dilatation of the cervix and descent of the presenting part.

Dilatation of the cervix

The cervical os cannot usually begin to dilate until the process of effacement is complete. Effacement and dilatation should be thought of as consecutive events in the nulliparous woman, but may occur simultaneously especially in the multiparous woman. Dilatation is expressed in centimetres between 0 and 10.

Dystocia

A dystocic labour is an abnormal or difficult labour.

Effacement of the cervix

Effacement refers to the process of inclusion of the length of the cervix into the lower segment of the uterus. It begins at the internal os and proceeds downward to the external os, at which time effacement is complete. This is a normal process in the last few weeks of pregnancy and is a necessary preparation for the onset of spontaneous labour (Fig. 9.40).

Engagement

This is when the widest diameter of the presenting part has passed through the pelvic brim. Engagement is assessed by abdominal examination and expressed in 'fifths palpable'.

Induction and augmentation of labour

A distinction is drawn between the attempt to artificially initiate the process of labour (induction) and to assist or accelerate labour that had already begun normally (augmentation). The two commonest procedures used for this are amniotomy and oxytocin.

Latent phase

This is a term used by some to describe a phase that precedes the active phase of labour. Use of the terms 'latent' and 'active' suffer from poor definitions and are therefore not helpful in the practical management of labour.

Malposition

This refers to the relationship between the denominator and the pelvis that makes spontaneous delivery unfavourable. Examples include occipito-posterior in a vertex presentation; sacro-posterior with a breech presentation; mento-posterior with a face presentation.

Malpresentation

This is any presentation other than the vertex. The most common is breech. Others include shoulder, brow or face.

Moulding

Under normal conditions of labour the fetal skull may change shape to adapt to the maternal pelvis during its passage. The bones of the vault of the skull are compressible, and the sutures allow some movement between the individual bones. The parietal bones usually tend to slide over the frontal bones and the occipital bones. One parietal bone can slip under

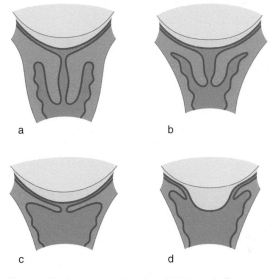

a   b

c   d

Figure 9.40 The process of cervical dilatation and effacement.

the edge of the other. Moderate moulding is not associated with any observable adverse effect on the underlying brain (Fig. 9.41). Severe moulding is a sign of cephalo-pelvic disproportion (CPD).

Oxytocin

This is a hormone produced naturally by the hypothalamus. It is uterotonic and the maternal serum levels rise throughout pregnancy. There are oxytocin receptors in the myometrium. Synthetic oxytocin can be given intravenously in labour. It can either be given to augment labour or to induce labour. Oxytocin infusions for augmenting and inducing labour are usually started at a dose of 2 mu/minute and can be increased to a maximum of 32 mu/minute.

Partogram

A partogram is the key record of events in labour on a single sheet of paper. Its most important feature is a graphical plot of progress in labour. This is measured by cervical dilatation in cm against time in hours.

Perineal body

The perineal body is a fibromuscular body receiving the attachments of the posterior ends of the bulbocavernous muscles, the medial ends of the superficial

and deep transverse perineal muscles and the anterior fibres from the external anal sphincter of the anal triangle (Fig. 9.42a and b). It is always involved with a 2° perineal tear or incised by an episiotomy.

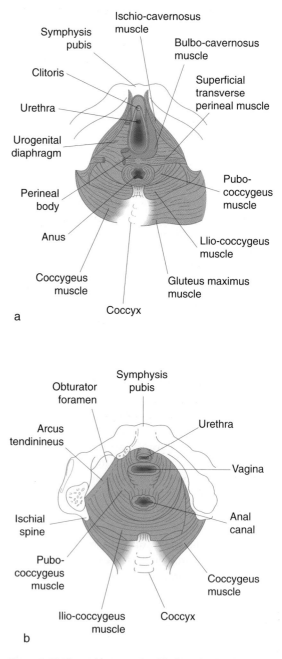

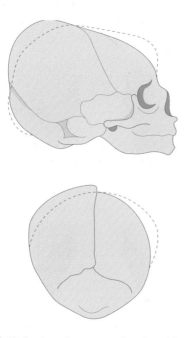

Figure 9.41 A schematic representation of moulding of the fetal skull.

Figure 9.42 The perineum, perineal body and pelvic floor from below showing superficial (a) and deeper (b) views. The pelvic floor muscles are made up of the levator ani which is in two portions; the pubo and ilio coccygeus.

Position

This describes the relationship which some selected part of the fetus (denominator) bears to a fixed part of the maternal pelvis. With a vertex presentation the denominator is the occiput, with a face presentation it is the chin (mentum) and with a breech presentation it is the sacrum. The occiput may be anterior or posterior, and right or left transverse. The occiput is sometimes described as being in-between these positions when a combination of left/right occipito-anterior/occipito-posterior is used.

Presenting part

This is the lowest part of the fetus palpable on vaginal examination and applied to the cervix. In a single cephalic pregnancy this may be vertex, face or brow depending on the attitude of the fetus. The normal presentation is the vertex, which indicates that the head is flexed. Any other presentation is known as a malpresentation.

Show

A show is a bloodstained plug of mucus passed from the cervix. In the presence of contractions it suggests, but is not conclusive of, a dynamic change in the condition of the cervix.

Station

This is the level of descent of the presenting part as assessed on vaginal examination. By convention when the lowest part of the presenting part has reached the level of the ischial spines the presenting part is at station 0. This occurs in most circumstances at the same time as engagement has taken place. The presenting part may be above or below the ischial spines and in this situation is by convention described by the number of centimetres it is either above or below the pelvis. The station is used as one of the five parameters making up the Bishop's score, which assesses the favourability of the cervix for induction.

Synclitism

This is the relationship of the sagittal suture to the plane of the inlet of the pelvis and to the sacrum posteriorly and the symphysis anteriorly when the fetal head is in the transverse position. There may be anterior asynclitism when the sagittal suture is closer to the symphysis and posterior asynclitism when it is closer to the sacrum. Severe asynclitism is associated with cephalo-pelvic disproportion.

Term

Term is defined as the period of gestation from 37 completed weeks (259 days) up to and including 41 completed weeks and 6 days (293 days).

Vertex

This is the area of the fetal skull bounded by the two parietal eminences and the anterior and posterior fontanelles. It is the part of the head that presents in normal labour.

References for further reading

O'Driscoll K, Meagher D, Boylan P. *Active Management of Labor, 3rd Edition*. Mosby, 1993.

Gibb D, Arulkumaran S. *Fetal Monitoring in Practice, 2nd Edition*. Oxford: Butterworth Heinemann, 1997.

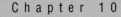
The puerperium

OVERVIEW

The puerperium refers to the six-week period following childbirth, when considerable adjustments occur before return to the pre-pregnant state. During this period of physiological change the mother is also vulnerable to psychological disturbances which may be aggravated by adverse social circumstances. Adequate understanding and support from her partner and family is crucial. Difficulty in coping with the newborn infant occurs more frequently with the first baby and vigilant surveillance is therefore necessary by the community midwife, general practitioner and health visitor. The degree of care provided by the health service varies from country to country. In the UK, a mother may be discharged from hospital within six hours of an uncomplicated birth, although she may request to stay longer. Irrespective of duration of hospital stay however, a midwife must visit her at least once daily for a minimum of ten days after delivery. Thereafter the health visitor takes on responsibility for continuing care particularly of the infant but the midwife may continue making home visits, if necessary, for up to four weeks after delivery. In the Netherlands a doctor or midwife provides care for the first five days but maternity aides are available to help mothers care for their older children and cope with household duties. In North America there is more dependence on private health care and very little organized care after discharge from hospital. There is therefore a lack of consensus as to what constitutes ideal postpartum care and protocols differ from one centre to the next.

Physiological changes

Uterine involution

Involution is the process by which the postpartum uterus, weighing about 1 kg, returns to its pre-pregnancy state of less than 100 g. Immediately after delivery the uterine fundus lies about 4 cm below the umbilicus or more accurately, 12 cm above the symphysis pubis. However within two weeks the uterus can no longer be palpable above the symphysis. Involution occurs by a process of autolysis whereby muscle cells diminish in size as a result of enzymatic digestion of cytoplasm. This has virtually no effect on the number of muscle cells and the excess protein produced from autolysis is absorbed into the blood stream and excreted in the urine. Involution appears to be accelerated by the release of oxytocin in women who are breastfeeding as the uterus is smaller than in those who are bottle-feeding. The

S | **Signs**

Causes of delayed involution
- Full bladder
- Loaded rectum
- Uterine infection
- Retained products of conception
- Fibroids
- Broad ligament haematoma

height of the uterine fundus is measured daily to ascertain the trend in involution.

A delay in involution in the absence of any other signs or symptoms, e.g. bleeding, is of no clinical significance.

Genital tract changes

Following delivery of the placenta, the lower segment of the uterus and cervix appear flabby and there may be small cervical lacerations. In the first few days the cervix can readily admit two fingers, but by the end of the 1st week it would become increasingly difficult to pass more than one finger and certainly by the end of the 2nd week the internal os would be closed. The external os however can remain open permanently giving a characteristic appearance to the parous cervix. In the first few days, the stretched vagina is smooth and oedematous but by the 3rd week rugae begin to reappear.

Lochia

Lochia is the bloodstained uterine discharge that is comprised of blood and necrotic decidua. Only the superficial layer of decidua becomes necrotic and is sloughed off. The basal layer adjacent to the myometrium is involved in the regeneration of new endometrium and this is complete by the 3rd week. During the first few days after delivery the lochia is red, which gradually changes to pink as the endometrium is formed and then ultimately becomes serous by the 2nd week. Persistent red lochia suggests delayed involution that is usually associated with infection or a retained piece of placental tissue. Offensive lochia, which may be accompanied by

pyrexia and a tender uterus, suggests infection and should be treated with a broad-spectrum antibiotic. Retained placental tissue is associated with increased red blood cell loss and clots and this may be suspected if the placenta and membranes were incomplete at delivery. (See postpartum haemorrhage, page 308.) Management includes use of antibiotics and evacuation of retained products under regional or general anaesthesia.

Puerperal disorders

Daily maternal observations include temperature, pulse, blood pressure, urinary function, bowel function, breast examination and feeding, assessment of uterine involution, appearance of lochia, perineal inspection, examination of legs and pelvic floor exercises. These observations should be made more frequently in high-risk women or if an abnormality has been detected, e.g. Caesarean Section, raised blood pressure, perineal infection, etc. In the UK it is traditional to check haemoglobin levels on day 3 unless otherwise indicated and most women who were particularly symptomatic would be transfused if their haemoglobin level was less than 8 g/dL. However, one study has shown that a haemoglobin level on day 7 is significantly higher and therefore may obviate the need for transfusions if it is more representative.

Perineal complications

Perineal discomfort is the single major problem for mothers and about 80 per cent complain of pain in the first three days after delivery, with a quarter continuing to suffer discomfort at day 10. Discomfort is greatest in women who sustain spontaneous tears or have an episiotomy, but especially following instrumental delivery. A number of non-pharmacological and pharmacological therapies have been used empirically with varying degrees of success. However, local cooling (with crushed ice, witch hazel or tap water) and topical anaesthetics such as 5 per cent lignocaine gel provide short-term symptomatic relief. Effective analgesia following perineal trauma can be achieved with paracetamol but a randomized study has shown that diclofenac suppositories (a non-steroidal anti-inflammatory agent) given at delivery followed by another 12 hours later are significantly more effective than placebo. Codeine derivatives are not preferable as they have a tendency to cause constipation.

Infections of the perineum are generally uncommon considering the risk of bacterial contamination during delivery, therefore when signs of infection (redness, pain, swelling and heat) occur, especially when associated with a temperature, it must be taken seriously. Swabs for microbiological culture must be taken from the infected perineum and broad-spectrum antibiotics (see below) should be commenced. If there is a collection of pus, drainage should be encouraged by removal of any skin sutures otherwise infection would spread with increasing morbidity and a poor anatomical result. Spontaneous opening of repaired perineal tears and episiotomies is usually the result of secondary infection. Surgical repair should never be attempted in the presence of infection. The wound should be irrigated twice daily and healing should be allowed to occur by secondary intention. If there is a large gaping wound secondary repair should only be performed when the infection has cleared, there is no cellulitis or exudate present and healthy granulation tissue can be seen.

Bladder function

Voiding difficulty and overdistension of the bladder are not uncommon after childbirth, especially if regional anaesthesia (epidural/spinal) has been used. It is now known that after epidural anaesthesia the bladder may take up to eight hours to regain normal sensation. During this time about 1 L of urine may be produced and therefore if urinary retention occurs, considerable damage may be inflicted on the detrusor muscle. Over-stretching of the detrusor muscle can dampen bladder sensation and make the bladder hypocontractile particularly with fibrous replacement of smooth muscle. In this situation overflow incontinence of small amounts of urine may erroneously be assumed as normal voiding. Fluid overloading prior to epidural analgesia, anti-diuretic effect of high concentrations of oxytocin during labour, increased postpartum diuresis, particularly in the presence of oedema and increased fluid intake by breastfeeding mothers all contribute to the increased urine production in the puerperium. Therefore an intake-output chart alone may not detect incomplete emptying of the bladder.

Women who have undergone a traumatic delivery such as, a difficult instrumental delivery, multiple/ extended lacerations or a vulvo-vaginal haematoma, may find it difficult to void because of pain or peri-urethral oedema. Other causes of pain, such as prolapsed haemorrhoids, anal fissures, abdominal wound haematoma or even stool impaction of the rectum may interfere with voiding. The midwife needs to be particularly vigilant after an epidural or spinal anaesthetic to avoid bladder distension. The distended bladder should either be palpable as a suprapubic cystic mass or it may displace the uterus laterally or upwards, thereby increasing the height of the uterine fundus. In order to minimise the risk of overdistension of the bladder in women undergoing a Caesarean Section under regional anaesthesia, a urinary catheter may be left in the bladder for the first 12 to 24 hours. The benefit of leaving a catheter *in situ* for about 12 hours after epidural insertion should be evaluated against a vigorously enforced postpartum voiding protocol and the small risk of urinary tract infection. However any woman who has not passed urine within four hours of delivery should be encouraged to do so before resorting to catheterization. In general, a clean catch specimen of urine should be sent for microscopy, culture and sensitivity and if the residual urine in the bladder is greater than 300 mL, a catheter should be left in to allow free drainage for 48 hours.

Although vaginal delivery is strongly implicated in the development of urinary stress incontinence, it rarely poses a problem in the early puerperium. Therefore any incontinence should be investigated to exclude a vesicovaginal, urethrovaginal or rarely an ureterovaginal fistula. Obstetric fistulae are rare in the UK but are a source of considerable morbidity in developing countries. Pressure necrosis of the bladder or urethra may occur following prolonged obstructed labour and incontinence usually occurs in the 2nd week when the slough separates. Small fistulae may close spontaneously after a few weeks of free bladder drainage; large fistulae will require surgical repair by a specialist.

Bowel function

Constipation is a common problem in the puerperium. This may be due to an interruption in the normal diet and possible dehydration during labour. Advice on adequate fluid intake and increase in fibre intake may be all that is necessary. However, constipation may also be the result of fear of evacuation due to pain from a sutured perineum, prolapsed haemorrhoids or anal fissures. Avoidance of constipation and straining is of utmost importance in women who have sustained a third or fourth degree tear. A large, hard bolus of stool in this situation would disrupt the repaired anal sphincter and cause anal incontinence. It is important to ensure that these women are prescribed lactulose and ispaghula husk (Fybogel, Regulan) or methylcellulose immediately after the repair, for a period of two weeks.

The high prevalence of anal incontinence and faecal urgency following childbirth has only recently been recognized. One prospective study using anal endosonography has identified evidence of occult anal sphincter trauma in one-third of primiparous women although only 13 per cent admitted to defaecatory symptoms by six weeks postpartum. Larger, retrospective short-term studies of parous women indicate a prevalence of between 6 and 10 per cent. Anal incontinence following primary repair of a third or fourth degree tear occurs in 20–50 per cent of women and anovaginal/rectovaginal fistulae occur in 2–4 per cent of these women (Fig. 10.1). It is therefore important to consider a fistula as a cause of anal incontinence in the postpartum period particularly if the woman complains of passing wind or stool per vaginam. Approximately 50 per cent of small anovaginal fistulae will close spontaneously over a period of six months but larger fistulae will require formal repair frequently with a covering colostomy.

Secondary postpartum haemorrhage (PPH)

This is defined as fresh bleeding from the genital tract between 24 hours and 6 weeks after delivery (see Chapter 20 for primary PPH). The most common time for secondary PPH is between days 7 and 14 and the cause is most commonly attributed to retained placental tissue. Associated features include crampy abdominal pain, uterus larger than appropriate, passage of bits of placental tissue or tissue within the cervix and signs of infection. The management of heavy bleeding includes an intravenous infusion, crossmatch blood, syntocinon, and an examination under anaesthesia and evacuation of the uterus. Antibiotics should be given if placental tissue is found even without evidence of overt infection. If blood loss is not excessive a pelvic ultrasound may be useful to exclude retained products. Other causes of secondary postpartum haemorrhage include endometritis, hormonal contraception, bleeding disorders, e.g. von Willebrand's disease and choriocarcinoma.

Genital haematoma

Genital haematomas usually occur following trauma, e.g. episiotomy or spontaneous tears. However, they may also occur without any evidence of external injury or bleeding and the mother presents with postpartum collapse. They are classified into

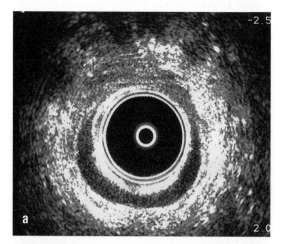
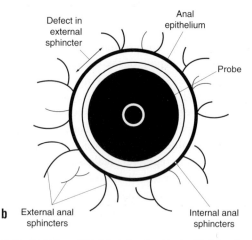

Figure 10.1 (a) Transanal ultrasound showing the anal mucosa, and anterior disruption of the internal anal sphincter (dark band) following a third degree tear at delivery. (b) Diagrammatic representation of part (a).

infralevator haematomas (vulval, perineal and low vaginal) and supralevator (broad ligament haematoma). Small infralevator haematomas (less than 5 cm) may be managed expectantly but, like larger haematomas, formal drainage will become necessary if the haematoma increases in size, there is worsening pain or an abscess develops. A supralevator haematoma can be difficult to recognize. Signs include shock, inappropriate pallor, pelvic pain, a mass in either iliac fossa or a boggy mass in the vaginal fornix displacing the uterus. These haematomas should be managed conservatively as it would be very difficult to identify the bleeding vessels following surgical exploration. If surgery becomes necessary the options include drainage and temporary packing, internal iliac artery ligation or hysterectomy.

Obstetric palsy

Obstetric palsy, or traumatic neuritis, is a condition where one or both lower limbs may develop signs of a motor and/or sensory neuropathy following delivery. Presenting features include sciatic pain, foot drop, parasthesia, hypoaesthesia and muscle wasting. The mechanism of injury is unknown and it was previously attributed to compression or stretching of the lumbosacral trunk as it crosses the sacroiliac joint during descent of the fetal head. It is now believed that herniation of lumbosacral discs (usually L4 or L5) can occur particularly in the exaggerated lithotomy position and during instrumental delivery. An orthopaedic opinion should be sought and management includes bedrest with a firm board beneath the mattress, analgesia and physiotherapy. Peroneal nerve palsy can occur when the nerve is compressed between the head of the fibula and the lithotomy pole resulting in unilateral foot drop. Until recently the development of urinary and faecal incontinence had been attributed largely to pudendal neuropathy following stretching of the pudendal nerve as it leaves Alcock's canal. However recent evidence indicates that structural damage to the sphincter muscle and supporting fascia is the major aetiological factor.

Symphysis pubis diastasis

Separation of the symphysis pubis can occur spontaneously in at least 1 in 800 vaginal deliveries.

Deliberate surgical separation of the pubis in labour (symphysiotomy) can be performed in cases of borderline cephalo-pelvic disproportion to increase the pelvic diameter. However, although it may be a safer option in underdeveloped countries (in preference to performing a Caesarean Section and risking a ruptured uterus in a subsequent pregnancy because of poor facilities for antenatal care) it is no longer practised in modern obstetrics. Spontaneous separation is usually noticed after delivery and has been associated with forceps delivery, rapid second stage of labour or severe abduction of the thighs during delivery. Common signs and symptoms include, symphyseal pain aggravated by weight-bearing and walking, a waddling gait, pubic tenderness and a palpable interpubic gap. Treatment includes bedrest, anti-inflammatory agents, physiotherapy and a pelvic corset to provide support and stability.

Thromboembolism

The risk of thromboembolic disease rises five-fold during pregnancy and the puerperium. The majority of deaths occurs in the puerperium and is more common after Caesarean Section. If deep vein thrombosis or pulmonary embolism is suspected, full anticoagulant therapy should be commenced and a bilateral venogram and/or lung scan should be carried out within 24 to 48 hours (see Chapter 20).

Puerperal pyrexia

Significant puerperal pyrexia is defined as a temperature of 38°C (100.4°F) or higher on any two of the first 10 days postpartum, exclusive of the first 24 hours (measured orally by a standard technique). A mildly elevated temperature is not uncommon in the first 24 hours but any pyrexia associated with tachycardia merits investigation. In about 80 per cent of women who develop a temperature in the first 24 hours following a vaginal delivery no obvious evidence of infection can be identified. The reverse holds true for women delivering by Caesarean Section when a wound infection should be considered. Common sites associated with puerperal pyrexia include chest, throat, breasts, urinary tract, pelvic organs, caesarean or perineal wounds and legs.

Chest complications

Chest complications are most likely to appear in the first 24 hours after delivery, particularly after general anaesthesia. Atelectasis may be associated with fever and can be prevented by early and regular chest physiotherapy. Aspiration pneumonia (Mendleson's syndrome) must be suspected if there is wheezing, dyspnoea, a spiking temperature and evidence of hypoxia.

Genital tract infection

Genital tract infection following delivery is referred to as puerperal sepsis and is synonymous with older descriptions of puerperal fever, milk fever and childbed fever. It was not realized until the mid-nineteenth century that the high maternal mortality and morbidity was due to poor hygiene of the birth attendants; the establishment of lying-in hospitals and overcrowding perpetuated the condition to epidemic proportions. Until 1937, puerperal sepsis was the major cause of maternal mortality. The discovery of sulphonamides in 1935 and the simultaneous reduction in the virulence of the haemolytic streptococcus, resulted in a dramatic fall in maternal mortality. Currently, the incidence of puerperal sepsis is approximately 3 per cent (range 1 to 8 per cent) and, excluding deaths after abortion, it accounts for 7 per cent of all direct maternal deaths (4 per million maternities).

Aetiology of genital tract infections

A mixed flora normally colonizes the vagina with low virulence. Puerperal infection is usually polymicrobial and involves contaminants from the bowel that colonize the perineum and lower genital tract. In one study of women with endometritis within 48 hours of delivery, two or more organisms were identified in more than 60 per cent of cases. The most frequently identified organisms were facultative Gram-positive cocci, particularly group B streptococcus, frequently co-existing with mycoplasma species. Following delivery, natural barriers to infection are temporarily removed and therefore organisms with a pathogenic potential (Table 10.1) can ascend from the lower genital tract into the uterine cavity. Placental separation exposes a large raw area equivalent to an open wound and retained products of conception and blood clots within the uterus can provide an excellent culture medium for infection. Furthermore, vaginal delivery is almost invariably associated with lacerations of the genital tract (uterus, cervix and vagina). Although these lacerations may not need surgical repair, they can become a focus for infection similar to iatrogenic wounds such as Caesarean Section and episiotomy.

Haemolytic streptococcus Lancefield Group A and *Staphylococcus aureus* are two exogenous organisms that can cause severe puerperal infection and have been associated with major epidemics and fatalities in the past. The infection usually originates from inpatients or birth attendants who may be asymptomatic carriers or who have an active infection. Transmission can occur by droplet infection, infected dust or by direct skin contact. The toxins produced by these organisms can result in a rapid deterioration into septicaemic shock and yet produce minimal local signs. With the advent of penicillin, serious infection is now rare although penicillin-resistant staphylococcus now poses a new threat.

Table 10.1 – Organisms commonly associated with puerperal genital infection

Aerobes
Gram-positive
Beta-haemolytic streptococcus, Groups A,B,D
Staphylococcus epidermis and aureus
Enterococci – Streptococcus faecalis
Gram-negative
Escherichia coli
Haemophilus influenzae
Klebsiella pneumonia
Pseudomonas aeruginosa
Proteus mirabilis
Gram-variable
Gardnerella vaginalis
Anaerobes
Peptococcus species
Peptostreptococcus sp.
Bacteroides – B. fragilis, B. bivius, B. disiens
Fusobacterium sp.
Miscellaneous
Chlamydia trachomatis
Mycoplasma hominis
Uroplasma urealyticum

👁 Signs of puerperal pelvic infection

- Pyrexia and tachycardia
- Uterus — boggy, tender and larger
- Infected wounds — Caesarean/perineal
- Peritonism
- Paralytic ileus
- Indurated adnexae (parametritis)
- Bogginess in pelvis (abscess)

S Symptoms of puerperal pelvic infection

- Malaise, headache, fever, rigors
- Abdominal discomfort, vomiting and diarrhoea
- Offensive lochia
- Secondary postpartum haemorrhage

Common risk factors for puerperal infecfion

- Antenatal intrauterine infection
- Caesarean Section
- Cervical cerclage for cervical incompetence
- Prolonged rupture of membranes
- Prolonged labour
- Multiple vaginal examinations
- Internal fetal monitoring
- Instrumental delivery
- Manual removal of the placenta
- Retained products of conception
- Non-obstetric, e.g. obesity, diabetes, HIV

Chlamydia trachomatis puerperal parametritis may develop in one-third of women who had pre-existing infection but presentation is usually delayed. Investigations for puerperal genital infections are shown in Table 10.2.

There are a number of factors that determine the clinical course and severity of the infection, namely the general health and resistance of the woman, the virulence of the offending organism, presence of haematoma or retained products of conception and timing of antibiotic therapy and associated risk factors. The common methods of spread of puerperal infection are outlined below.

1. An ascending infection from the lower genital tract or primary infection of the placental site may spread via the Fallopian tubes to the ovaries giving rise to a salpingo-oophoritis and pelvic peritonitis. This could progress to a generalized peritonitis and the development of pelvic abscesses.

2. Infection may also spread by contiguity directly into the myometrium and the parametrium giving rise to a metritis or parametritis, also referred to as pelvic cellulitis. Pelvic peritonitis and abscesses may also occur.

3. Infection may also spread to distant sites via lymphatics and blood vessels. Infection from the uterus can be carried by uterine vessels into the inferior vena cava via the iliac vessels or, directly, via the ovarian vessels. This could give rise to a septic thrombophlebitis, pulmonary infections or a generalized septicaemia and endotoxic shock.

In contrast to pelvic inflammatory disease unrelated to pregnancy, tubal involvement in puerperal sepsis is in the form of perisalpingitis, which rarely causes tubal occlusion and consequent infertility.

Table 10.2 – Investigations for puerperal genital infections

Investigations	Abnormalities
Full blood count	Anaemia, leucocytosis, thrombocytopaenia
Urea and electrolytes	Fluid and electrolyte imbalance
High vaginal swabs and blood culture	Infection screen
Pelvic ultrasound	Retained products, pelvic abscess
Clotting screen (haemorrhage or shock)	Disseminated intra-vascular coagulation
Arterial blood gas (shock)	Acidosis and hypoxia

Tubo-ovarian abscesses are also a rare complication of puerperal sepsis.

Mild to moderate infections can be treated with a broad-spectrum antibiotic, e.g. Co-amoxiclav, or a cephalosporin such as Cephalexin plus Metronidazole. Depending on severity, the first few doses should be given intravenously.

With severe infections, there is a release of inflammatory and vasoactive mediators in response to the endotoxins produced during bacteriolysis. The resultant local vasodilation causes circulatory embarrassment and hence poor tissue perfusion. This phenomenon is known as septicaemic/septic/endotoxic shock and delay in appropriate management could be fatal (see Obstetric Emergencies, Chapter 20).

Necrotizing fasciitis is a rare but frequently fatal infection of skin, fascia and muscle. It can originate in perineal tears, episiotomies and Caesarean Section wounds. Perineal infections can extend rapidly to involve the buttocks, thighs and lower abdominal wall. A variety of bacteria can be involved but anaerobes predominate and *Clostridium perfringens* is usually identified. In addition to general signs of infection there is extensive necrosis, crepitus and inflammation. In addition to measures taken in the management of septic shock, wide debridement of necrotic tissue under general anaesthesia is absolutely essential to avoid mortality. Split-thickness skin grafts may be necessary at a later date.

Prevention of puerperal sepsis

Increased awareness of principles in general hygiene, good surgical approach and use of aseptic techniques have contributed to the decline in severe puerperal sepsis. However the risk of sepsis is higher following Caesarean Section particularly when performed after the onset of labour. There is now overwhelming evidence that prophylactic antibiotics during emergency Caesarean Section reduce the risk of postoperative infection, namely wound infection, metritis, pelvic abscess, pelvic thrombophlebitis and septic shock. A single intra-operative dose of antibiotics (amoxiclav or cephalosporin plus metronidazole) should be given after clamping of the umbilical cord to avoid unnecessary exposure of the baby to antibiotics. The benefit of prophylaxis for elective Caesarean Sections would be of greater significance in units where the background infectious morbidity is high (Table 10.3).

The breasts

Anatomy

The breasts are largely made up of glandular, adipose and connective tissue (Fig. 10.2). They lie superficial to the pectoralis major, external oblique and serratus anterior muscles extending between the second and sixth rib from the sternum to the axilla. A pigmented area called the areola, which contains sebaceous glands, surrounds the nipple. During pregnancy the areola becomes darker and the sebaceous glands become prominent (Montgomery's tubercles). The breast comprises of 15 to 25 functional units arranged radially from the nipple and each unit is made up of a lactiferous duct, a mammary gland lobule and alveoli. The lactiferous ducts dilate to form a lactiferous sinus before converging to open in the nipple. Contractile myoepithelial cells surround the ducts as well as the alveoli.

Physiology

The human species is unique in that most of the breast development occurs at puberty and is therefore primed to produce milk within two weeks of hormonal stimulation. It is hypothesized that unlike

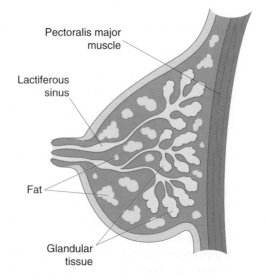

Figure 10.2 The breast during lactation.

Table 10.3 – Investigations for puerperal genital infections

Symptoms	Diagnosis	Special investigations	Management
Cough Purulent sputum Dyspnoea	Chest infection Pneumonia	Sputum M,C&S Chest X-ray	Physiotherapy Antibiotics
Sore throat Cervical lymphadenopathy	Tonsillitis	Throat swab	Antibiotics
Headaches Neck stiffness (epidural/spinal anaesthetic)	Meningitis	Lumbar puncture	Antibiotics
Dysuria Loin pain and tenderness	Pyelonephritis	Urine M,C&S	Antibiotics
$2°$ PPH Tender bulky uterus	Metritis Retained placental tissue	Pelvic ultrasound	Antibiotics Uterine evacuation
Pelvic/calf pain/tenderness Chest pain	Deep vein thrombosis Pulmonary embolism	Dopplers/venogram of legs Lung perfusion scan angiogram Chest X-ray and blood gases	Heparin
Painful engorged breasts	Mastitis Abscess	Milk M,C&S	Express milk Antibiotics Incision and drainage

animals, female breasts have an erotic role to attract the male to procreate. The control of mammary growth and development is not fully understood and many hormones may contribute to this process. In general, oestrogens stimulate proliferation of the lactiferous ducts (possibly with adrenal steroids and growth hormones) while progesterone is responsible for the development of the mammary lobules. During early pregnancy lactiferous ducts and alveoli proliferate, while in later pregnancy the alveoli hypertrophy in preparation of secretory activity. The lactogenic hormones, prolactin and human placental lactogen probably modulate these changes during pregnancy.

Colostrum

Colostrum is a yellowish fluid secreted by the breast that can be expressed as early as the 16th week of pregnancy but is replaced by milk during the second postpartum day. Colostrum has a high concentration of proteins but contains less sugar and fat than breast milk although it contains large fat globules. The proteins are mainly in the form of globulins, particularly Immunoglobulin (Ig) A, which plays an important role in protection against infection. Colostrum is also believed to have a laxative effect, which may help empty the baby's bowel of meconium.

Breast milk

The major constituents of breast milk are lactose, protein, fat and water (Table 10.4). The composition of breast milk however is not constant; early lactation differs from late lactation, one feed differs from the next and the composition can even change during a feed. Artificial infant formulas cannot therefore be identical to breast milk. Compared to cow's milk, breast milk provides slightly more energy, has less protein but more fat and lactose. The major protein fractions are lactalbumin, lactoglobulin and caseinogen. Lactalbumin is the major protein in breast milk whereas caseinogen forms 90 per cent of the protein in cow's milk. The mineral content is much higher in cow's milk, particularly sodium, and can therefore be dangerous if given to a baby who is dehydrated from gastroenteritis. In addition to Ig A, breast milk contains small amounts of Ig M and Ig G and other factors such as lactoferrin, macrophages, complement and lysozymes. Although breast milk contains a lower concentration of iron, its absorption is better than from cow's milk or iron-supplemented infant formula (>75 per cent, 30 per cent and 10 per cent respectively). The improved bioavailability may be related to lactoferrin, an iron-binding glycoprotein, which also inhibits bacterial growth. With the exception of vitamin K, all other vitamins are found in breast milk and therefore vitamin K is given to the baby to minimize the risk of haemorrhagic disease.

Prolactin

Prolactin is a long-chain polypeptide produced from the anterior pituitary and levels rise up to twenty-fold during pregnancy and lactation. Peak levels of prolactin are reached within 45 minutes of suckling but return to normal immediately after weaning and in non-breastfeeding mothers. The exact mechanism of action is not fully understood but prolactin appears to have a direct action on the secretory cells to synthesize milk proteins. Prolactin is essential for lactation and it is hypothesized that nipple stimulation prevents release of prolactin-inhibiting factor from the hypothalamus, thereby initiating the production of prolactin by the anterior pituitary. This theory is supported by the fact that lactation can be

Table 10.4 – Comparison between human and cows' milk

	Human breast milk	Cow's milk
Energy (kcal/mL)	75	66
Lactose (g/100mL)	6.8	4.9
Protein (g/100mL)	1.1	3.5
Fat (g/100mL)	4.5	3.7
Sodium (mmol/L)	7	22
Water (mL/100mL)	87.1	87.3

arrested with bromocryptine, a dopamine agonist, which inhibits prolactin. A similar phenomenon occurs following pituitary necrosis (Sheehan's syndrome) when prolactin production ceases.

Oxytocin

Once milk has been produced under the influence of prolactin it has to be delivered to the infant. The milk-ejection or let-down reflex is initiated by suckling which stimulates the pulsatile release of oxytocin from the posterior pituitary. Oxytocin contracts the myoepithelial cells surrounding the alveoli as well as the myoepithelial cells lying longitudinally along the lactiferous ducts thereby aiding expulsion of milk. Oxytocin release can also be stimulated by visual, olfactory or auditory stimuli, e.g. hearing the baby cry, but can be inhibited by stress. Oxytocin can also stimulate uterine contractions giving rise to the 'after pains' of childbirth.

Breastfeeding

Women who opt to breastfeed tend to decide before or very early in their pregnancy. This decision is usually based on previous experience, influence of family or friends, culture and custom. A new mum who is unprepared for breastfeeding may find it a frustrating task and turn to bottle-feeding. There is now evidence to suggest that antenatal classes and literature on breastfeeding given antenatally may be beneficial.

The most common reasons mothers give for abandoning breastfeeding are inadequate milk production or sore and cracked nipples. Both these problems can be overcome by correct positioning of the baby on the breast (Fig. 10.3). The mouth should be placed over the nipple and areola so that suction created within the baby's mouth draws the breast tissue into a teat which extends as far back as the junction of the soft and hard palate. The tongue applies peristaltic force to the underside of the teat against the support of the hard palate. In this way there should be no to and fro movement of the teat in and out of the baby's mouth thus minimizing friction. The mother should also be taught how to implement the rooting reflex. When the skin around the baby's mouth is touched the mouth begins to gape. At this point the mother should reposition the baby so the lower rim of the baby's mouth fits well below the nipple allowing a liberal mouthful of breast tissue. When the baby is properly attached, breastfeeding should be pain free. The use of creams and ointments for cracked nipples has not been shown to be beneficial and the use of a nipple shield merely reduces milk production.

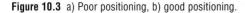

a Poor positioning

b Good positioning

Figure 10.3 a) Poor positioning, b) good positioning.

Although no study has identified the threshold of the critical time limit for successful breastfeeding, early suckling appears to be beneficial. However this should not be rushed and perhaps should be done initially under supervision when the mother is comfortable and in the privacy of the couple.

There is no scientific evidence to justify a rigid breastfeeding schedule. Babies should be fed on demand and left on the breast until feeding finishes spontaneously. An imposed time limit on feeding can have a deleterious effect on calorie intake.

Supplementary feeds of formula, glucose or water are often given to breastfed infants in the belief that the baby is still hungry or thirsty. However this is a misconception as this practice merely increases the risk of total abandonment of breastfeeding.

Test-weighing infants before and after a feed to establish the ideal quantity of milk intake is an archaic practice that should be abandoned as inappropriate action could prove hazardous.

There is evidence to suggest that dopamine receptor blockers, e.g. metoclopramide, sulpiride and domperidone, may be used to treat women who are temporarily unable to breastfeed. Sublingual or buccal oxytocin may also be used to augment lactation with good effect.

Non-breastfeeding mothers

There are various reasons as to why a woman may choose not to breastfeed ranging from personal choice to stillbirth. The United Nations has issued recommendations intended to discourage women infected with HIV from breastfeeding. In 1997, of the 600 000

🔑 Key Points

Advantages of breastfeeding

- Readily available at the right temperature and ideal nutritional value
- Cheaper than formula feed
- Associated with a reduction in:
  childhood infective illnesses, especially gastroenteritis
  fertility with amenorrhoea
  atopic illnesses, e.g. eczema and asthma
  necrotizing enterocolitis in preterm babies
  juvenile diabetes
  childhood cancer, especially lymphoma
  pre-menopausal breast cancer

HIV-infected children worldwide, up to one-third became infected through breastfeeding. Non-breast-feeding mothers may therefore suffer considerable engorgement and breast pain. Fluid restriction and a tight brassiere have been shown to be equally effective as bromocriptine usage by the 2nd week. Oestrogens are effective but not used frequently because of abnormal vaginal bleeding and increased risk of thromboembolism. Dopamine receptor stimulants, such as bromocriptine and cabergoline, inhibit prolactin and thus suppress lactation. Comparative studies of a single dose of cabergoline versus a twice daily dose of bromocriptine for 14 days have shown that cabergoline is more effective, associated with fewer side effects and less rebound lactation. It is therefore the drug of choice for suppression of lactation.

Breast disorders

Bloodstained nipple discharge

Bloodstained nipple discharge of pregnancy is typically bilateral and believed to be due to epithelial proliferation. It usually occurs in the second or third trimester of pregnancy and rarely persists beyond two months postpartum. As the condition is self-limiting no investigation or treatment is necessary and the woman should be reassured.

Painful nipples

The nipple can become very painful if the covering epithelium is denuded or if a fissure develops giving rise to 'cracked nipples'. The cause is usually attributed to poor positioning of the baby on the breast although thrush (candidiasis) may also cause soreness. Cracked nipples are also associated with an increased risk of a breast abscess developing. Treatment involves resting the affected nipple and manually expressing milk. Breastfeeding should then be reintroduced gradually.

Galactocele

A galactocele is a retention cyst of the mammary ducts following blockage by inspissated secretions. It is identified as a fluctuant swelling with minimal pain and inflammation. It usually resolves spontaneously but may also be aspirated; with increasing discomfort surgical excision may become necessary.

Breast engorgement

Engorgement of the breasts usually begins by the 2nd or 3rd postpartum day and if breastfeeding has not been effectively established, the over-distended and engorged breasts can be very uncomfortable. Breast engorgement may give rise to puerperal fever of up to 39° in 13 per cent of mothers. Although the fever rarely lasts more than 16 hours, other infective causes must be excluded. A number of remedies for treatment of breast engorgement, such as manual expression, firm support, applying an ice bag and an electric breast pump, have all been recommended in the past, but allowing the baby easy access to the breast is the most effective method of treatment and prevention.

Mastitis

Inflammation of the breast is not always due to an infective process. Mastitis can occur when a blocked duct obstructs the flow of milk and distends the alveoli. If this pressure persists, the milk extravasates into the perilobular tissue initiating an inflammatory process. The affected segment of the breast is painful and appears red and oedematous (Fig. 10.4). Flu-like symptoms develop associated with a tachycardia and pyrexia. In the first few postpartum days about 15 per cent of women will develop a temperature of up to 39°, lasting less than 24 hours, due to breast engorgement. By contrast, in infective mastitis the pyrexia develops later and persists for longer. In general, suppurative mastitis usually presents at the 3rd to 4th postpartum week and is usually unilateral. Symptoms include rigors, fever, pain and reddened swollen breasts. The most common infecting organism is *Staphylococcus aureus*, which is found in 40 per cent of women with mastitis. Other bacteria include coagulase negative staphylococci and *Streptococcus viridans*. The most frequent source of infection is from the baby's nose or throat and secondly from an infected umbilical cord. Management includes isolation of mother and baby, ceasing

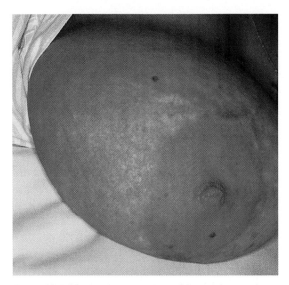

Figure 10.4 Mastitis demonstrating redness, oedema and engorged veins.

breastfeeding from the affected breast, expression of milk either manually or by electric pump and microbiological culture and sensitivity of a sample of milk. Flucloxacillin can be commenced while awaiting sensitivity results.

About 10 per cent of women with mastitis develop a breast abscess. Treatment is by a radial surgical incision and drainage under general anaesthesia.

Contraception

The exact mechanism of lactational amenorrhoea is poorly understood but the most plausible hypothesis is that during lactation there is inhibition of the normal pulsatile release of luteinizing hormone from the anterior pituitary. Breastfeeding therefore provides a contraceptive effect, but it is not totally reliable as up to 10 per cent of women can conceive during this period. However it has recently been shown that a mother who is still in the phase of postpartum amenorrhoea while fully breastfeeding her baby has a less than 2 per cent chance of conceiving in the first six months. Although this is comparable to some of the other methods of contraception (see Chapter 6 in *Gynaecology by Ten Teachers 17E*), most women in developed countries would use some form of additional contraception such as barrier methods. If an intra-uterine contraceptive device is preferred it is best to wait at least four weeks to allow for involution. Care needs to be exercised in breastfeeding mothers, as there have been reports of increased rates of uterine perforation with the Lippes loop but not with the T-shaped devices. The combined oral contraceptive pill enhances the risk of thrombosis in the early puerperium and can have an adverse effect on the quality and constituents of breast milk. The progesterone-only pill (the minipill) is therefore preferable and should be commenced about day 21 following delivery, prior to which there may be puerperal breakthrough bleeding. Injectable contraception, such as Depot medroxyprogesterone acetate (Depo provera) given three-monthly or Norethisterone oenanthate (Noristerat) given two-monthly, are also very effective. However, injectable contraception given within 48 hours of delivery for convenience can cause breakthrough bleeding and therefore it is preferable to be given five to six weeks postpartum. Sterilization can be offered to mothers who are certain that they have completed their family. Tubal ligation can be performed during Caesarean Section or by the open method (mini-laparotomy) in the first few postpartum days. However, it is better delayed after six weeks postpartum when it can be done by laparoscopy. This allows the mother to spend more time in comfort with her newborn baby and furthermore laparoscopic clip sterilization is less traumatic and associated with a lower failure rate.

Women who are not breastfeeding should commence the pill within four weeks of delivery as ovulation can occur by six weeks postpartum.

Pelvic floor exercises

It is a widespread belief that pelvic floor exercises tone up muscles of the pelvic floor and should therefore be advocated in the postpartum period. However, large randomized trials to evaluate its benefit in preventing genital prolapse, urinary incontinence or anal incontinence are lacking. There is also no evidence that antenatal exercises prevent incontinence or prolapse. However, as general exercise is known to strengthen striated muscle and pelvic floor exercises are unlikely to be harmful, women are still taught postnatal exercise. This should also serve to cultivate a feeling of pelvic floor awareness so women with pelvic floor dysfunction may seek medical help sooner.

Perinatal death

- Stillbirth: a baby born with no sign of life.
- Perinatal death: stillbirth ≥ 24 weeks' gestation or death within 7 days of birth.
- Live birth: any baby which shows sign of life irrespective of gestation.

Counselling and bereavement following perinatal death requires special expertise and is best left to a senior clinician and a trained bereavement counsellor. Inappropriate management of this traumatic period can have a devastating effect on the woman's emotional and marital life. Effective communication and support are crucial and women should be encouraged to make contact with organizations such as SANDS (Stillbirth and Neonatal Death Society). The grieving process can be facilitated by practices such as, seeing and holding the dead baby, naming the baby, taking hand/foot prints and photographs. Coming to terms with a perinatal death of a twin is even more difficult because the mother has to mourn one baby and celebrate the arrival of the other.

A postmortem is the most important diagnostic test even though there may be no positive findings. Couples who decline a postmortem may do so because of religious reasons or they may fear mutilation. In this situation a partial postmortem should be discussed whereby an autopsy of a single organ or a tissue biopsy can be performed. A full body X-ray or preferably MRI may be useful in some cases (Table 10.5).

If the baby was stillborn then a stillbirth certificate should be completed by the attending doctor. Otherwise the paediatrician should complete the certificate. The certificate should be given to the parents to register the death with Registrar of Births and Deaths. Funeral arrangements can be made privately or arranged by the hospital.

Every mother who has lost a baby should have the six-week postnatal visit at hospital.

The postnatal examination

This is carried out at about six weeks postpartum by the general practitioner or by the obstetrician if delivery had been complicated. The examination includes an assessment of the woman's mental and physical health as well as progress of the baby. In particular, direct questions must be asked about urinary, bowel and sexual function. Incontinence and dyspareunia are embarrassing issues that women do not volunteer readily. Weight, urine analysis and blood pressure are checked and a complete general, abdominal and pelvic examination is performed. If a cervical smear is due it can be taken although it is preferable to take one after three months postpartum. Contraception and pelvic floor exercises are also discussed.

Table 10.5 Investigations into perinatal death

Investigations	Reason
Full blood count	Anaemia, leucocytosis
Clotting screen	Disseminated intravascular coagulation
Kleihauer test	Fetomaternal transfusion
Virology, Infection screen	Cytomegalovirus, parovirus
Autoantibody screen (anticardiolipin and lupus anticoagulant)	Antiphospholipid syndrome, systemic lupus erythematosus
Blood and placenta culture	Infections such as *Listeria*
Antibodies in Rhesus-negative women	Haemolytic disease
Toxoplasma antibodies	Toxoplasmosis
Skin biopsy/cardiac blood/placental biopsy	Chromosome analysis
Full body X-ray or MRI	To identify congenital defects

CASE HISTORY

A 42-year-old woman who delivered vaginally four days previously, presents with heavy fresh vaginal bleeding and clots. She admits to feeling unwell and experiencing cramp-like abdominal pains.

On examination she has a temperature of 38.2°C and there is mild suprapubic tenderness. Vaginal examination revealed blood clots but no products of conception. The cervix admitted only the tip of a finger and the uterus was slightly tender and measured 18 weeks in size. Looking back at her delivery notes it was noted that the placental membranes were ragged at delivery.

What is the most likely diagnosis?

Secondary postpartum haemorrhage due to infected retained products of conception.

How should the patient be managed?

- Blood cultures.
- Intravenous broad-spectrum antibiotics, e.g. cephalosporin and metronidazole.
- Although a pelvic ultrasound may confirm the diagnosis, it is not a prerequisite when the diagnosis is obvious.
- Surgical evacuation of retained products in the uterus

Key Points

- The puerperium refers to the six-week period following childbirth
- Care during this transition period is crucial before the woman returns to her pre-pregnant state
- Perineal discomfort is a major complaint following vaginal delivery and therefore adequate analgesia should be pre-scribed
- Common disorders include puerperal sepsis, thromboem-bolism, bowel and bladder dysfunction

References for further reading

Sultan AH, Monga AK, Stanton SL. The pelvic floor sequelae of childbirth. *Br J Hosp Med* 1996; **55(9):** 575-9.
Bryon CC, Brost B. Emergency management of sudden puerperal fever. *Obstet Gynecol Clin N Am.* 1995; **22(2):** 357-67.

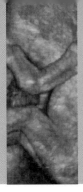

Chapter 11

Disorders of placentation

OVERVIEW

As stated in Chapter 3, the Confidential Enquiry into Maternal Mortality has repeatedly identified pre-eclampsia and eclampsia as leading causes of maternal death in pregnancy. In addition, pre-eclampsia is responsible for the 'medicalization' of many pregnancies, with extra hospital visits and admissions inflicting a high cost on women, families and the Health Service. Fetal growth restriction is a major determinant of perinatal and neonatal morbidity. Although fetal growth is determined by a number of factors including genetic predisposition, maternal nutritional status and ability of the placenta to allow nutrient exchange, it is now apparent that the origins of both pre-eclampsia and much of the fetal growth restriction seen in clinical practice lie in defective placentation. A further condition frequently related to impaired trophoblast invasion is abruptio placentae or premature separation of a normally sited placenta, which is usually of sudden onset and associated with a high fetal mortality and substantial maternal mortality and morbidity. A knowledge of the early events in the invasion of the maternal uterine wall by placental trophoblast cells is therefore helpful in understanding the aetiology of these important clinical conditions.

THE PLACENTA

The placenta is usually regarded as a fetal organ, although it contains maternal and fetal vascular beds that are juxtaposed. It receives the highest blood flow of any fetal organ (40 per cent of fetal cardiac output) and towards the end of pregnancy competes with the fetus for maternal substrate consuming the major fraction of glucose and oxygen taken up by the gravid uterus.

The functional unit of the placenta is the fetal cotyledon and the mature human placenta has about 120 cotyledons, which are grouped into visible lobes. Each cotyledon contains a primary villus stem arising from the chorionic plate and supplied by primary branches of fetal vessels. The primary stems divide to form secondary and tertiary stems from which arise the terminal villi, where maternal–fetal exchange takes place. The fetal cotyledons appear to develop around the entries of the maternal spiral arteries from the decidual plate and the centre of each cotyledon is hollow, where the pulsatile jet of blood from the spiral artery enters the intracotyledonary space (Fig. 11.1). Blood from the spiral arteries rises high to the chorionic plate, then disperses laterally between and over the surface of the terminal villi, becoming increasingly desaturated of oxygen and nutrients and picking up CO_2 and waste products. The blood then filters into narrow venous channels between the cotyledons before falling back to the maternal decidual plate, where the maternal veins return the desaturated blood to the maternal circulation (Fig. 11.2). Maternal and fetal blood are separated by three microscopic tissue layers: trophoblastic tissue, connective tissue and the endothelium of the fetal capillaries. However, microscopic examination of the terminal villi, surrounding the intracotyledonary space, shows numerous vasculosyncytial membranes where the fetal capillaries and trophoblast fuse to form a very thin membrane, where most of the transfer of nutrients and blood gases takes place (Fig. 11.3).

Normal placentation

The maternal blood flow to the placenta increases throughout pregnancy from 50 mL/min in the first trimester to 600 mL/min at term. This twelve-fold increase in perfusion can only be accomplished by an anatomical conversion of the maternal spiral arteries by trophoblast, from narrow tortuous muscular vessels to wide-bored flaccid vessels. In the first 12 weeks the decidual segments of the spiral arteries are invaded and replaced by trophoblast and fibrinoid. At the end of this period, the trophoblast plugs, which occupy the lumen of the spiral arteries, are released and this is associated with a sudden increase

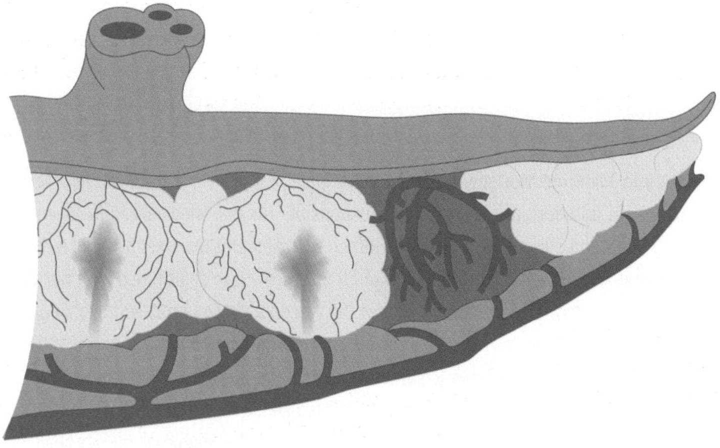

Figure 11.1 Diagram of placenta showing arrangement of fetal cotyledons and the maternal and fetal vascular system.

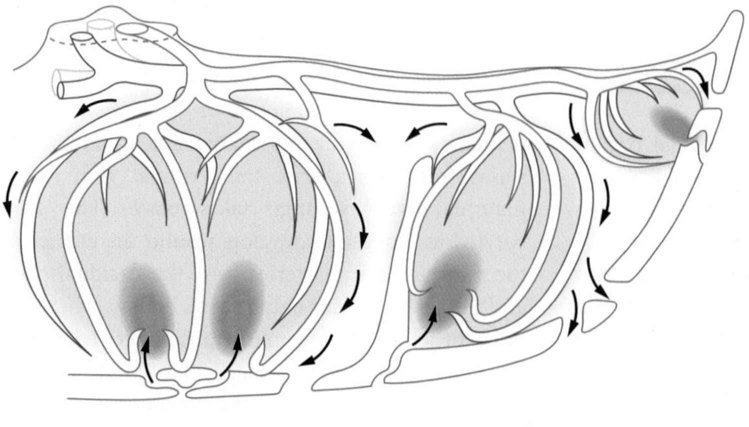

Figure 11.2 Diagram showing the direction of maternal flow through the fetal cotyledons.

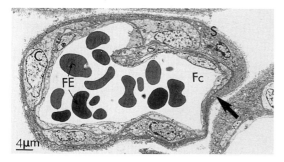

Figure 11.3 A terminal villus in cross section. Vasculo-syncytial membrane is illustrated (arrow).

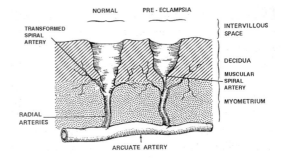

Figure 11.4 The transformation of spiral arteries.

in blood flow to the intervillous space. Following this, the trophoblast invasion of the intramyometrial segment of the spiral arteries occurs, which further reduces resistance to blood flow to the placenta and is associated with a mid-trimester fall in the maternal blood pressure. This process should be complete by 20 weeks. These flaccid transformed spiral arteries not only permit increased perfusion, but because they lack smooth muscle, they are less likely to respond to vaso-active compounds (Fig. 11.4).

Abnormal placentation

Pre-eclampsia, intrauterine growth restriction (IUGR) and abruptio placentae are clinical manifestations of total or patchy failure of trophoblast invasion of the myometrial segments of the spiral arteries. In terms of the aetiology of the condition, there are still more questions than answers. It is still not clear why trophoblast

invasion fails and why this pathological maladaption can produce a pregnancy with either pre-eclampsia or IUGR or abruptio placentae, or all three. It is likely that the more complete the failure of trophoblast invasion, the more likely that pre-eclampsia will supervene. There are other general conditions associated with impaired perfusion of the placenta such as collagen vascular disease, antiphospholipid syndrome, severe diabetes mellitus and chronic hypertension. All of these result in a small placenta with gross morphological changes. The most serious of these changes are:

- infarcts (Fig. 11.5);
- basal haematomas (Fig. 11.6).

An infarct represents an area of ischaemic necrosis of a cotyledon resulting from spiral artery occlusion, usually by thrombosis. A placenta with multiple infarcts is significantly associated with intrauterine fetal death and growth restriction. Closely associated with infarcts are placental haematomas, which consist of a mass of blood in the centre of the fetal

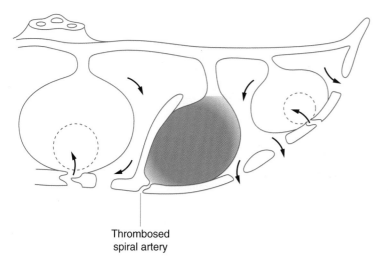

Thrombosed spiral artery

Figure 11.5 Diagram showing how an infarct occurs due to thrombosis of spiral artery.

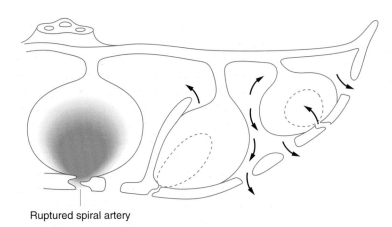

Figure 11.6 Diagram showing the formation of a massive haematoma.

Ruptured spiral artery

cotyledon due to rupture of a damaged spiral artery. This lesion is also associated with maternal hypertension and increased perinatal mortality. These serious pathological lesions should not be confused with calcification or fibrin deposition in the placenta, which can often give it an 'unhealthy' appearance, but are benign.

Definitions

Historically many terms referring to hypertension in pregnancy have been used interchangeably. This has led to difficulty in comparing studies on treatments, or outcomes, in different populations.

Normal blood pressure

Blood pressure normally falls in pregnancy, with the lowest recordings at 14–20 weeks' gestation, before rising towards pre-pregnancy values by term. This is an important concept, as definitions that rely on changes in blood pressure during pregnancy will depend on when the initial reading was taken.

Pre-eclampsia

A diastolic blood pressure exceeding 90 mmHg, on at least two occasions in the second half of pregnancy, where the blood pressure was previously normal, accompanied by significant proteinuria (>300 mg/24 h). Traditionally the presence of peripheral oedema has been included in the definition, however this is a common finding in otherwise normal pregnancy and its absence does not preclude the diagnosis.

Eclampsia

When the above picture is complicated by tonic–clonic seizures not caused by coincidental

neurological disorders. With improved management of antenatal pre-eclampsia, most cases of eclampsia seen in the UK present either intra- or postpartum.

Gestational hypertension (pregnancy-induced hypertension)

An exaggerated increase in blood pressure in the second half of pregnancy without the development of proteinuria. In general this does not have important maternal or fetal consequences and may even be associated with an increased birth weight.

Chronic hypertension

Hypertension which is apparent prior to, in the first half of, or persisting more than six weeks after pregnancy. The definition of superimposed pre-eclampsia in the presence of chronic hypertension can be difficult to make, but is usually associated with a worsening of the hypertension and the development, or worsening, of proteinuria.

PRE-ECLAMPSIA

Incidence and epidemiology

The incidence of pre-eclampsia varies between 5 and 10 per cent depending on the exact definition used and the population studied. It is more common in primigravid women and at the extremes of reproductive age. The recurrence rate for pre-eclampsia, with the same male partner, is approximately 20 per cent, and usually becomes apparent at a later gestation

Risk factors

Predisposing factors for the development of pre-eclampsia include:

- conditions where the placenta is enlarged (multiple gestation, diabetes, hydrops)
- pre-existing hypertension
- pre-existing vascular disease (such as in diabetes or autoimmune vasculitis)
- sickle cell disease

than in the first pregnancy. A new partner increases an individual woman's risk of recurrence.

Prolonged exposure to paternal antigens (e.g. through unprotected sex) prior to conceiving and cigarette smoking appear to reduce the incidence of pre-eclampsia.

Aetiology

Pre-eclampsia is often referred to as the disease of theories, with many mechanisms proposed to account for the clinical picture. Serum from women with pre-eclampsia is able to activate and damage vascular endothelial cells *in vitro*, and investigators believe a poorly perfused trophoblast may release a 'factor X' which enters the maternal circulation and damages her vascular beds. The nature of this factor has not yet been defined. Other theories include abnormal lipid metabolism; reduced anti-oxidant status; altered catecholamine homeostasis; abnormal dietary calcium, magnesium, or selenium content; reduced production of nitric oxide and an abnormal immune response to pregnancy.

Whilst abnormalities in these processes are undoubtedly present in established pre-eclampsia, it has been difficult to demonstrate which, if any, precede the endothelial activation, a prerequisite for establishing cause and effect. As changes in many of these pathways are seen in clinically normal pregnancies, the clinical picture of pre-eclampsia may be observed only when endothelial-compensating mechanisms fail.

Whilst vascular dysfunction is important in the pathophysiology of pre-eclampsia, the aetiology appears to be due to abnormal trophoblast invasion. Pre-eclampsia has been described in pregnancies lacking a fetus (molar pregnancies) and in the

absence of a uterus (abdominal pregnancies), suggesting the trophoblast is of paramount importance. Approximately 100–150 spiral arteries supply the maternal surface of the placenta. Placental bed biopsies have demonstrated that in pre-eclampsia trophoblast invasion is patchy, and the spiral arteries retain their muscular walls. This is thought to prevent the development of a high flow, low impedance utero-placental circulation. The reason why trophoblast invades less effectively in these pregnancies, and why a first pregnancy is subsequently protective, is not understood. Extravillous trophoblast cells from placental bed biopsies taken from pre-eclamptic pregnancies do not show the normal adhesion molecule switch characteristic of invasive trophoblast, although the reason for this also remains poorly understood.

Pathophysiology

There is now abundant evidence that the clinical picture of pre-eclampsia is due to an activation, or dysfunction, of vascular endothelial cells and co-existent platelet activation. The plasma concentration of cell surface markers for endothelial cell damage and platelet activation (including fibronectin, adhesion molecules and von Willebrand factor) are increased, as is the concentration of platelet degranulation products.

Normal pregnancy is characterized by marked peripheral vasodilatation, resulting in a fall in total peripheral resistance and a reduction in blood pressure despite an increase in cardiac output and circulating volume. This peripheral vasodilatation is accomplished through a reduced vascular sensitivity to vasoconstrictors such as angiotensin, and possibly by enhanced vasodilator production by vascular endothelial cells. A strong candidate for this latter role is nitric oxide. In pre-eclampsia the insensitivity to vasoconstrictors is lost and vessels *in vivo* and *in vitro* show reduced sensitivity to vasodilators and enhanced sensitivity to vasoconstrictors.

A reduction in the synthesis of vasodilatory nitric oxide (NO) and prostacyclin (PGI_2), and an increased production of endothelin by the vascular endothelium in pre-eclampsia could account not just for the characteristic vasospasm, but also the activation of circulating platelets (NO and PGI_2 stabilize these cells). Vasospasm and endothelial cell dysfunction, with subsequent platelet activation and micro-aggregate formation account for many of the pathological features of pre-eclampsia.

In the kidney a highly characteristic lesion (called glomeruloendotheliosis) is seen. This consists of endothelial and mesangial cell swelling, basement membrane inclusions but little disruption of renal epithelial podocytes. This is relatively specific for pre-eclampsia and is associated with the development of proteinuria, reduced renal clearance of uric acid and oliguria. It is not seen with hypertension due to other causes.

In the liver, subendothelial fibrin deposition is associated with Elevation of Liver enzymes. This can be associated with Haemolysis and a Low Platelet count due to platelet consumption (and subsequent widespread activation of the coagulation system). The presence of these findings is called the HELLP syndrome. The HELLP syndrome is a particularly severe form of pre-eclampsia. It occurs in approximately 2–4 per cent of women with pre-eclampsia and is associated with a fetal loss rate of up to 60 per cent if occurring antenatally and a maternal mortality of up to 24 per cent.

Vasospasm and cerebral oedema have both been implicated in the cerebral manifestations of pre-eclampsia and the progression to eclampsia. Retinal haemorrhage, exudates and papilloedema are characteristic of hypertensive encephalopathy and are rare in pre-eclampsia, suggesting the hypertension per se is not responsible for the cerebral pathology. It

S **Symptoms of pre-eclampsia**
• may be asymptomatic
• headache
• visual disturbance
• epigastric and right upper abdominal pain
• oedema (progressive)

is therefore likely that endothelial cell function can again be implicated.

Within the vasculature of the placental bed the characteristic lesion seen in pre-eclampsia is acute atherosis of the spiral arteries, with platelet micro-aggregates and larger thromboses.

Screening tests

Over 100 screening tests have been proposed, which will identify women at increased risk of subsequently developing pre-eclampsia. These have included tests that exploit the altered vascular sensitivity in pre-eclampsia and tests that detect plasma or urine metabolites of vasoactive mediators, renal markers or markers of endothelial damage. Other tests have been suggested that use ultrasound to detect high-resistance uterine artery Doppler waveforms or a waveform with a notch that implies inadequate or incomplete trophoblast invasion of the spiral arteries (see Chapter 11). This test has the advantage of being quick and immediate and will identify a cohort of women at high risk of pre-eclampsia. For example, notching on both uterine arteries at 24 weeks' gestation will identify over 80 per cent of women who will subsequently develop pre-eclampsia with a false positive rate of only 5 per cent. If performed before 24 weeks the false positive rate will be higher, but delaying preventive therapy until 24 weeks may reduce the effectiveness of treatment. Screening has also been criticized on the basis that it will cause unnecessary alarm in pregnant women at a time when prevention of pre-eclampsia has not yet been proven. The most commonly used preventive therapy is low dose aspirin (at 100 mg daily) on the basis that this dose will inhibit platelet activation and the release of vasoactive compounds such as thromboxanes without impairing the synthesis of vasodilating prostaglandins produced by the vascular endothelium. Two large placebo-

Organ-specific changes associated with pre-eclampsia

Cardiovascular:	generalized vasospasm
	increased peripheral resistance
	reduced central venous/pulmonary wedge pressures
Haematological:	platelet activation and depletion
	coagulopathy
	decreased plasma volume
	increased blood viscosity
Renal:	proteinuria
	decreased glomerular filtration rate
	decreased urate excretion
Hepatic:	periportal necrosis
	subcapsular haematoma
Central nervous:	cerebral oedema
	cerebral haemorrhages

Signs of pre-eclampsia

- elevation of blood pressure
- fluid retention (non-dependent oedema/ rapid weight gain)
- brisk reflexes
- ankle clonus (more than three beats)
- uterus (and fetus) may feel small for gestational age

controlled studies have failed to show any significant benefit of aspirin therapy in preventing pre-eclampsia. There is evidence however that aspirin may be more effective if given to a more targeted group at high risk of developing the disease and if given in doses that affect bleeding times (e.g. 150 mg daily). This is why the development of early and effective screening tests for this condition is so important. There are other reasons for developing such tests. Assigning low- and high-risk groups allows the former to have more community-based antenatal care; high-risk groups are useful for trials of preventive or therapeutic intervention and screening tests are usually based on hypothesis relating to the aetiology or pathophysiology of the condition. Testing such hypotheses potentially helps our understanding of the condition.

Treatment

The mainstay of treatment for pre-eclampsia remains ending the pregnancy by delivering the fetus (and the placenta). This can be a significant problem for the baby if pre-eclampsia occurs at 24–28 weeks' gestation, thus many treatments have been proposed to delay the need for delivery.

Diagnosis of pre-eclampsia usually requires admission of the patient for bedrest and more intensive monitoring of her condition. When diastolic blood pressure is relatively normal (90–95 mmHg) and proteinuria is mild (trace or 1+ on clinic testing with indicator sticks) it may be possible to monitor the patient's condition as an outpatient, attending a feto-maternal assessment regularly. With higher blood pressure values, or greater proteinuria admission is mandatory.

Methyldopa is the maintenance antihypertensive most commonly used in the UK. This is not because it is the best agent, but rather that so much use in pregnancy has suggested its safety. It is important to

realize that treating the maternal hypertension does not affect the disease itself, which can still progress. Indeed lowering the blood pressure too aggressively can further reduce uterine blood flow and lead to fetal distress. Treating the blood pressure above diastolic values of 105 mmHg reduces the likelihood of maternal cerebrovascular accident. Other antenatal therapies, including aspirin, nitric oxide donors, plasmapheresis, oxygen therapy and restoring the circulating volume by massive intravenous transfusion with central venous monitoring remain unproven by large prospective, randomized trials.

Pre-eclampsia may first present during labour. If this is the case, or where blood pressure increases during labour for an established pre-eclamptic, an intravenous infusion of hydralazine is the most commonly used antihypertensive. This allows the dosage to be titrated rapidly against change in blood pressure. Epidural anaesthesia is encouraged where there is no abnormality in clotting studies as it has a hypotensive effect. Ergometrine is avoided in the management of the third stage of labour as it can significantly increase blood pressure.

After delivery maternal blood pressure can be treated more aggressively, with more modern drugs. Most of the maternal deaths related to pre-eclampsia are due to a failure to recognize a deteriorating condition after delivery and result from multiple organ failure including disseminated intravascular coagulation, adult respiratory distress syndrome and renal

Investigations for pre-eclampsia

These investigations will be repeated at intervals dependent on the overall clinical picture.

- urinalysis by dipstick (quantitatively inaccurate)
- 24 h urine collection (total protein and creatinine clearance)
- full blood count (platelets and haematocrit)
- blood chemistry (renal function, protein concentration)
- plasma urate concentration
- liver function
- coagulation profile if delivery is indicated
- ultrasound assessment:
    fetal size
    amniotic fluid volume
    maternal and fetal
    Dopplers

CASE HISTORY - PRE-ECLAMPSIA

Mrs A A

41-year-old married doctor, non-smoker. Weight 90 kg. Gravida 1. No past history of note. Booked for antenatal care at 11 weeks. Well. BP 120/75 mmHg.

Ultrasound nuchal screening for Down's syndrome, confirmed dates, low-risk aneuploidy

Normal antenatal course to 30 weeks' gestation when BP found to be 150/95 mmHg and urinalysis revealed ++ proteinuria.

Discussion

How should this patient be managed?

This woman has a positive screen for pre-eclampsia in the clinic. She should have her blood pressure taken again several times to ensure it is not simply related to attending the clinic. She should also be screened for a urinary tract infection, a common cause of proteinuria. Assuming her blood pressure is elevated she should be admitted for bedrest, 24 h urine collection (quantify protein and creatinine clearance), baseline platelet count and renal and hepatic function, and she should have a scan to assess fetal growth, liquor volume and possibly fetal Doppler studies.

Should she be commenced on medications?

At this blood pressure there is no proven advantage to commencing antihypertensives. This situation is not analogous to chronic elevated blood pressure and the only aim of treatment is the prevention of an acute episode such as cerebrovascular accident (CVA). As she is overweight and has been admitted for bedrest she should be commenced on heparin prophylaxis against thromboembolism. As she may require delivery in the near future she should be given a course of dexamethasone to promote fetal lung maturation.

If delivery is the main treatment for pre-eclampsia when should this be carried out?

The decision to deliver must balance the beneficial effect on the mother's health against detrimental effects on the baby's prognosis. Many women with pre-eclampsia run a chronic course and prolonging gestation will improve fetal maturity. There is no correct answer to this question. The decision to deliver must be based on frequent repetition of investigations into maternal and fetal health, and will occur at a time when it is felt that either maternal health is becoming compromised by further delay to delivery, or that the fetus can be better looked after *ex utero* than *in utero*.

failure. The importance of involving clinicians from other specialities (Intensive Care, Haematology) cannot be overstated.

The treatment for eclampsia is resuscitation of the mother (Airway, Breathing, Circulation), diazepam treatment (intravenously) to bring the initial convulsion under control and then magnesium sulphate therapy (intravenously or intramuscularly) to prevent further convulsions. The efficacy of this latter drug for preventing a second convulsion has now been proven conclusively by prospective randomized trials. It is used extensively in the USA for preventing eclampsia (i.e. preventing the first convulsion). Its prophylactic role is currently being assessed prospectively in several studies.

Additional points in management

Iatrogenic premature delivery of the fetus is often required in severe pre-eclampsia. This necessitates optimizing the fetal condition prior to delivery. Dexamethasone (12 mg i.m., twice, 12 h apart) should be given to the mother to reduce the chance of neonatal pulmonary insufficiency. If the patient's condition permits she should be transferred to a tertiary centre prior to delivery, to improve both her own management and the facilities for her baby. Delivery before term is usually by Caesarean Section. Such patients are at particularly high risk for thromboembolism and should be given prophylactic subcutaneous heparin and issued with anti-thromboembolic stockings.

New developments

Several groups are investigating the genetics of pre-eclampsia, although the variable phenotype of the condition within a couple suggests the cause is unlikely to relate to a single gene. Several studies investigating whether nitric oxide donors can prevent, or be used to treat pre-eclampsia are now in progress. Similar studies on the therapeutic role of vitamins C and E (major anti-oxidants), and on dietary supplementation in areas of calcium deficiency will also report in the near future.

Mrs KK

26-year-old woman recently arrived in the UK from Bangladesh was seen in the Accident and Emergency department of the hospital. With the help of her husband, who spoke some English, she gave a history of severe headache, and epigastric pain, for two days. The husband also informed the triaging nurse that his wife was six months pregnant. The nurse found her blood pressure to be 190/125 mmHg. Whilst the casualty doctor was being informed of these findings the patient had a generalized convulsion.

What is the diagnosis?

In situations where a complete history is unavailable and previous obstetric or antenatal notes are missing, or have never been produced, only a differential diagnosis is possible. The most likely diagnosis in this pregnant, hypertensive patient is eclampsia, although after initial management other differential diagnoses such as epilepsy, CVA, space-occupying lesion in the head and drug reaction must all be considered.

What is the initial management?

Several steps need to be taken in managing an eclamptic convulsion. It is usually unnecessary to try to stop the initial convulsion, which typically lasts for only 60–90 seconds. Diazepam is often given acutely, but can cause apnoea and cardiac arrest if given too quickly. Maternal injury should be prevented by rolling the patient on to her left side, applying suction to foam and secretions from her mouth and adequate oxygenation should be maintained. This can be by face mask oxygen supplementation. Difficulty in maintaining respiration and aspiration pneumonia are rare in the post-ictal phase, but are more likely if diazepam has been given, or if objects have been forced into the mouth to prevent tongue biting. The drug of choice to prevent a further convulsion is magnesium sulphate. This is given as an initial intravenous bolus of 4–6 g over 15 minutes. The higher dose will maintain therapeutic anti-convulsant concentrations for longer, but will be closer to toxic levels. A second convulsion will occur in 10–15 per cent of women after loading with magnesium, and a further bolus of 2 g should be given. Maternal acidaemia should also be corrected, if necessary, with intravenous sodium bicarbonate. At systolic blood pressures exceeding 170 mmHg and diastolic pressures above 110 mmHg there is a risk of CVA. Antihypertensive therapy should therefore be given. In the UK this is likely to be either a calcium channel blocker (10–20 mg sublingual nifedipine), or an intravenous bolus of hydrallazine (5 mg), followed by an infusion titrated against the blood pressure.

What is the subsequent management?

After initial resuscitation the patient should have a size 16 G venflon inserted into a peripheral vein and blood should be sent to the laboratories for determination of haemoglobin concentration, platelet count, renal and hepatic function, uric acid concentration, coagulation studies and blood group. A urinary catheter should be passed and the urine stick tested for protein. Once the mother is stabilized the health of the fetus can be assessed. If the baby is still alive it is necessary to estimate gestation by ultrasound and assess wellbeing by Doppler and cardiotocography. Although at extremely premature gestations several series from the USA have advocated intensive monitoring of maternal health in the hope of improving fetal outcome by increasing gestation at delivery, the practice in most UK centres is to deliver the baby, regardless of gestation, after the mother's condition has been optimized.

The principles of postnatal management for an eclamptic patient are attention to fluid balance, blood pressure and renal, hepatic and CNS function. Blood pressure can be more aggressively controlled after delivery of the baby as the possibility of utero-placental hypoperfusion, with subsequent fetal distress, is removed. Magnesium sulphate therapy is usually maintained for 48 h, at 1 g/h IV. Toxicity is assessed clinically by a loss of deep tendon reflexes and respiratory depression, and biochemically by measuring the plasma magnesium concentration (therapeutic range 2–5 mg/dL). As these patients are often delivered by caesarean section they are at risk of venous thromboembolism. They should therefore be given compression stockings and commenced on subcutaneous heparin prophylaxis.

What is the prognosis for future pregnancies?

The recurrence risk for pre-eclampsia/eclampsia in a large series from the USA was 20 per cent. In the majority of women the condition was milder, and the incidence of recurrent eclampsia was 0.9 per cent. In this series a higher than otherwise expected incidence of pre-eclampsia (25 per cent) and eclampsia (3 per cent) was seen in the daughters of women who had developed eclampsia. The incidence of these two complications in the sisters of women who had developed eclampsia was respectively 37 per cent and 4 per cent.

ECLAMPSIA

Eclampsia is a serious complication of pre-eclampsia as it has a relatively increased maternal and fetal mortality. The incidence of eclampsia is one per 1–2000 deliveries, depending on the population studied and complicates 1–2 per cent of pregnancies with pre-eclampsia. In the UK most cases are intrapartum or postpartum. This may reflect less optimum care at these times, or may be an increased release of the placental factor responsible for pre-eclampsia during delivery. It is important to be aware of the features that may precede the convulsion. These are features of extreme vasospasm and include severe headache, irritability, visual disturbance, restlessness and twitching, drowsiness, epigastric pain, oliguria and tachycardia. Although there is usually no difficulty with the diagnosis in a patient known to be pregnant and suffering from pre-eclampsia, other causes of coma or convulsion must be considered when the blood pressure is not elevated, which has been described in one fifth of cases. Depending on local facilities maternal and fetal mortality rates of 20–40 per cent have been described.

The principles of treatment for eclampsia are to prevent further convulsions and provide general life support while vascular endothelial dysfunction resolves (allowing a resolution of vasospasm, impaired organ perfusion and vascular permeability). The patient should receive individualized nursing care, in a darkened, quiet room with adequate monitoring facilities. As large fluid shifts between body compartments can occur, monitoring intravascular (circulating) volume by measuring the central venous pressure (CVP), or pulmonary wedge pressure (with a Swann-Ganz catheter) is necessary. Accurate fluid balance can only be assessed by strict measurement of urine output, and a urinary catheter is, therefore, warranted. Eclamptic women are prone to both thromboembolism, and to the development of disseminated intravascular coagulation (DIC). Measures must therefore be taken to prevent the former (subcutaneous heparin prophylaxis, compression stockings) and diagnose and treat the latter (in conjunction with the Haematologist this might require replacement of clotting factors as fresh frozen plasma and platelet infusions, particularly if the patient is actively bleeding). Other organ failure (such as hepatic failure) requires intensive supportive treatment, often in a specialized unit. Psychological support after the patient has recovered is also vital. It is now appreciated that traumatic childbirth is a significant cause of post-traumatic stress disorder, and both the patient and her partner should receive expert counselling.

Intrauterine growth restriction (IUGR)

This considers fetuses which are small due to a congenital anomaly, including fetal infection and chromosomal abnormality. However the majority of fetuses which appear to be small are either constitutionally small (i.e. born to small parents and are fulfilling their genetic potential) or are small secondary to abnormal placental function.

Significance of IUGR

IUGR is a major cause of neonatal morbidity and mortality. It has a significant cost in terms of the facilities required to look after these infants. In addition, there is a growing appreciation that certain adult diseases (including hypertension and diabetes) are related to IUGR.

Definitions and incidence

IUGR is defined as failure of the fetus to achieve its genetic growth potential. This usually results in a fetus that is small for gestational age (SGA) and babies born below a particular centile weight for gestation (e.g. below the 3rd or 5th centile) are frequently classified as IUGR. While this is convenient and makes it simple to calculate the incidence of IUGR (3 per cent if the 3rd or 5 per cent if the 5th centile is chosen), the terms SGA and IUGR are not synonymous. The term SGA implies that the fetus or neonate is below a certain defined centile of weight or size for a particular gestational age and some SGA fetuses are constitutionally small due to normal genetic influences. IUGR indicates that a particular pathological process is operating to modify the intrinsic growth potential of the fetus by reducing its growth rate. Indeed some IUGR fetuses may not fall into any definition of SGA, but will have failed to achieve their full growth potential.

Aetiology

There are many causes of IUGR (Table 11.1). They are best grouped into two main categories: factors that directly affect the intrinsic growth potential of the fetus and external influences that reduce the support for fetal growth. Postnatal 'catch up' growth is more likely to occur in fetuses in the latter category than in the former (Fig. 11.7).

Chromosome abnormalities, genetic syndromes, infections and drugs can alter intrinsic fetal growth potential. Many chromosome abnormalities, such as trisomy 18 and triploidy and single gene defects such as Seckel's syndrome will alter the genetic potential of the fetus, as will some multi-factorial structural abnormalities such as anencephaly and renal agenesis. Viral infections, such as cytomegalovirus and rubella, and protozoal infections such as toxoplasmosis can also affect fetal growth potential.

External influences that affect fetal growth can be subdivided into maternal systemic factors and placental insufficiency. Maternal under-nutrition is globally the major cause of IUGR and even in developed countries, it is now recognized that maternal eating disorders, such as anorexia or bulaemia, can significantly affect fetal growth. Low maternal oxygen saturation, which can occur with cyanotic heart disease, chronic respiratory disease or at high altitude will reduce fetal PO_2 levels and fetal metabolism. Smoking, by increasing the amount of carboxy-haemoglobin in the maternal circulation, effectively reduces the amount of available oxygen to the fetus, thus causing growth restriction. A wide variety of drugs other than tobacco can affect fetal growth; alcohol, marijuana, heroin and cocaine are all associated with fetal growth restriction, probably through multiple mechanisms affecting fetal enzyme systems, placental blood flow and maternal substrate levels.

In developed countries, the most common cause of IUGR is poor placental function, secondary to inadequate trophoblast invasion of the uterine decidua and myometrial spiral arteries. This results in reduced perfusion of the intra-cotyledonary space, which leads to abnormal development of the terminal villi and impaired transfer of oxygen and nutrients to the fetus. Less frequently reduced perfusion can occur from other conditions, such as a severe diabetes mellitus, the antiphospholipid syndrome, and sickle cell disease. Multiple gestation usually results in a sharing of the uterine vascularity, which causes a relative reduction in the blood flow to each placenta. On the fetal side of the placental circulation, abnormalities of the umbilical cord, such as a

Table 11.1 – Causes of IUGR

Investigations	Cause
Reduced fetal growth potential	Chromosome defects, e.g. Trisomy 18, triploidy
	Single gene defects, e.g. Seckel's syndrome
	Structural abnormalities, e.g. renal agenesis
	Infections, e.g. CMV, toxoplasmosis
Reduced fetal growth support	*Maternal factors*
	Undernutrition, e.g. poverty, eating disorders
	Maternal hypoxia, e.g. altitude, cyanotic heart disease
	Drugs, e.g. cigarette smoke, alchohol, cocaine
	Placental factors
	Reduced utero-placental perfusion, e.g. inadequate trophoblast invasion, antiphospholipid syndrome, diabetes mellitus, sickle cell disease, multiple gestation
	Reduced feto-placental perfusion, e.g. single umbilical artery, twin–twin transfusion syndrome

Doppler:

L.Uterine Artery:	RI	0.71	
	Notch		
R.uterine Artery:	RI	0.86	
	Notch		
Umbilical Artery:	PI	1.34	
	RI	0.78	
	End diastolic flow: positive		
Fetal Aorta	PI	2..29	
	End diastolic flow: positive		
Middle Cerebral Artery	PI	1.15	
	RI	0.07	
	End diastolic flow: positive		
Ductus Venosus	PIV	0.880	

Diagnosis: Stable moderate redistribution. Increased DV PI.

Figure 11.7 This figure illustrates the growth pattern of an IUGR fetus. Note the relative brain sparing effect with head circumference less affected than the abdominal circumference or femur length. The Doppler chart demonstrates high resistance and notches in the uterine artery. There is fetal hypoxia as demonstrated by low resistance waveforms in the fetal brain (low pulsatility index) and probable acidaemia due to the high pulsatility in the ductus venosus.

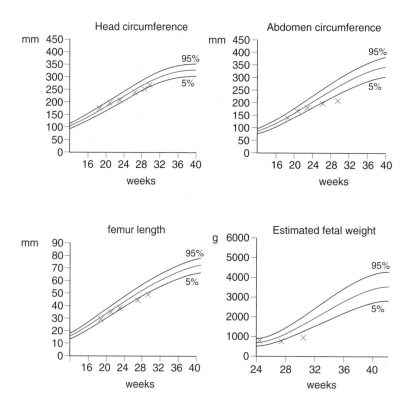

Pathophysiology

IUGR fetuses are frequently described as symmetric or asymmetric in terms of their body proportions. Symmetrically small fetuses are usually associated single umbilical artery, is associated with IUGR as are the intra-placental vascular connections found in monochorionic twinning.

with factors that directly impair the intrauterine growth potential of the fetus (i.e. chromosome abnormalities, viral infections, etc.), while asymmetric growth restriction is classically associated with utero-placental insufficiency. The cause of fetal asymmetry follows upon the reduced oxygen transfer to the fetus and impaired excretion of CO_2 by the placenta. The resulting fall in PO_2 and rise in PCO_2 in the fetal blood will induce a chemoreceptor response in the fetal carotid bodies with resulting vasodilatation in the fetal brain, myocardium and adrenal glands and vasoconstriction in the kidneys, splanchnic vessels, limbs and subcutaneous tissues. The liver circulation is also severely reduced; normally 50 per cent of the well-oxygenated blood in the umbilical vein passes to the right atrium through the ductus venosus eventually to reach the fetal brain, with the remainder going to the portal circulation in the liver. When there is fetal hypoxia, more of the well-oxygenated blood from the umbilical vein is diverted through the ductus venosus, which means that the liver receives less. The result of all these circulatory changes is an asymmetric fetus with relative brain sparing, reduced abdominal girth and skin thickness. The vasoconstriction in the fetal kidneys results in impaired urine production and oligohydramnios. The fetal hypoxaemia also leads to severe metabolic changes in the fetus reflecting intrauterine starvation. Antenatal fetal blood sampling has shown reduced levels of nutrients, such as glucose and amino acids (especially essential amino acids) and hormones such as thyroxine and insulin. There are increased levels of corticosteroids and catecholamines, which reflect the increased perfusion of the adrenal gland. Haematological changes also reflect the chronic hypoxia with increased levels of erythropoietin and nucleated red blood cells.

The fetal hypoxia eventually leads to fetal acidaemia, both respiratory and metabolic, which if prolonged can lead to intrauterine death if the fetus is not removed from its hostile environment. IUGR fetuses are especially at risk from profound asphyxia in labour due to the further compromise of the utero-placental circulation caused by the uterine contractions.

Investigation

The prediction and detection of the IUGR fetus is a principal aim of antenatal care and the earlier the diagnosis is made, the better the chance of improving the outlook for the fetus. On the premise that most IUGR fetuses are SGA, most antenatal screening programmes for IUGR judge their efficacy on the ability to predict the birth weight of an infant below the 5th centile birth weight for gestation. The detection of an SGA infant contains two elements: firstly, the accurate assessment of gestational age and secondly, the recognition of fetal smallness. As described in Chapter 6, early measurement of the fetal crown–rump length before 12 weeks

or the biparietal diameter between 12 and 20 weeks is routinely carried out in most hospitals and provides the most accurate assessment of gestational age. If there is any discrepancy between the assessments made at 12 weeks and 20 weeks, then the prediction from the earlier measurement should be accepted. The most precise method of detecting fetal smallness is by ultrasound biometry, in particular, measurement of the biparietal diameter, head circumference, abdominal circumference and femur length. It is logistically impossible to repeat these measurements in all pregnancies, so serial ultrasound biometry is usually performed on the following groups:

1. Pregnant mothers, who have had a previous SGA fetus, who are of low pre-pregnancy weight (<40 kg), who are heavy smokers, drug abusers, have a medical condition such as hypertension, antiphospholipid syndrome or diabetes, or who give a history of eating disorders or persistent hyperemesis.
2. Pregnancies where twins have been diagnosed at the first or second trimester scan.
3. Pregnancies where there are abnormal uterine artery waveforms at the mid-pregnancy scan (this is only performed in a few hospitals).
4. Pregnancies where the symphysis–fundal height measurement, which is made at each visit to the antenatal clinic, is more than 3 cm below the expected size for the gestational age.

When a diagnosis of SGA has been made, the next step is to establish whether this represents IUGR or whether the fetus is 'small normal'. A careful ultrasound scan of the fetal anatomy should be made to detect whether there are any fetal abnormalities to explain fetal smallness that may have been missed on the 2nd trimester scan. Even if the anatomy is normal, if the fetal head and femur are disproportionately small or if there is an increased amount of amniotic fluid, this would raise the suspicion of a fetal genetic defect and, under these circumstances, an amniocentesis and rapid fetal karyotype should be offered. Features suspicious of uteroplacental insufficiency would be an asymmetric fetus with a relatively small abdominal circumference, oligohydramnios and a high umbilical artery resistance.

Management

At present there are no widely accepted treatments available for growth restriction related to placental

Ms K I

17 years old, unemployed, smoked 10 cigarettes per day. Gravida 1. No past history of note. Booked for antenatal care at 12 weeks' gestation. Early pregnancy ultrasound scan confirmed a single fetus gestational age and the crown–rump length confirmed this. The nuchal translucency measurement gave a low risk for trisomy 21. At 20 weeks' gestation she attended for an anomaly scan which was normal, but at 20 weeks' and at 24 weeks' gestation, bilateral notches in the uterine artery Doppler waveforms were identified. On this basis she attended for regular ultrasound scans and fetal Doppler assessments and was reviewed weekly in the antenatal clinic. At 29 weeks' gestation she was found to have an elevated blood pressure but no proteinuria. In view of the poor fetal growth and reduced amniotic fluid volume, with fetal Doppler showing absent diastolic flow in the umbilical artery and suggesting centralisation of blood flow to the fetal brain and heart, Ms K I was admitted and given a course of dexamethasone injections. She continued to be monitored with daily fetal cardiotocographs, twice-weekly Doppler and regular (1–2 weekly) growth scans (see Fig. 11.7). At 31 weeks' gestation the decision was taken to deliver the baby by Caesarean Section, when the fetal cardiotocographs became suboptimal. At Caesarean Section a baby boy weighing 1.15 kg was delivered. The arterial cord pH was 7.22. After spending four weeks on the special care baby unit, he was discharged in good condition.

What antenatal risk factors for growth restriction did Ms K I exhibit?

Fetal growth restriction is more common at the extremes of reproductive age. It is also more common if the mother is unemployed, or employed in high stress occupations. Although there is strong epidemiological evidence that smoking reduces the incidence of pre-eclampsia, smoking is strongly associated with fetal growth restriction. Pre-eclampsia and chronic hypertension are both correlated with fetal growth restriction, but an increase in blood pressure in the third trimester of pregnancy, without accompanying proteinuria is not associated with IUGR. The role of abnormal uterine artery Doppler waveforms in predicting subsequent growth restriction is controversial. Whilst there is no doubt that women with bilateral notches in these waveforms are at greater risk of both IUGR and pre-eclampsia, widespread introduction of this test has not yet occurred due to lack of training and equipment and a belief that this false positive rate is too high.

What therapeutic interventions might have been of benefit in this case?

In the presence of an identifiable medical cause (such as diabetes mellitus, or systemic lupus erythematosus) treatment of the underlying condition should be optimised (e.g. diabetic control should be tightened, aspirin and heparin should be instituted for antiphospholipid syndrome). In the absence of such a cause no pharmacological treatment has been proven to be of benefit. Aspirin, GTN, dietary supplementation and oxygen therapy have all been reported as successful in either anecdotal cases, or small series, but their widespread use has not been implemented. Stopping smoking and reducing alcohol and other recreational drug consumption increases weight gain in growth restricted fetuses. The rationale for bedrest is to try to improve utero-placental blood flow where this is felt to be the cause of the IUGR. There is conclusive evidence that antenatal administration of dexamethasone reduces respiratory distress syndrome and intraventricular haemorrhage in preterm infants.

What are the complications of being born at 31 weeks?

The immediate complications of being born at 31 weeks include difficulties with feeding, maintaining blood glucose concentrations and body temperature and respiratory distress syndrome. Necrotizing enterocolitis and cerebral intraventricular haemorrhage are also increased in frequency. In the longer term there may be residual respiratory problems and an increased incidence of non-progressive neurological impairment. Maternal bonding may be impaired with a prolonged period spent on a special care baby unit, as may emotional and psychological development, manifest particularly during early school years. An association between IUGR and the incidence of adult diseases (such as hypertension and diabetes) is now also becoming apparent.

dysfunction. Obvious adverse factors such as smoking, alcohol and drug abuse should be stopped and the health of the woman should be maximized (optimize control of diabetes, thyroid dysfunction, etc).

When growth restriction is severe, and the fetus is considered too immature to be delivered, bedrest in hospital is usually advised in an effort to maximize placental blood flow. The aim of these interventions is to gain as much maturity as possible before delivering the fetus, thereby reducing the morbidity associated with prematurity. A growth-restricted baby weighing 1 kg and delivered at 32 weeks' gestation usually has a less stormy neonatal course than does a normally grown baby delivered at 28 weeks' gestation with the same birth weight.

Timing delivery to maximize gestation without the baby dying *in utero* involves intensive fetal surveillance. The most widely accepted methods of monitoring the fetus are discussed in Chapter 6. In brief, serial ultrasound scans are performed to establish that some fetal growth is maintained; cessation of fetal growth may be an indication in itself for delivery. However, fetal biometry cannot give meaningful estimates of growth rate at intervals less than two weeks so dynamic tests of fetal wellbeing such as Doppler ultrasound and fetal cardiotocography are now the principle means of determining fetal wellbeing. Absence of blood flow in the umbilical artery during fetal cardiac diastole or reversed flow (i.e. back towards the heart) requires delivery in the near future as it reflects high placental resistance and is usually a pre-terminal event. When this situation is seen at peri-viable gestations (24–28 weeks), more complicated fetal arterial and venous Doppler studies are used in some tertiary centres in an attempt to delay delivery. Unlike the umbilical artery Doppler, the role of other fetal Doppler studies has not yet been proven by large prospective trials.

No effective drug therapy for IUGR has yet been found. Small studies have suggested that aspirin, nitric oxide donors or anti-oxidants may be helpful in some cases. These drugs may act by reducing platelet activation in the utero-placental circulation, or may be acting directly as vasodilators. Larger, prospective, placebo-controlled studies are awaited to assess the use of these agents in either prevention, or treatment, of IUGR.

Prognosis

The main danger to the baby is intrauterine death, due either to failure in making the diagnosis, or excessive delay prior to delivery. Some babies will suffer morbidity, or die, as a result of premature delivery. The long-term prognosis for survivors is good, with low incidences of mental or physical handicap. Whilst height and weight curves for these infants remain slightly below the 50th centile, most infants with IUGR secondary to placental insufficiency show 'catch up' growth after delivery, when feeding can be optimized. Where IUGR is related to a congenital infection, or chromosomal anomaly, subsequent development of the child willl be determined by the precise abnormality present.

A link between IUGR and the adult incidence of both hypertension and diabetes has now been established. It remains to be seen whether other associations will be found in the future.

Placental abruption

Definition

This is uterine bleeding following premature separation of a normally sited placenta. It is concealed in approximately one-third of cases (i.e. no blood loss is seen per vaginam) and revealed in two-thirds of cases.

Incidence

This has been documented as between 0.5–2.0 per cent of pregnancies, but varies depending on the criteria used for diagnosis. Where diagnosis is based on histological examination of the placenta, the incidence has been reported to be as high as 4 per cent.

Aetiology

This is unknown in the majority of cases, although there is evidence for an association with defective trophoblastic invasion, as with pre-eclampsia and growth restriction. Other associations include direct abdominal trauma (e.g. road traffic accidents, assault, external cephalic version), high parity, uterine overdistension (polyhydramnios and multiple gestation), sudden decompression of the uterus (e.g. after delivery of the first twin or release of polyhydramnios) and smoking. The association with hypertension may reflect a direct cause, or may be a manifestation of poor trophoblastic invasion.

Clinical presentation

The classical presentation is that of abdominal pain, vaginal bleeding, and uterine contractions. The vaginal bleeding is usually dark and non-clotting, however as the bleeding may be concealed its absence does not preclude the diagnosis. Abruptio placentae often occurs close to term and frequently during labour. Although abdominal pain is a common feature, and is probably due to extravasation of blood into the myometrium, 'silent' abruptions have also been described. Some patients present additionally with nausea, restlessness and faintness.

If blood loss is significant there may be signs of hypovolaemic shock, with increased pulse rate, hypotension and signs of peripheral vasoconstriction. Abdominal palpation reveals a tender uterus that is often described as being 'woody hard'. The uterus may be larger than gestation suggests and the fetus is often difficult to palpate. Depending on the size of the abruption, and the area of placental separation, the fetus may be dead, in distress or be unaffected. Vaginal examination may reveal blood or cervical dilatation if the abruption has precipitated labour.

Diagnosis

This is usually made on clinical grounds. Where abruption has not been severe the diagnosis may only be made by inspection of the placenta after the third stage of labour is complete. Ultrasound can be helpful in some cases, demonstrating retro-placental clot and excluding placenta praevia. Ultrasound examination is also important where abruption is managed conservatively (see effects on the fetus, below). The differential diagnosis of placental abruption can be broadly divided into two groups; other causes of vaginal bleeding and other causes of abdominal pain in pregnancy.

Placental abruption: effects on the mother

Hypovolaemic shock
There is a tendency to underestimate the amount of blood loss. This is due to some haemorrhage being concealed behind the placenta and within the uterine wall. In addition some patients will have been hypertensive prior to the abruption, masking the hypotensive effect of blood loss. CVP measurement is extremely helpful both in assessing the degree of blood loss, and in accurate fluid replacement.

Disseminated intravascular coagulation
Disseminated intravascular coagulation (DIC) is always a secondary phenomenon following a trigger to generalized activation of coagulation systems. Consumption of fibrin, clotting factors and platelets occurs, resulting in continued bleeding and further depletion of these factors. The triggers known to precipitate DIC include tissue thromboplastin release, endothelial damage to small vessels and pro-coagulant phospholipid production secondary to intravascular coagulation. The incidence is very variable, but serious DIC probably affects about 0.1 per cent of pregnancies. Laboratory investigations include measuring the thrombin time (estimating clottable fibrinogen in whole blood), fibrin degradation products (FDPs) and platelet count. These tests should be repeated at regular intervals as resuscitation takes place. In cases of significant DIC it is vital to involve the Haematologist in the early care of the woman.

Acute renal failure
This is a consequence of poor renal perfusion, secondary to hypovolaemia, hypotension and DIC (microthrombi in the kidneys). The patient initially becomes oliguric and may develop acute tubular necrosis if the reduced renal perfusion is prolonged. After adequate fluid replacement and treatment of the DIC the patient may become polyuric, during which phase the plasma urea and creatinine concentrations may continue to rise. Fluid, acid-base and electrolyte balance must be carefully monitored. Dialysis may be required. In general the prognosis for acute renal failure after placental abruption, in women who are adequately resuscitated, is excellent.

Postpartum haemorrhage
Postpartum haemorrhage (PPH) can be due to coagulation failure, a poorly contracting 'Couvelaire' uterus (bruised due to extravasation of blood into the myometrium) and predisposing factors for PPH, including polyhydramnios and multiple gestation.

Feto-maternal haemorrhage
This can lead to sensitization of the mother to fetal

A 28-year-old woman in her third pregnancy attended the labour ward at 32 weeks' gestation with a two-hour history of severe lower abdominal pain followed by minimal vaginal bleeding. The patient also reported excessive fetal movements since the onset of the pain. Her gestation had been confirmed by ultrasound scanning in the first trimester. Her previous pregnancies had been uncomplicated and resulted in vaginal deliveries of normally grown infants. Her 20 week anomaly scan had shown the placenta to be fundally sited.

On examination the patient was in obvious distress. Her pulse rate was 120 bpm and her blood pressure was 120/60 mmHg. She was vasoconstricted, with cool, clammy skin and a clinically low jugular venous pressure. Abdominal palpitation revealed a tender, hard uterus with a symphysis–pubis height of 36 cm. Fetal palpation was difficult but a portable ultrasound scan on labour ward revealed a single fetus with cephalic presentation and a fetal heart rate of 80 bpm. Vaginal examination revealed a closed cervix.

What is the immediate management?

This patient has had a major placental abruption, compromising both her own circulation and fetal health. Despite the normal blood pressure, she should be regarded as being in shock as the blood pressure may reflect previous hypertension. Initial management is to resuscitate the woman. Venous access should be achieved with one (or two) 16 G venflons. Blood should be taken and sent for X-match (4–6 units), full blood count for haemoglobin and platelet concentrations, clotting studies and renal function. Fluid resuscitation with a mixture of crystalloid (such as normal saline), colloid and if necessary group O negative blood should be instituted. As excessive replacement is a risk, central venous monitoring of circulating volume is

valuable. When maternal condition is stabilized as far as possible delivery of the fetus can be considered.

What complications may occur?

These can be divided into maternal and fetal. She is at risk of further haemorrhage and developing DIC. Prompt delivery will reduce the risk of the latter, but if it develops her management should be in conjunction with the Haematology department. DIC is self-correcting after delivery as the source of thromboplastin causing fibrin, clotting factors and platelets to be consumed is removed. Where DIC is associated with on-going bleeding, fresh blood or clotting factors (in the form of fresh frozen plasma or cryo-precipitate) should be transfused. If other organ failure occurs management of the woman should be in an Intensive Care setting. The fetus has been active, but now has a bradycardia. It is likely that some degree of fetal compromise has occurred. As the uterine cervix is closed vaginal delivery will not be imminent. Delivery should therefore be by caesarean section. Even if born alive, the degree of fetal compromise sustained *in utero* may result in varying levels of infant morbidity or even neonatal death.

What longer term follow-up would be appropriate in this case?

Emergency admission with a pregnancy complication necessitating immediate delivery eight weeks before the EDD is a very stressful experience. If this is further complicated by medical problems in the mother, or by a child with handicap, post-traumatic stress syndrome can occur in the mother and her partner. They will have questions about what happened and why, and possibly about the likelihood of recurrence in future pregnancies. It is part of the management of abnormal pregnancy to see couples again, usually 6–8 weeks after the event, to address all their questions. This approach has been demonstrated.

blood group antigens. This is particularly important for the Rhesus D blood group, and all mothers who are D-negative should have a Kleihauer test to quantify the size of the feto-maternal haemorrhage and an appropriate dose of anti-D immunoglobulin.

Maternal mortality

Successive Confidential Enquiries into Maternal Mortality continue to record placental abruption as a significant cause of death, usually as a consequence of the complications listed above.

Recurrence

After a single episode of abruption the recurrence rate is approximately 10 per cent, increasing to 25 per cent after two episodes.

Placental abruption: effects on the fetus

Perinatal mortality

Abruption is a significant cause of fetal and neonatal loss. Perinatal mortality rates are influenced by size of abruption, interval to delivery, gestational age at which the abruption and delivery have occurred, and other associated factors such as growth retardation related to poor placentation.

Intrauterine growth restriction

This probably has two main components. The first cause is probably inadequate trophoblast invasion of the maternal decidua and spiral arteries, as with the increased risk of pre-eclampsia. Where abruption is chronic, or recurrent, the area of placenta available for nutrient and waste exchange between the fetus and the mother is reduced. This may also contribute to fetal growth restriction.

Management of placental abruption

Once the diagnosis has been made the management depends on the severity, the gestational age and the fetal and maternal conditions. As outlined in the clinical case above, for all but the most minor degrees of placental abruption the amount of blood lost from the maternal circulation is likely to be significant. For this reason the plasma volume should be monitored by CVP measurements and strict fluid balance, with urine output being measured hourly after urethral catheterization, should be performed. Where abruption has resulted in fetal death, maternal resuscitation followed by induction of labour, aiming for a vaginal delivery, is the usual management. When the fetus is still alive the decision on how best to deliver may be difficult. Immediate delivery by Caesarean Section may prevent both intrauterine death and the increased neonatal morbidity associated with delayed delivery. However, some patients will present in labour and where rapid delivery is anticipated

vaginal delivery may be acceptable, avoiding the increased complications of abdominal delivery where clotting disorders may supervene. In this latter situation close electronic monitoring of the fetal heart rate, with rapid resort to Caesarean Section is vital.

Where smaller degrees of abruption have occurred and there is no evidence of fetal distress, particularly where gestational age favours delaying the delivery to allow greater fetal maturity, conservative management may be instituted. This will require close monitoring of fetal wellbeing, using ultrasound scans of fetal growth, amniotic fluid volume, umbilical artery Doppler and cardiotocography. As with many complicated obstetric problems timing of delivery will be when the perceived risks of leaving the fetus undelivered outweigh the risk of premature delivery, and the decision is best taken in conjunction with either local Paediatricians, or with the Regional Neonatal Unit.

Risk factors for placenta abruption

- Hypertension
- Smoking
- Trauma to the abdomen
- Crack cocaine usage
- Anticoagulant therapy
- Polyhydramnios
- Low socio-economic
- IUGR

Clinical features

- Tender, tense uterus
- Tachycardia and hypotension out of proportion to vaginal bleeding
- Renal compromise
- Coagulation disorders: possibly DIC

🔑 Key Points

- Abnormal trophoblast invasion in the first trimester of pregnancy will not enable a low-resistance utero-placental circulation to develop
- The mechanism for this is not known, but its presence can be detected non-invasively by uterine artery Doppler ultrasound in the second trimester: 'notched' uterine artery waveforms indicate high resistance to flow before any problem is manifest
- The consequences of abnormal trophoblast invasion are pre-eclampsia, intrauterine growth restriction, placental abruption and intrauterine death
- The search for effective prophylaxis of these conditions has to date been only partially successful, and remains a major aim of perinatal medicine for the future.

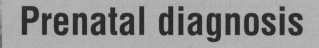

Chapter 1 2

Prenatal diagnosis

OVERVIEW

The term congenital abnormality refers to fetal malformations or disorders conferred by birth, rather than 'inherited' as is typically assumed. Although, there are numerous congenital abnormalities, the overall prevalence of disorders is approximately 2 per 100 pregnancies. The classification and incidence of common congenital abnormalities is shown in Table 12.1. The prenatal detection of congenital malformation is an essential part of routine antenatal care. This chapter presents an overview of prenatal testing in pregnancy.

The early prenatal detection of congenital abnormality allows both parents and medical carers to plan the management for the pregnancy. Where the fetal condition is untreatable or is associated with significant handicap, the parents may wish to terminate the pregnancy. Alternatively, the time, mode and place of delivery may be planned in order to ensure the optimal prognosis for the neonate. Parental decisions in prenatal diagnosis are dependent on their prior beliefs and expectations. Accurate provision of information regarding the incidence, likely outcome, screening and diagnosis of congenital abnormalities is an essential part of pregnancy care.

Prenatal screening and diagnostic tests

The distinction between screening and diagnosis is often blurred in common usage (Table 12.2). Screening tests are performed on all women in order to identify a subset of patients who are at high risk of a disorder. They do not confer any risk to the pregnancy and are performed for disorders with a relatively high prevalence and for which there are accurate prenatal diagnostic tests. Diagnostic tests on the other hand are carried out on pregnancies

that have been identified as high-risk by a prior screening test. They are usually invasive and carry a small risk of miscarriage. Inevitably the risks of being affected by the condition are severe enough to warrant consideration for a diagnostic test.

Invasive diagnostic tests

A number of different tests exist to enable sampling material of fetal origin (Table 12.3). The sample obtained can be used for cytogenetic, biochemical,

Table 12.1 – Classification and prevalence of common congenital abnormalities

Congenital abnormality	Example	Incidence per1000 births
Structural	Congenital heart disease	4–6
	Neural tube defects	2–6
	Cleft lip/palate	1–2
	Talipes equinovarus	1
Chromosomal	Trisomy 21 (Down's syndrome)	1.5
	Monosomy X (Turner's syndrome)	0.3
	Other trisomies (13 and 18)	0.3
Genetic	Cystic fibrosis	0.5
	Sickle cell disease	(depends on ethnicity)
Miscellaneous	Viral infection	0.2

Table 12.2 – Difference between prenatal screening and diagnostic tests

	Screening	Diagnostic tests
Population tested	All women	Women at 'high risk'
Purpose of test	Select a 'high-risk' group	To diagnose abnormality
Usual method of testing	Maternal history	Ultrasound
	Maternal biochemistry	Amniocentesis
	Maternal virology	Chorion villus sampling
	Ultrasound	Cordocentesis
Prerequisite to test	Diagnostic test available	Patient aware of potential risks
Risk of test	Anxiety of a 'screen positive' result	Small risk of miscarriage from invasive test

enzymatic or DNA analysis to give a prenatal diagnosis. Generally these tests are invasive in nature and carry a small risk of miscarriage.

Amniocentesis
A thin needle is passed transabdominally under ultrasound guidance into the amniotic cavity (Fig. 12.1). A small amount of amniotic fluid is removed, which contains fetal fibroblasts. This test is usually performed at or after 15 weeks' gestation. The procedure-related miscarriage rate for this test is 1 per cent. Although, it is technically possible to do amniocentesis at earlier gestations, this is generally avoided, as it is associated with a higher rate of miscarriage, neonatal talipes and respiratory difficulties.

Chorion villus sampling (CVS)
A thin needle is passed transabdominally or transcervically under ultrasound guidance into the placenta (chorionic plate) (Fig.12.1). Chorionic villi, which are fetoplacental in origin, are aspirated or biopsied through this needle. This test is usually performed at or after 10 weeks' gestation. Although the miscarriage rate after CVS is thought to be higher (2–3 per cent), this is because the background spontaneous miscarriage rate of pregnancy is higher at 10 weeks. The procedure-related miscarriage rate of CVS is the same as amniocentesis, 1 per cent. Although, it is technically possible to do CVS at earlier gestations, this is generally avoided, as it is associated with a higher rate of cleft lip/palate and digital amputation abnormalities.

Table 12.3 – Details of prenatal diagnostic procedures

	Amniocentesis	Chorion villus sampling	Cordocentesis
Gestation	15–40 weeks	10–40 weeks	20–40 weeks
Route	Transabdominal	Transabdominal/transcervical	Transabdominal
Cells sampled	Fetal fibroblasts	Trophoblast cells	Fetal white blood cells
Procedure-related risk of miscarriage	1%	1%	1%
Direct karyotype result	None	24–48hrs	Not needed
Culture karyotype result	2–3 weeks	1–2 weeks	24–48hrs
Mosaicism rate on karyotype	None	1%	None

Cordocentesis

A thin needle is passed transabdominally under ultrasound guidance into the umbilical cord to sample fetal blood (Fig. 12.1). This test is usually performed at or after 20 weeks' gestation. The procedure-related miscarriage rate for this test is 1 per cent. Although, it is technically possible to do this test at earlier gestations, this is generally avoided, as it is associated with a higher rate of miscarriage.

Laboratory analysis

Cytogenetic analysis

Cells obtained from invasive prenatal diagnostic tests are cultured until enough cells in mitosis are available to make a cytogenetic diagnosis. The more rapidly the tissue divides, the quicker the results are available. Hence the time for diagnosis for amniocentesis, CVS and cordocentesis is 2–3 weeks, 1–2 weeks and 24–48 hours, respectively. With CVS, the sampled chorionic villi have so many cells already in mitosis, that a 'direct' result may be available in 24–48 hours. In this instance, the quality of the diagnosis is adequate to exclude an aneuploidy (abnormal number of chromosomes). The direct preparation is usually not of sufficient quality to permit G-banding, hence chromosomal aberrations such as deletions or inversions cannot be effectively excluded.

DNA analysis

Fetal DNA obtained from invasive tests can be used for DNA probe (sickle cell disease and cystic fibrosis),

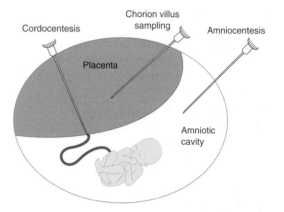
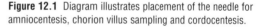

Figure 12.1 Diagram illustrates placement of the needle for amniocentesis, chorion villus sampling and cordocentesis.

polymerase chain reaction (PCR) (fragile X syndrome, congenital toxoplasmosis and cytomegalovirus) or linkage analysis (fragile X syndrome).

Biochemical and enzymatic analysis

When DNA analysis is not possible, biochemical or enzymatic assays can be performed for specific diseases (congenital adrenal hypoplasia and mucopolysaccharidoses).

Chromosomal abnormality

The most common chromosomal abnormalities can be classified as either aneuploidies (usually trisomies) or sex chromosome abnormalities.

Aneuploidies

Trisomies occur in the majority of cases due to non-dysjunction in meiosis. This abnormality of gameto-genesis is known to occur more frequently with advancing maternal age. Rarely, trisomies may occur due to unbalanced translocations (6 per cent) or mosaicism (4 per cent). Although any chromosome may be affected, the majority of trisomies result in first trimester miscarriage except for trisomies 13 (Patau's), 18 (Edward's) and 21 (Down's). Down's syndrome is associated with characteristic mental and physical features (Table 12.4). Trisomies 13 and 18 are associated with such major structural defects that their diagnosis is usually suspected on antenatal ultrasound. Since trisomies 13 and 18 have a very high intrauterine lethality (90–95 per cent), screening programmes are geared mainly towards the antenatal detection of Down's syndrome, which is the commonest chromosomal abnormality at birth.

Sex chromosome abnormalities

The prevalence of sex chromosome abnormalities does not change with maternal age, unlike trisomies. The cumulative prevalence of Turner's (monosomy X or 45XO), Klinefelter's (47XXY) and other sex chromosome abnormalities is greater than Down's syndrome. Turner's syndrome individuals are infertile females of normal intellect and short stature. Klinefelter's syndrome individuals are infertile males with slightly reduced IQ, testicular dysgenesis and tall stature. As many of the characteristics of these conditions are mild, many affected individuals remain undiagnosed throughout their lifetime. Routine screening for these conditions is not available and the diagnosis is often made incidentally.

Fragile X

Fragile X syndrome is the most common inherited cause of mental retardation, explaining the excess of males affected by non-specific mental retardation in the population. The fragile X gene (FMR1) becomes hypermethylated and inactivated multiple (>200) repeats. The estimated prevalence of the condition is 1:4000 males. Prenatal diagnosis is possible using PCR and Southern analysis, but only on male fetuses at present. As screening for fragile X in pregnancy is not feasible, prenatal testing is reserved for families where one of the parents is known to be a carrier by virtue of a previous affected pregnancy.

Screening tests for Down's syndrome

Maternal history

The prevalence of Down's syndrome increases with advancing maternal age, therefore women over 35 years are routinely screened (Fig. 12.2). However, 90 per cent of pregnant women are younger than 35 years and despite being at lower risk they give birth to 75–80 per cent of Down's syndrome babies. Women who have already had a pregnancy affected by Down's syndrome are also offered prenatal diagnosis, based on the finding that their background risk for trisomy is slightly increased.

Table 12.4 – Characteristic features of Down's syndrome

Intrauterine lethality	40% at 12–40 weeks
Mental effects	Mental retardation, deafness, short-sightedness
Physical effects	Flat facies, macroglossia, cardiac septal defects (40%), intestinal atresias
Postnatal outcome	Premature ageing, reduced immunity, leukaemia, reduced life-span

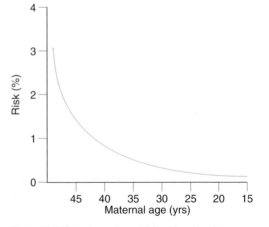

Figure 12.2 Down's syndrome risk and maternal age.

Maternal serum biochemistry

Measurement of maternal serum hormones at 15–22 weeks' gestation offers an alternative method of screening. The two main hormones of fetal origin that are commonly assayed are alpha-fetoprotein (AFP) and human chorionic gonadotrophin (hCG). In Down's syndrome these levels are decreased and increased, respectively. Based on maternal age, gestation and variation in hormone levels, an algorithm predicts the individual's risk for Down's syndrome.

Nuchal translucency

A newer screening test for Down's syndrome involves the sonographic measurement of a translucent space on the neck of the fetus at 10–13 weeks' gestation. The nuchal translucency measurement is increased in the majority of aneuploid fetuses in the first trimester of pregnancy (Fig.

12.3a and b and Table 12.5). Based on maternal age, gestation and nuchal translucency measurement, an algorithm predicts the individual's risk for Down's syndrome. The advantage of early screening being that the termination of pregnancy, if required, may be performed as a day case surgical procedure rather than by induction of labour as is often required after maternal serum biochemistry which takes place at 15–22 weeks.

Structural abnormality

Structural abnormalities constitute the majority of congenital abnormalities encountered in clinical practice. Fetal neural tube and cardiac defects have established screening programmes and are discussed in detail in this section. The remainder of fetal

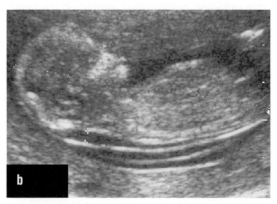

Figure 12.3 First trimester measurement of fetal nuchal translucency. (a) Normal, (b) 3.5 mm (increased) suggestive of chromosome abnormality.

Table 12.5 – Screening tests for Down's syndrome

	Maternal age	Maternal serum biochemistry	Nuchal translucency
Method	History	Blood test	Ultrasound scan
Gestation	Any	15–22 weeks	10–13 weeks
False-positive rate	5–10%	5%	5%
Sensitivity	25%	60–75%	75–80%
Advantages	Simple	Cheap	Early test
		Operator-independent	Screens for all aneuploidy
Disadvantages	Poor sensitivity	Late test	Operator-dependent
		Specific for Down's	
		Requires dating scan	

structural malformations occurs less commonly and is sporadic in nature.

Neural tube defects

Neural tube defects (NTDs) are among the most common major malformations in most countries. NTDs occur due to defects in the formation of the neural tube during embryogenesis. The aetiology is multifactorial with well-defined environmental, genetic, pharmacological and geographical factors implicated.

The majority of NTDs affect the cranial vault, presenting as anencephaly or encephalocoele. The former is universally lethal, while the prognosis from encephalocoele is inversely related to the size of the defect. The remainder of NTDs, termed spina bifida, usually affects the spinal cord at the caudal end. The local effects of spina bifida (paralysis of the legs, urinary and faecal incontinence) depend on the spinal level and the number of spinal segments affected in the lesion. Spina bifida has previously been associated with impaired intellect due to progressive hydrocephalus and infection of ventriculo-peritoneal shunts. With modern imaging techniques and antibiotics, the intellectual prognosis for this condition is much improved.

Prenatal screening and diagnosis of NTDs

When a parent or previous sibling has had an NTD, the risk of recurrence is 5–10 per cent. Mid-trimester maternal serum AFP levels are increased in pregnancies affected by open NTDs, with the risk being related to the AFP level. These were once used as the established screening tests for NTDs, with screen pos-

itive women being referred for amniocentesis. The presence of acetyl-cholinesterase, a CNS neurotransmitter, in amniotic fluid was taken as being diagnostic of an open NTD. The need for a two-step screening/diagnosis process was quickly superseded by the development of high-resolution ultrasound. Anencephaly and encephalocoeles are detectable on first trimester ultrasound, if an adequate examination of the cranial vault is performed at the same time (Fig. 12.4). Spina bifida on the other hand requires the systematic detailed examination of the fetal spine (Fig. 12.5a and b) at the routine 20-week anomaly scan. The diagnosis may be suspected from the visualization of the 'lemon' (shape of the skull) and 'banana' (absent cerebellum) signs in the fetal brain at this examination (Fig. 12.6a and b). The sensitivity of ultrasound for both open and NTDs is greater than 95 per cent. Other CNS abnormalities (not strictly NTDs), such as hydrocephalus, can also be detected at the 20-week scan (Fig. 12.7 and Table 12.6).

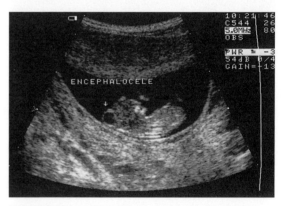

Figure 12.4 Fetal encephalocoele detected at 12 weeks' gestation.

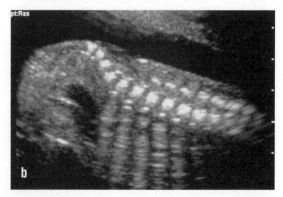

Figure 12.5 (a) Normal fetal spine showing posterior spinous process. (b) Abnormal fetal spine with spinous process absent in the sacral and 5th lumbar segments.

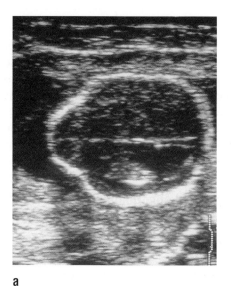

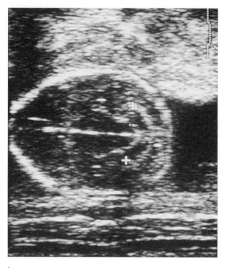

a   b

Figure 12.6 (a) Lemon-shaped skull, (b) curved (banana) cerebellum, which are typical cranial signs of spina bifida.

Prevention of NTDs

Folate deficiency and drugs that interfere with folate metabolism (i.e. anti-epileptics) are implicated in about 10 per cent of NTD cases. Periconceptual folate supplementation of the maternal diet reduces by about half the risk of developing these defects. Folic acid should be given for at least three months prior to conception and for the first trimester of pregnancy. The dosage of folic acid is 400 µg for primary prevention and 4 mg in women wishing to prevent a recurrence of an NTD.

Congenital heart defects

Abnormalities of the heart and great arteries are the most common congenital abnormalities. About half are either lethal or require major surgery and the remainder are asymptomatic. The aetiology of congenital heart defects (CHDs) is heterogeneous and

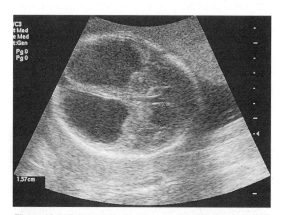

Figure 12.7 Enlarged cerebral ventricles at 22 weeks, diagnostic of hydrocephalus.

includes genetic factors, environmental factors (e.g. diabetes mellitus, drugs (e.g. lithium) and viral infections (e.g. rubella). Gene mutations and chromosomal abnormalities account for less than 5 per cent of cases.

Table 12.6 – Some major structural abnormalities detectable by ultrasound at the mid-trimester scan

The abnormalities with an asterisk can frequently be detected at the first trimester scan

Body system	Example
Cranium	Anencephaly*
	Encephalocoele*
	Hydrocephalus
Skeleton	Spina bifida
	Kyphoscoliosis
Thorax	Congenital heart disease
	Cystic adenomatoid malformation
	Diaphragmatic hernia
Abdomen	Gastroschisis
	Exomphalos*
	Renal agenesis
	Multi/polycystic disease
	Hydronephrosis
Limbs	Talipes equinovarus
	Polydactyly*

Prenatal screening for CHDs

When a previous sibling or father is affected by CHD, the risk is 2 per cent. When two siblings or the mother has CHD, the recurrence risk is 10 per cent. The second major group considered to be at high risk is maternal diabetes mellitus, where the incidence of CHD is doubled. However, more than 90 per cent of fetuses with CHD are from pregnancies without such risk factors.

Prenatal diagnosis of CHDs

Although in specialist centres 90 per cent of major CHDs may be detected antenatally, in most general units performing routine 20-week anomaly scans this figure is closer to 30 per cent. As specialist fetal echocardiography cannot be performed on all pregnancies, the limiting factor in diagnosis is selection of cases for referral to these specialist units (Fig. 12.8a and b).

Other structural abnormalities

Cleft lip/palate

The typical cleft lip appears as a linear defect extending from the lip to the nostril, with the majority of cases (75 per cent) being unilateral. In about 50 per cent of cases, both the lip and palate are defective, in the remainder either the lip or palate is involved. Cleft lip (+/- palate) is identifiable on ultrasound, whereas the diagnosis of isolated cleft palate is difficult. Associated abnormalities are found in about 15 per cent of fetuses with cleft lip/palate, usually because genetic or chromosomal abnormalities are implicated in the aetiology. Postnatally, because of cosmetic, feeding and respiratory problems, early surgical correction is usually advocated.

Talipes equinovarus

In talipes equinovarus, also known as clubfoot, the forefoot is supinated and the ankle is plantar flexed. The deformity is bilateral in 50 per cent of cases and affects twice as many males as females. The aetiology is sporadic and the condition is neurological in origin,

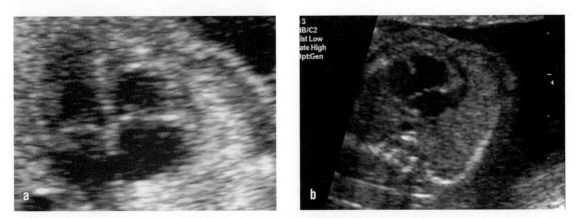

Figure 12.8 (a) Normal four chamber fetal heart, (b) abnormal heart with atrio-ventricular and septal defect.

with the skeletal malformation being secondary. The diagnosis is reliably established on ultrasound, except in positional talipes, a temporary malformation secondary to oligohydramnios. Talipes equinovarus is lethal in about 20 per cent of cases because of associated malformations, most commonly spina bifida.

Genetic disorders

There are numerous congenital abnormalities that exhibit a classical mendelian pattern of inheritance. The commonest of these, cystic fibrosis and the haemoglobinopathies, are discussed below. Additionally numerous genetic syndromes exist, the majority of which are sporadic but some with recessive, dominant or sex-linked patterns of inheritance. The latter have a relatively low frequency and are only screened for after the family has undergone genetic counselling regarding the disease, likelihood of recurrence, diagnostic tests and possible therapeutic interventions.

Cystic fibrosis

Cystic fibrosis is an autosomal recessive condition and the most common lethal genetic disease in Caucasians. The cystic fibrosis gene has been isolated to the long arm of chromosome 7 and there are over 700 mutations identified to this region that are responsible for the disease. The commonest of these mutations is ΔF508, which is present in 68 per cent of cases. Multiple gene mutations and the cost of DNA testing for the population are the major reasons why effective parental screening has not been effective to date. At present prenatal diagnosis is offered only to parents who are known carriers, usually because they have had an affected child already.

Haemoglobinopathies

Sickle cell anaemia and thalassaemia are both autosomal recessive conditions with considerable disease heterogeneity. The carrier frequency may be as high as 20 per cent, especially in African (sickle cell disease) and Mediterranean (thalassaemia) populations. Screening of at-risk populations is possible by haemoglobin electrophoresis. Sickle cell mutations are limited in number and fairly well characterized,

hence prenatal diagnosis is usually possible. As there are numerous thalassaemia mutations, parental studies are a prerequisite to establish whether a fetal diagnosis is possible. Prenatal diagnosis is made on fetal DNA, which can be obtained by any of the invasive techniques. As the risk of an affected pregnancy is high (25 per cent) for parents who are carriers, early testing through CVS is advocated.

Congenital viral and parasitic infections

Fetal infection with rubella, cytomegalovirus (CMV), toxoplasmosis and parvovirus are known to have potentially serious deleterious effects (Table 12.7) and these are discussed in detail in Chapter 15. Maternal viral infections in pregnancy are relatively infrequent, with the likelihood of transplacental transfer and fetal infection increasing with gestational age. Most infected fetuses (>95 per cent), however, remain unaffected. The risk of a congenitally infected fetus being affected is inversely proportional to the gestational age. Hence, although the chance of fetal infection is low in early pregnancy, if infected the fetus is likely to be seriously affected and the pregnancy is doomed to miscarriage. Therefore, the most susceptible pregnancies are those infected at 12–18 weeks' gestation, when infected fetuses are likely to be seriously affected and yet survive.

Screening for congenital viral and parasitic infections

There is an established screening programme for rubella in pregnancy. Rubella-susceptible women are advised to avoid antenatal exposure to the virus and are vaccinated in the puerperium. Screening is not advocated for maternal CMV or toxoplasmosis infections in pregnancy because of the low incidence, the high false-positive rates and the miscarriage rate of prenatal diagnosis to confirm fetal infection. Additionally, confirming fetal infection does not necessarily indicate that the fetus has been affected.

Prenatal diagnosis of congenital viral and parasitic infections

In cases of confirmed maternal viral infection, regular fetal ultrasound to detect the characteristic features of congenital infection is advocated. There is limited evidence that treatment of toxoplasmosis-infected mothers with spiramycin may prevent

Table 12.7 – Characteristics of congenital viral infection

	Rubella	Cytomegalovirus	Toxoplasmosis	Parvovirus
Source	Infected individuals	Infected individuals	Cat litter Undercooked meat	Infected children
Features of congenital infection	Cataracts Heart defects Growth restriction Hepatomegaly Thrombocytopenia Mental retardation	Microcephaly Ventriculomegaly Cerebral calcification Heart defects Growth restriction Hepatomegaly Thrombocytopenia Mental retardation	Microcephaly Ventriculomegaly Cerebral calcification Heart defects Growth restriction Hepatomegaly Thrombocytopenia Mental retardation	Aplastic anaemia Hydrops

congenital fetal infection. Congenital parvovirus infection may result in a temporary fetal aplastic anaemia and hydrops. Supportive therapy with fetal intrauterine blood transfusions in these cases dramatically improves the prognosis.

Future developments in prenatal diagnosis

Fetal cells in the maternal circulation
The presence of fetal cells in maternal blood is an established phenomenon. The methods for their isolation, identification and genetic analysis continue to be refined. Most investigators are focused on the isolation of fetal nucleated red blood or trophoblastic cells. The validation of a reliable technique for the safe, non-invasive acquisition of fetal cells will revolutionize prenatal diagnosis.

Fluorescent *in situ* hybridization (FISH)
Rapid FISH analysis of interphase cells has become an essential part of routine cytogenetics in prenatal diagnosis. A variety of DNA probes are available for use, ranging from chromosome-specific to single-gene copy probes. The use of FISH analysis has significantly decreased the time between sampling and a reliable cytogenetic diagnosis. Amniocentesis, which is a technically simpler procedure than CVS, now can produce results to exclude specific genetic diagnosis in a few days. The accuracy of these results is similar to that of direct results after CVS.

Preimplantation genetic diagnosis (PGD)
Couples at high risk of having pregnancies with inherited diseases may benefit from PGD in the early stages of human zygote/embryo development. The development of PGD allows parents to avoid the decision to terminate a pregnancy. PGD has evolved from the development of safe and effective techniques for embryo biopsy and the appropriate methods of genetic diagnosis by FISH or PCR.

3-D ultrasound
Advanced imaging technology has permitted the real-time 3-D reconstruction of data acquired by specially adopted ultrasound machines. This technology permits the increased resolution required for certain fetal malformations such as cleft lip/palate. Routine 2-D ultrasound requires the sonographer to 'reconstruct' the third dimension in a mental image. The real practical value of 3-D ultrasound technology is the potential to allow the remote acquisition of ultrasound data by technicians that can latter be analysed by appropriate experts.

Fetal magnetic resonance imaging (MRI)
The uses of prenatal MRI are being evaluated increasingly. The development of ultra-fast MRI sequences to overcome fetal movement artefact has resulted in significant improvement in the quality and usefulness of the image. MRI has the potential to become a powerful adjunct to the evaluation of the abnormal fetus discovered on ultrasound.

References for further reading

Milunsky A. (ed.) *Genetic disorders and the fetus: diagnosis, prevention and treatment.* London: John Hopkins Press Ltd, 1998.

Pilu G, Nicolaides KH. (eds) *Diagnosis of fetal abnormalities: the 18-23 week scan.* London: Parthenon Publishing, 1999.

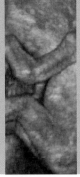

Multiple gestation

OVERVIEW

In 1–2 per cent of pregnancies there is more than one fetus. The chances of miscarriage, fetal abnormalities, poor fetal growth, preterm delivery and intrauterine or neonatal death are considerably higher in twin than in singleton pregnancies. In about two-thirds of twins the fetuses are non-identical, or dizygotic, and in one-third they are identical, or monozygotic. In all dizygotic pregnancies there are two separate placentas (dichorionic). In two-thirds of monozygotic twins there are vascular communications within the two placental circulations (monochorionic) and in the other one-third of cases there is dichorionic placentation. Monochorionic, compared to dichorionic twins have a much higher risk of abnormalities and death. The maternal risks are also increased in multiple gestations including adverse symptoms such as nausea and vomiting, tiredness and discomfort, and risks of serious complications including hypertensive and thromboembolic disease and antepartum and postpartum haemorrhage.

Types of multiple gestation

Multiple gestation results from the ovulation and subsequent fertilization of more than one oocyte. In such cases the fetuses are genetically different (dizygotic or non-identical). Multiple gestation can also result from the splitting of one embryonic mass to form two or more genetically identical fetuses (monozygotic).

Dizygotic twins have their own amniotic sac (diamniotic), and placenta (dichorionic). In monozygotic twins, there may be sharing of the same placenta (monochorionic), amniotic sac (monoamniotic) or even fetal organs (conjoined or Siamese). When the single embryonic mass splits into two

within three days of fertilization, which occurs in one-third of monozygotic twins, each fetus has its own amniotic sac and placenta (diamniotic and dichorionic). When embryonic splitting occurs after the 3rd day following fertilization, there are vascular communications within the two placental circulations (monochorionic). Embryonic splitting after the 9th day following fertilization results in monoamniotic monochorionic twins and splitting after the 12th day results in conjoined twins.

Incidence and epidemiology

Twins account for about 1 per cent of all pregnancies with two-thirds being dizygotic and one-third monozygotic (Fig. 13.1). The incidence of twins varies with:

- ethnic group (up to 5 times higher in certain parts of Africa and half as high in parts of Asia);
- maternal age (2 per cent at 35 years);
- parity (2 per cent after four pregnancies);
- method of conception (20 per cent with ovulation induction);
- family history.

The incidence of monozygotic twins is similar in all ethnic groups and does not vary with maternal age, parity or method of conception.

The incidence of spontaneous multifetal (more than two) pregnancies can be derived from Hellin's rule (1 in 80^{n-1} pregnancies). In recent years assisted reproduction techniques, such as ovulation induction and *in vitro* fertilization, have become very important causes of multiple gestations and about 20 per cent of assisted reproduction pregnancies are multiple.

Determination of zygosity and chorionicity

Zygosity can only be determined by DNA fingerprinting. Prenatally, such testing would require an invasive procedure to sample amniotic fluid (amniocentesis), placental tissue (chorion villus sampling), or fetal blood (cordocentesis).

Chorionicity can be determined by ultrasound and relies on the assessment of fetal gender, number of placentas, and characteristics of the membrane between the two amniotic sacs. Different-sex twins are dizygotic and therefore dichorionic, but in about two-thirds of twin pregnancies the fetuses are of the same sex and these may be either monozygotic or dizygotic. Similarly, if there are two separate placentas the pregnancy is dichorionic, but in the majority of cases the two placentas are adjacent to each other and there are often difficulties in distinguishing between dichorionic-fused and monochorionic placentas. In dichorionic twins the inter-twin membrane is composed of a central layer of chorionic tissue sandwiched between two layers of amnion, whereas in monochorionic twins there is no chorionic layer. Consequently, the inter-twin membrane is thicker and more echogenic in dichorionic than monochorionic pregnancies but this is a subjective and poorly reproducible feature.

The best way to determine chorionicity is by an ultrasound examination in the first trimester of pregnancy. In dichorionic twins there is an extension of placental tissue into the base of the inter-twin membrane, referred to as the 'lambda' sign, whereas in monochorionic twins this sign is absent (Fig. 13.2).

Pregnancy complications according to chorionicity

Miscarriage and severe preterm delivery

The most important complication of any pregnancy is delivery before term and especially before 32 weeks (Fig. 13.3). Almost all babies born before 24 weeks die and almost all born after 32 weeks survive. Delivery between 24 and 32 weeks is associated with a high chance of neonatal death and survivors are usually handicapped. In a singleton pregnancy the chance of delivery between 12 and 23 weeks (miscarriage) is about 1 per cent, and the chance of delivery between 24 and 32 weeks is also about 1 per cent. In dichorionic twins the chance of miscarriage is 2 per cent and of delivery at 24–32 weeks is 5 per cent. In monochorionic twins the chances are 12 per cent and 10 per cent respectively. The average gestation at delivery for twins is 37 weeks and therefore about half of twins deliver preterm. As in singleton pregnancies, neither bedrest nor prophylactic administration of tocolytics are useful in preventing preterm delivery.

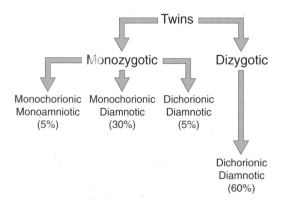

Figure 13.1 Incidence of monozygotic and dizygotic twins.

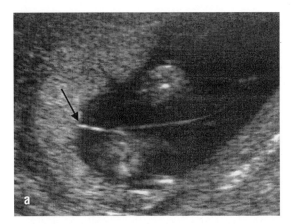
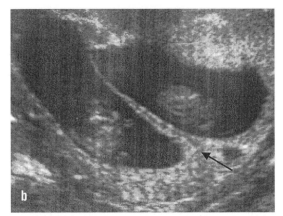

Figure 13.2 Ultrasound appearance of monochorionic (a) and dichorionic (b) twin pregnancies at 12 weeks' gestation. Note that in both types there appears to be a single placental mass but in the dichorionic type there is an extension of placental tissue into the base of the inter-twin membrane forming the lambda sign.

Perinatal mortality in twins

The perinatal mortality rate in twins is around six times higher than in singletons. This high rate is almost entirely due to prematurity-related complications and it is therefore twice as high in monochorionic than dichorionic twin pregnancies. In

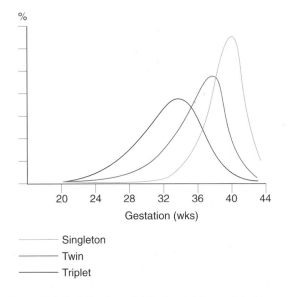

Figure 13.3 Gestational age distribution at delivery of singleton, twin and triplet pregnancies.

monochorionic twins, an additional complication to prematurity is twin-to-twin transfusion syndrome.

Intrauterine growth restriction

In singleton pregnancies the birth weight is below the 5th centile for gestation in about 5 per cent of babies. In dichorionic twins the chances of low birth weight is double for each baby than in singletons and therefore the risk that at least one of the fetuses will suffer poor growth is about 20 per cent. In monochorionic twins the chance of poor fetal growth is almost double that of dichorionic twins.

In singleton pregnancies where it is presumed that utero-placental insufficiency is the cause of fetal growth restriction, the main aims of antenatal care are to predict the severity of impaired fetal oxygenation and to select the appropriate time for delivery. This is done by balancing the relative risks of intrauterine death with the expectant management and risk of neonatal death or handicap from preterm delivery. In extreme cases of placental insufficiency, delivery may be undertaken as early as 26–28 weeks.

In dichorionic twin pregnancies where one fetus has intrauterine growth restriction, the condition of both fetuses needs to be considered since the potential benefit of delivery for the small fetus must be weighed against the risk of prematurity-related complications in the normally grown twin. In general, delivery should be avoided before 32 weeks even if there is evidence of imminent intrauterine death of the smaller twin. Such a policy may not be applicable in the management of monochorionic twins since death of one fetus may result in death or handicap of its co-twin because of complications arising from the presence of placental vascular anastamoses between the two circulations.

Monitoring for fetal growth and wellbeing in twins is by ultrasound scan to assess fetal measurements, fetal activity and amniotic fluid volume. When one or both fetuses are small the condition of the fetuses can be monitored by cardiotocography and Doppler assessment of the fetal circulations.

Fetal abnormalities

The prevalance of structural abnormalities, such as spina bifida, for each fetus in a dichorionic twin pregnancy is the same as in singleton pregnancies and therefore the chance that in such twin pregnancies at least one of the fetuses would be affected is twice as high as in singleton pregnancies. In monochorionic twin pregnancies the risk for abnormalities for each fetus is four times as high as in singleton pregnancies.

Multiple gestations showing abnormality in one fetus can essentially be managed expectantly or by selective fetocide of the abnormal twin. In cases where the abnormality is non-lethal but may well result in handicap, the parents need to decide whether the potential burden of a handicapped child is enough to risk the loss of the normal twin from fetocide-related complications. In cases where the abnormality is lethal it may be best to avoid such risk to the normal fetus, unless the condition itself threatens the survival of the normal twin. Anencephaly is a good example of a lethal abnormality that can threaten the survival of the normal twin because in more than 50 per cent of pregnancies affected by fetal anencephaly there is polyhydramnios which can cause severe preterm delivery of the abnormal, and also the normal, co-twin. See Table 13.1.

Chromosomal defects and twinning

In monozygotic twin pregnancies, chromosomal abnormalities, such as Down's syndrome, affect either none or both fetuses. The risk for chromosomal abnormalities, as in singleton pregnancies, increases with maternal age.

In dizygotic twins, the maternal age-related risk for chromosomal abnormalities for each twin may also be the same as in singleton pregnancies. Therefore, the chance that at least one fetus is affected by a chromosomal defect is twice as high as in singleton pregnancies of the same maternal age. However, the rate of dizygotic-twinning increases with maternal age, and in addition, with the more widespread availability of assisted reproductive techniques the mean maternal age in dizygotic twins is increasing. Consequently, the overall prevalence of chromosomal defects in dizygotic twins is higher than in singletons.

The relative proportion of spontaneous dizygotic to monozygotic twins in the UK is about 2:1 and therefore the prevalence of chromosomal abnormalities affecting at least one fetus in twin pregnancies overall would be about 1.6 times that in singletons.

If the pregnancy is dichorionic, the parents can be counselled that the risk of one fetus developing a chromosomal abnormality is about twice that in singleton pregnancies. The risk that both fetuses would be affected can be derived by squaring the singleton risk ratio. For example, in a 40-year-old woman with a risk for Trisomy 21, based on maternal age, of about 1 in 100, in a dizygotic twin pregnancy the risk that one fetus would be affected is 1 in 50 (1 in 100 plus 1 in 100). However, the risk that both fetuses would be affected is 1 in 10,000 (1 in 100 x 1 in 100).

Tests for detection of Trisomy 21 using maternal serum biochemistry (see Chapter 12) are not effective in multiple gestations. The best method of screening in twins is by measurement of fetal nuchal translucency thickness in each fetus by ultrasound at 10–14 weeks. If invasive prenatal diagnosis is required (see Chapter 12), this may be carried out by amniocentesis or chorion villus sampling, but since it is essential that both fetuses are sampled and that the results correspond to the correct fetus, this should always be carried out in specialist centres.

Death of one fetus in a twin pregnancy

Intrauterine death of a fetus in a twin pregnancy may be associated with a poor outcome for the co-twin but the type and degree of risk is dependent on chorionicity. Second or third trimester intrauterine death of one fetus may be associated with the onset of labour in dichorionic twins, and acute hypotensive episodes in monochorionic twins leading to death or handicap of the co-twin in about 25 per cent of cases. The mechanism is acute haemodynamic shifts from the live to the dead fetus.

Following intrauterine death and retention of the fetus in singleton pregnancies maternal complications such as disseminated intravascular coagulation have been reported, but in twin pregnancies the incidence of this complication is very low.

Complications unique to monochorionic twinning

In all monochorionic twin pregnancies there are placental vascular anastamoses present which allow communication of the two fetoplacental circulations. In some monochorionic twin pregnancies, imbalance in the net flow of blood across the placental vascular arterio-venous communications from one fetus, the donor, to the other, the recipient, results in twin-to-twin transfusion syndrome (TTTS). The development of mild, moderate or severe TTTS depends on the net flow. The precise underlying mechanisms by which a select population of monochorionic pregnancies with vascular communications that develop TTTS is not fully understood.

The donor fetus suffers from both hypovolaemia due to blood loss and hypoxia due to placental insufficiency. There is a compensatory redistribution in the fetal circulation with preferential perfusion of the brain at the expense of the viscera. This fetus becomes growth restricted and oliguric. The recipient fetus exhibits hypervolaemia, leading to polyuria and polyhydramnios, and high output cardiac failure. Severe disease becomes apparent at 18–24 weeks of pregnancy, with the mother complaining of a sudden increase in abdominal girth associated with extreme discomfort. On clinical examination there is tense polyhydramnios and ultrasound examination reveals polyhydramnios in the recipient fetus and oligohydramnios in the growth-restricted donor fetus.

More than 90 per cent of pregnancies complicated by TTTS end in miscarriage or severe preterm delivery, due to the polyhydramnios or intrauterine death of one or both fetuses. A common method of treatment is amniocentesis every 1–2 weeks and drainage of large volumes of amniotic fluid; this treatment improves survival by prolonging the pregnancy. A more recent method involves the introduction of a thin endoscope into the uterus and the use of laser to coagulate the placental blood vessels that connect the circulations of the two fetuses; in about 70 per cent of pregnancies one or both babies survive.

Clinical features

The clinical features of multiple gestations are related to firstly, the increased uterine size for a given gestation, and secondly, the increased production of pregnancy-related hormones, which leads to exaggeration of the normal maternal responses in pregnancy (see Chapter 5). In a twin pregnancy, compared to a singleton, the maternal cardiac output, pulmonary tidal volume, glomerular filtration rate, gastrointestinal changes and haematological changes, due to increase in plasma volume, are greater.

Table 13.1 – Common pregnancy complications in twin pregnancies according to chorionicity, compared with singleton pregnancies

Complication	Singleton	Twins	
		Dichorionic	Monochorionic
Miscarriage at 12–23 wks	1%	2%	12%
Delivery at 24–32 wks	1%	5%	10%
Growth restriction	5%	10%	20%
Fetal defects	1%	2%	8%

Key Points

Diagnosis of multiple gestation

History
- Assisted conception
- Family history of multiple gestation
- Increased 'symptoms of pregnancy'
- Abdomen larger than expected for gestation

Clinical examination
- Uterus larger than expected for gestation
- More than two fetal poles present
- Two fetal heart beats (at different rates) present

Investigations
- Ultrasound examination

Routine antenatal care of multiple gestations

In view of the increased risk of complications, these pregnancies should be managed in hospital obstetric units by a consultant-led team and require additional surveillance as well as the routine antenatal care given to all women. Ideally they should be seen in a specialist clinic where advice is available regarding practical aspects of preparation for caring with two or more babies at once, as well as providing specialist medical care. Mothers should be given the option to contact parent support groups such as TAMBA (Twin and Multiple Birth Association) early in the pregnancy. Visits should be four weekly until 28 weeks, twice weekly to 32 weeks, then weekly, with increased frequency if complications develop.

In multiple gestations ultrasound examination plays a major role in management. In the first trimester it is used to diagnose the number of fetuses, determine chorionicity, accurately date the pregnancy (especially important because of the risk of preterm delivery), and detect major fetal abnormalities. In the second trimester it is used to detect fetal abnormalities, in the third trimester to monitor fetal growth and wellbeing, and in labour, to determine presentation and position of the fetuses. Additional ultrasound examinations are needed in monochorionic pregnancies to detect the development of TTTS, and in all cases if complications occur.

Pregnancy complications and their management

Hyperemesis gravidarum

Increased placental hormone production, especially human chorionic gonadotrophin, may lead to severe vomiting in the first trimester. All cases of hyperemesis should therefore undergo an ultrasound scan to diagnose multiple gestation (and other causes such as hydatidiform mole). This complication is managed the same way as in singletons (see Chapter 14).

Hypertensive disease

Pregnancy-associated hypertension occurs about three to five times more commonly in multiple gestations than singletons, and may occur at an earlier gestation and be more severe. Management principles are the same as in singletons (see Chapter 11).

Gestational diabetes

The increased levels of diabetogenic placental hormones in multiple gestation result in a greater prevalence of gestational diabetes and routine screening should be carried out according to local policy (see Chapter 16).

Anaemia

Increased plasma volume expansion and increased feto-placental demand for iron and folic acid lead to an increased prevalence of anaemia which may require dietary supplementation.

'Minor' symptoms of pregnancy

Gastro-oesophageal reflux, abdominal discomfort, back pain, leg swelling, bladder symptoms and haemorrhoids are all more common and/or severe in multiple gestation due to the increased size of the uterus and the increased placental hormone levels. Management is symptomatic, as for singletons.

Antepartum haemorrhage (placenta praevia, placental abruption)

Antepartum haemorrhage is a major contributor to perinatal mortality and the prevalence of antepartum haemorrhage is increased in multiple gestations both due to the larger placental area and increase in other complications, such as hypertensive disease, which may lead to placental abruption.

Thromboembolic disease

The more marked prothromboembolic physiological alterations and the increased effect of uterine pelvic venous compression leads to increased risk of thromboembolic disease and appropriate prophylaxis and treatment should be given (see Chapter 14).

Labour and delivery

Malpresentations

The presentation of the first twin will be vertex in about 70 per cent of twin pregnancies but the prevalence of malpresentations is increased, presumably due to uterine crowding preventing fetal movement. In such cases there are the associated risks of any malpresentation, such as cord prolapse. The position and presentation of the second twin is essentially irrelevant until after delivery of the first since it will move to occupy the available space. The second twin may therefore present as a breech, compound or shoulder much more commonly than in singletons and manipulation, either external or internal version with or without ultrasound guidance, is often required for delivery of the second twin. Fetal heart rate monitoring should be continued throughout the delivery of both twins. Oxytocin may be required if uterine contractions decrease following delivery of the first twin, although there is no urgency to deliver the second twin within a set time period providing both mother and baby remain well.

A specific complication, rarely seen in practice, of twin pregnancies delivery vaginally is 'locked twins' in which the first is a breech presentation and the second a vertex, and during delivery of the

presenting twin the two heads become locked, necessitating operative delivery.

Mode of delivery

If the first twin is presenting by the vertex and there are no other complications, many obstetricians will allow a vaginal delivery with the same contraindications as for singletons. However, since in some twin vaginal deliveries there may be complications in delivery of the second twin which require an instrumental or operative intervention, some obstetricians prefer to deliver most multiple gestations by elective Caesarean Section. Ultimately, the decision in each case must be based on the previous obstetric history, the presentation, presence or absence of other complications, and maternal preferences.

In the presence of a previous lower segment Caesarean Section the contraindications for trial of vaginal delivery are the same as in singletons.

Anaesthesia

Since operative or instrumental assistance to deliver the second twin is much more likely than in singletons it may be recommended that an epidural is sited during labour which will provide pain relief and allow for rapid additional anesthesia should operative intervention be required.

Labour management

An IV line should be sited since operative intervention may be required and there is increased risk of antepartum and postpartum haemorrhage. A twin cardiotocography machine and portable ultrasound machine should be available, and it is essential that two resuscitation trolleys, two obstetricians and two paediatricians are available for the delivery and that the special care baby unit is informed well in advance of the delivery.

Postpartum haemorrhage

Due to the large placental site and excessive uterine distention with consequent lack of uterine muscle tone, the risk of postpartum haemorrhage is increased in twin pregnancies. Management is as for singletons, but all multiple gestations should have an IV line sited and blood grouped and saved during labour, and an oxytocin infusion is often commenced following delivery (see Chapter 19).

Embryo reduction in higher order multiple gestations

A consequence of the widespread introduction of assisted reproductive techniques has been an exponential increase in the prevalence of multifetal pregnancies, which are associated with increased risk of both miscarriage and perinatal death, primarily as a consequence of severe preterm delivery. The objective of iatrogenic embryo reduction is to improve pregnancy outcome by reducing this complication and has now become one of the established options in the management of such pregnancies and is an efficient and safe way of improving outcome for quadruplets or higher order.

Iatrogenic fetal death is achieved by the ultrasound-guided puncture of the fetal heart and injection of potassium chloride. During the months following reduction there is gradual resorption of the dead fetuses and their placentas. Although it is technically feasible to perform reduction from as early as seven weeks' gestation it is usually preferable to delay until around 11 weeks to allow for spontaneous reduction, to diagnose major fetal abnormalities and screen for chromosomal defects in order to determine which fetuses should be reduced. As with any uterine needling procedure, there are associated risks, the overall risk of miscarriage being about 10 per cent. The risk of subsequent miscarriage and severe preterm delivery increases with the number of fetuses reduced.

CASE HISTORY

Miss PO

Aged 32, single supported research scientist

Otherwise fit and well

Para 0

Subfertility requiring clomiphene ovarian stimulation

Triplet pregnancy noted on transvaginal scan at 8 weeks

Now 13 weeks: trichorionic, triamniotic triplet pregnancy; all fetuses appear structurally normal and all have nuchal measurements that represent a considerable reduction in her age-related risk of Down's.

What obstetric risks does Miss O face?

The risks of miscarriage, and more particularly severe preterm delivery are far higher with a triplet pregnancy. The mean gestation at delivery is approximately 34 weeks and perinatal morbidity and mortality is much increased over a singleton pregnancy. In addition, pre-eclampsia and venous thromboembolism are slightly more frequent in multiple gestation. She will suffer much more from the 'minor' conditions of pregnancy; backache, varicose veins, heartburn and anaemia particularly.

Might embryo reduction be considered?

This is an option, but is usually reserved for higher order multiple gestation or twins/triplets where there is a fetal abnormality. The risks of embryo reduction are an increased miscarriage and preterm delivery rate.

Is there any way of predicting her risk of severe preterm labour?

There is some evidence that transvaginal ultrasound cervical length assessment at 20–24 weeks is useful in this scenario. A very short cervix (<15 mm) might warrant cervical suture insertion.

How often should Miss O be seen at the hospital?

She should be booked for full care in the hospital under the supervision of a consultant conversant with the management of multiple gestation. She will require a detailed structural ultrasound survey of all three fetuses at 20–24 weeks, and growth scans every three weeks thereafter.

What other antenatal measures should be taken?

Many would argue that iron supplements should be given routinely to women with multiple gestation due to their increased requirements. It might be appropriate to arrange a joint neonatal/obstetric consultation at 24–26 weeks in view of the high likelihood that these babies will need some degree of neonatal care after delivery.

New developments

- Cervical length screening at 20–24 weeks may predict severe preterm delivery
- Antenatal steroids are sometimes given routinely at 24–26 weeks in view of the preterm delivery risk
- The increased uptake of assisted conception has increased the background level of multiple gestation, especially in older women
- It has become apparent in the last few years that the use of tocolytics such as beta-adrenergic agonists can be especially hazardous in women with multiple gestation; they must be used with great caution

Key Points

- Twins account for about 1 per cent of pregnancies
- Perinatal mortality rate in twins is about five times higher than in singletons
- Most complications are related to chorionicity
- Serious maternal complications, including pre-eclampsia, antepartum and postpartum haemorrhage, and thromboembolic disease, are increased in multiple gestation

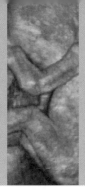

Antenatal obstetric complications

OVERVIEW

The physiological changes of pregnancy exacerbate many irritating symptoms that in the normal non-pregnant state would not require specific treatment. These so-called 'minor' problems of pregnancy are not in any way dangerous to the mother but can be troublesome on a day-to-day basis; most are considerably improved by simple treatments. The more major fetal and maternal complications that may arise directly due to pregnancy are also discussed including malpresentation, Rhesus disease, thromboembolism, abnormalities of amniotic fluid production and antepartum haemorrhage.

The 'minor' problems of pregnancy

Backache

Backache is due to the laxity of spinal ligaments and weight of the pregnancy causing an exaggerated lumbar lordosis. Pregnancy can exacerbate the symptoms of a prolapsed intervertebral disc, occasionally leading to complete immobility. Advice should include maintenance of correct posture, avoiding lifting heavy objects (including children), avoid high-heels, regular physiotherapy and simple analgesia (paracetamol or paracetamol-codeine combinations). Women often find swimming very soothing.

Symphysis pubis dysfunction (SPD)

An excruciatingly painful condition usually occurring in the third trimester. The symphysis pubis joint becomes 'loose', causing the two halves of the pelvis to rub on one another when walking or moving. The condition will only improve after delivery and the management revolves around simple analgesia and, under the physiotherapist's direction, a low stability belt may be worn.

Constipation

Constipation is usually blamed on the effect of progesterone in slowing gut motility, but the physical weight of the gravid uterus on the rectum may contribute, as may concomitantly administered iron tablets. A high-fibre diet should be encouraged, and a mild (non-stimulant) laxative such as lactulose may be suggested.

Hyperemesis gravidarum

Nausea and vomiting is often most pronounced in the first trimester but by no means confined to it, and is otherwise erroneously called morning sickness. It is worse in a molar or multiple gestation and is probably related to high circulating human chorionic gonadotrophin levels. Severe symptoms may lead to Mallory-Weiss tears, haematemesis, dehydration and even malnutrition. In this situation, admission to hospital is mandatory and anti-emetics such as metoclopramide or prochlorperazine are given on a regular basis. In addition, intravenous hydration support should be administered as long as the woman is vomiting. In the severest cases, total parenteral nutrition (TPN) is given and parenteral B complex vitamins including thiamine are reported to reduce the mortality of the condition. A tapering course of steroids has been used with encouraging results in uncontrolled studies. In the very worst cases, termination of pregnancy may be considered if the mother is becoming malnourished and dehydrated.

Heartburn

This is very common. The symptoms are of burning in the chest or discomfort often on lying down. Heartburn is caused by the weight effect of the pregnant uterus preventing stomach emptying, and the general relaxation of the oesophageal sphincter due to progesterone. Management includes liquid antacid preparations, stopping smoking, reducing alcohol intake, frequent light meals and lying with the head propped up at night. Severe, refractory dyspeptic symptoms warrant gastroenterology referral just in case a stomach ulcer or hiatus hernia is being overlooked.

Varicose veins and piles

These both become worse in later pregnancy. Both are thought to be due to the relaxant effect of progesterone on vascular smooth muscle, and the dependent venous stasis caused by the weight of the pregnant uterus on the inferior vena cava.

Neither condition should be treated surgically in pregnancy; piles may be improved with local anaesthetic/anti-irritant creams and a high-fibre diet. Never overlook the 'warning' symptoms of tenesmus, mucus, blood mixed with stool and back passage discomfort that may suggest rectal carcinoma; a rectal digital examination should be carried out if these symptoms are suggested.

Varicose veins of the legs may be symptomatically improved with support stockings, avoidance of standing for prolonged periods and simple analgesia. Thrombophlebitis may occur in a large varicose vein, more commonly after delivery. A large superficial varicose vein may bleed profusely if traumatized; the leg must be elevated and direct pressure applied. Vulval and vaginal varicosities are uncommon but symptomatically troublesome; trauma at the time of delivery (episiotiomy, tear, instrumental delivery) may also cause considerable bleeding.

Carpal tunnel syndrome

Compression neuropathies occur in pregnancy due to increased soft tissue swelling. The most common of these is carpal tunnel syndrome. The median nerve, where it passes through the fibrous canal at the wrist before entering the hand, is most susceptible to compression. The symptoms include numbness, tingling and weakness of the thumb and forefinger, and often quite severe pain at night. Diuretics are not advised; simple analgesia and splinting of the affected hand usually helps although there is no realistic prospect of cure until after delivery. Surgical decompression is very rarely performed in pregnancy.

Oedema

This is common, occurring to some degree in most pregnancies. There is generalized soft tissue swelling and increased capillary permeability, which allows intravascular fluid to leak into the extravascular compartment. The fingers, toes and ankles are usually worst affected and the symptoms are aggravated by hot weather. Oedema is best dealt with by advising frequent periods of rest with leg elevation; occasionally support stockings are indicated. Excessively swollen fingers may necessitate removal of rings and jewellery before they get stuck! It is important to remember that oedema may be a feature of pre-eclampsia, so remember to check the woman's blood pressure and urine for protein. More rarely, severe oedema may suggest underlying cardiac impairment or nephrotic syndrome.

Other common 'minor disorders'

- Itching
- Urinary incontinence
- Nose-bleeds
- Thrush (vaginal candidiasis)
- Headache
- Fainting
- Breast soreness
- Tiredness
- Altered taste sensation
- Insomnia
- Leg cramps
- Striae gravidarum and chloasma

🔑 Key Points

The most common 'minor' disorders of pregnancy
- Backache: usually low back, aggravated by movement
- Heartburn: worst on lying down, better for sitting up
- Varicose veins and piles: often co-exist, worse if pre-existing
- Carpal tunnel syndrome: worse at night, may require splint
- Oedema: worse in hot weather and for walking, better for resting with feet up

---

Problems due to abnormalities of the pelvic organs

Fibroids (leiomyomata)

Fibroids are compact masses of smooth muscle that either lie in the cavity of the uterus (submucous), within the uterine muscle (intramural) or on the outside surface of the uterus (subserous). They may enlarge in pregnancy, and in so doing present problems later on in pregnancy or at delivery (Fig. 14.1). A large fibroid at the cervix or in the lower uterine segment may prevent descent of the presenting part and obstruct vaginal delivery.

Red degeneration is one of the commonest complications of fibroids in pregnancy. The fibroid, as it

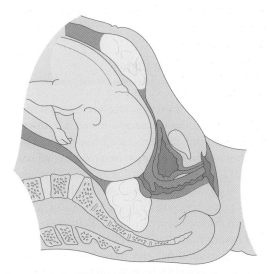

Figure 14.1 Fibroids complicating pregnancy. The tumour in the anterior wall of the uterus has been drawn up out of the pelvis as the lower segment was formed, but the fibroid arising from the cervix remains in the pelvis and will obstruct labour.

Problems associated with fibroids

Antenatal	Labour	Puerperium
subfertility	malpresentation	secondary PPH
miscarriage	obstructed labour	necrosis and infection (particularly if submucous)
preterm labour	primary PPH	
red degeneration	difficult Caesarean Section	
unstable lie		

grows, may outgrow its arterial supply and at the same time obstruct the venous outflow. The net effect is ischaemia of the fibroid, which manifests itself clinically by causing acute pain, tenderness over the fibroid, and frequent vomiting. If these symptoms are severe, it may precipitate uterine contractions causing miscarriage or preterm labour. Red fibroid degeneration requires treatment in hospital, with potent analgesics (usually opiates and intravenous fluids). The symptoms will usually settle within a few days. The differential diagnosis of red degeneration includes acute appendicitis, pyelonephritis/urinary tract infection, ovarian cyst accident and placental abruption.

A subserous pedunculated fibroid may tort in the same way that a large ovarian cyst can. When this happens, acute abdominal pain and tenderness may make the two difficult to distinguish from one another. In this scenario, a pertinent history followed by ultrasound scan (transvaginal in the first trimester, transabdominal in the second and third) will clinch the diagnosis.

Retroversion of the uterus

Fifteen percent of women have a retroverted uterus. In pregnancy, the uterus grows and a retroverted uterus will normally 'flip' out of the pelvis and begin to fill the abdominal cavity, as an anteverted uterus would. In a small proportion of cases, the uterus remains in retroversion and eventually fills up the entire pelvic cavity; as it does so, the base of the bladder and the urethra are stretched. Retention of urine may occur, classically at 12–14 weeks, and this is not only very painful but may cause long-term bladder damage if the bladder becomes overdistended. In this situation, catheterization is essential until the position of the uterus has changed.

Congenital uterine anomalies

The shape of the uterus is embryologically determined by the fusion of the Muellerian ducts. Abnormalities of fusion may give rise to anything from a subseptate uterus, through to a bicornuate uterus and even (very rarely) to a double uterus with two cervices. These findings are often discovered incidentally at the time of a pelvic operation such as a laparoscopy, or an ultrasound scan.

Problems associated with bicornuate uterus are:
- miscarriage;
- preterm labour;
- preterm prelabour rupture of membranes (PPROM);
- abnormalities of lie and presentation;
- higher Caesarean Section rate.

Ovarian cysts in pregnancy

Ovarian cysts are common in pregnant women; fortunately the incidence of malignancy is uncommon in women of childbearing age. The most common types of pathological ovarian cyst are serous cysts and benign teratomas. Physiological cysts of the corpus luteum may grow to several centimetres but rarely require treatment, therefore asymptomatic cysts may be followed up by clinical and ultrasound examination but large cysts (for example, dermoids) may require surgery in pregnancy.

Surgery is usually postponed until the late second or early third trimester, when there is the potential that if the baby were delivered, it would be able to survive. The major problems are of large (>8 cm) ovarian cysts in pregnancy, which may undergo torsion, haemorrhage or rupture, causing acute abdominal pain. The resulting pain and inflammation may lead to a miscarriage or preterm labour. Symptomatic cysts, most commonly due to torsion, will require an emergency laparotomy and ovarian cystectomy or even oophorectomy if the cyst is torted. A full assessment must include a family history of ovarian or breast malignancy, tumour markers (although these are of limited value in pregnancy) and detailed ultrasound investigation of both ovaries. Surgery is normally performed through a midline or paramedian incision; a low transverse suprapubic incision would not allow access to the ovary as it is drawn upwards in later pregnancy.

Cervical cancer

Good pre-conception screening includes ensuring that a mother-to-be is up to date on cervical smears. Cervical abnormalities are much more difficult to deal with in pregnancy partially because the cervix itself is more difficult to visualize at colposcopy, and also because any biopsy will cause considerable bleeding. Cervical carcinoma may most commonly arise in a woman with previous abnormal smears, or in a poor attender for cervical screening. The disease may be asymptomatic, but a common presenting feature is vaginal bleeding (especially post-coital). Examination may reveal a friable or ulcerated lesion with bleeding and purulent discharge. The terrible prospect of cervical carcinoma in pregnancy leads to complex ethical and moral dilemmas over whether the pregnancy must be terminated (depending upon the stage it has reached) and Wertheim hysterectomy performed. Cervical cancer is dealt with in greater detail in Chapter 12 of *Gynaecology by Ten Teachers, 17th edition.*

Urinary tract infection (UTI)

UTIs are common in pregnancy. Eight per cent of women have asymptomatic bacteruria; if this is untreated it may progress to UTI or even pyelonephritis with the attendant associations of low birth weight and preterm delivery.

Predisposing factors:
- history of recurrent cystitis;
- renal tract abnormalities: duplex system; scarred kidneys; ureteric damage and stones;
- diabetes;
- bladder emptying problems, e.g. multiple sclerosis.

The symptoms of UTI may be different in pregnancy; occasionally UTI presents as low back pain and general malaise with flu-like symptoms. The classic presentation of frequency, dysuria and haematuria is not often seen. On examination, tachycardia, pyrexia, dehydration and loin tenderness may be present. Investigations should include a full blood count and mid-stream specimen of urine (MSU) sent for urgent microscopy, culture and sensitivities. If there is a strong clinical suspicion of UTI, treatment with antibiotics should start straight away. The woman should drink plenty of clear fluids, and take a simple analgesia such as paracetamol.

The commonest organism for UTI is *Escherichia coli,* less commonly streptococci, proteus, pseudomonas and klebsiella are implicated. If $>10^5$ organisms are present at culture, this confirms a diagnosis of UTI. The commonly reported 'heavy mixed growth' is often associated with UTI symptoms and may be treated, or MSU repeated after a week, depending on the clinical

scenario. The first line antibiotics for UTI are amoxycillin or oral cephalosporins.

Pyelonephritis is characterized by dehydration, a very high temperature ($>38.5°C$), systemic disturbance and occasionally shock. This requires urgent treatment including intravenous fluids, opiate analgesia, intravenous antibiotics (such as cephalosporins or gentamicin). In addition, renal function should be determined with at least baseline urea and electrolytes and the baby must be monitored with cardiotocography. An ultraound scan may reveal a growth restricted baby with oligohydramnios if the course of the infection has been subacute. It is a mistake, however, to deliver the baby without first resuscitating and treating the mother because an anaesthetic might be dangerous in these circumstances, and fetal condition may improve as a result of treating the mother. The woman may require intensive therapy unit management, including inotropic support and oxygen should overwhelming sepsis occur. In this situation, fetal wellbeing is a secondary consideration.

Recurrent UTIs in pregnancy require MSU specimens to be sent to the microbiology lab at each antenatal visit, and low dose prophylactic oral antibiotics may be prescribed. Investigation should take place after delivery, unless frank haematuria or other symptoms suggest that an urgent diagnosis is essential. Investigations might include a renal ultrasound scan, renal DMSA function scan, creatinine clearance, intravenous urogram and cystoscopy.

Oligohydramnios, polyhydramnios and PPROM

Amniotic fluid is produced almost exclusively from fetal urine from the second trimester onwards. It serves a vital function in protecting the developing baby from pressure or trauma, allowing limb movement, hence normal postural development, and permitting the fetal lungs to expand and develop through breathing.

Oligohydramnios

Too little amniotic fluid (oligohydramnios) is commonly defined as amniotic fluid index <5th centile for gestation. Amniotic fluid index (AFI) is an ultrasound estimation of amniotic fluid derived by adding together the deepest vertical pool in four quadrants of the abdomen. The AFI (in cm) is therefore given to some degree of error. In general, however, it is possible to differentiate subjectively on ultrasound between 'too much', 'too little' and 'normal looking'.

Oligohydramnios may be suspected antenatally following a history of clear fluid leaking from the vagina; this may represent preterm prelabour rupture of the membranes (PPROM). Clinically, on abdominal palpation, the fetal poles may be very obviously felt and 'hard' with a small-for-dates uterus. The possible causes of oligohydramnios and anhydramnios (no amniotic fluid) are described in the box below.

The fetal prognosis depends on the cause of oligohydramnios, but both pulmonary hypoplasia and limb deformities (contractures, talipes) are common to severe early onset (<24 weeks) oligohydramnnios. Renal agenesis and bilateral multicystic kidneys carry a lethal prognosis as life after birth is impossible without functioning kidneys. In this situation, the fetal lungs would likely be hypoplastic; this may also be true of severe urinary tract obstruction. Oligohydramnios due to intrauterine growth restriction/utero-placental insufficiency is usually of a less severe degree and less commonly causes limb and lung problems.

Preterm prelabour rupture of the membranes (PPROM)

A distinction must be drawn between spontaneous rupture of the membranes (SROM) at term, and preterm prelabour rupture of the membranes (PPROM). Whereas SROM may occur prior to a normal term labour, PPROM is a pathological occurrence and has major implications for both mother and baby. PPROM is rupture of the membranes between 24–37 weeks' gestation, and occurs in approximately 2 per cent of all pregnancies in the UK. The major causative factors are thought to be infection (for example bacterial vaginosis) and cervical weakness; this is more classically associated with late miscarriage but is also implicated in early gestation PPROM. Most of the risk factors for preterm labour (see Chapter 18) also apply to PPROM.

Clinical features of PPROM from the history normally include comments such as the woman feeling a 'gush of fluid' vaginally or 'leaking in dribbles'. This must be distinguished from leaking urine (ask about frequency, urgency, leakage and dysuria) as a UTI may present in a similar way, with slight urine leakage. Fetal movements may be reduced with PPROM, and occasionally contractions may start.

On examination, the woman may be flushed and her temperature and pulse rate increased, particularly if there is any evidence of infection. Abdominally, the findings may be of oligohydramnios (see above). The definitive diagnosis can only be made by performing a sterile speculum examination; a pool of amniotic fluid in the posterior vagina is diagnostic. It is also important at this point to visualize the cervix and establish whether there is dilatation. A vaginal swab must be sent for microscopy, culture and sensitivities and it is common practice to use a nitrazine stick to define the presence of amniotic fluid (it turns black, though false positives occur with blood, semen and even urine).

Further investigation must include regular

Possible causes of oligo- and anhydramnios

Too little production	Diagnosed by
Renal agenesis	Ultrasound: no renal tissue, no bladder
Multicystic kidneys	Ultrasound: enlarged kidneys with multiple cysts, no visible bladder
Urinary tract abnormality/obstruction	Ultrasound: kidneys may be present, but urinary tract dilatation
IUGR and placental insufficiency	Clinical: reduced SFH, reduced fetal movements, possibly abnormal CTG
	Ultrasound: IUGR, fetal Dopplers show hypoxia or acidaemia
Maternal drugs (NSAIDs)	Witholding NSAIDs may allow amniotic fluid to reaccumulate
Post-dates pregnancy	
Leakage	**Diagnosed by**
PPROM	Speculum examination: pool of amniotic fluid on posterior blade

assessment of the mother's state (blood pressure, pulse rate and temperature). Blood tests must include a full blood count (white cell count important), C-reactive protein (raised in infection) grouped and saved, and clotting studies if there is a hint of infection. A cardiotocograph must be obtained, and ultrasound of the fetus will give valuable information about the lie, presentation, amount of amniotic fluid and estimated fetal weight. Amniocentesis is sometimes performed in PPROM to establish whether there is intrauterine infection (chorio-amnionitis); a sample of amniotic fluid is sent for Gram stain, microscopy and culture. There is, however, a risk of stimulating preterm labour by performing an invasive test, and amniocentesis can be technically very difficult if there is virtually no amniotic fluid.

Further management must be directed at making the mother comfortable (rehydration and simple analgesia initially) and informing her and her partner about the risks of the condition to her and the baby. As PPROM frequently (50 per cent of cases) predates preterm labour, liaison with neonatologists, determining mode of delivery and administration of steroids to the mother are important. There has been controversy over the role of prophylactic antibiotics in PPROM; the neonatal/obstetric consensus probably favours their use. A combination of a penicillin (e.g. amoxyl) or erythromycin and metronidazole is acceptable.

The outlook for PPROM depends largely on what gestation it has occurred at, and the degree of residual amniotic fluid accumulation. PPROM at 24 weeks with frank anhydramnios carries a much worse prognosis than a 'hindwater' leak at 32 weeks with some residual amniotic fluid remaining. The presence of infection at presentation is always a bad sign and usually means that delivery should be expedited to save the mother becoming systemically septic (a very dangerous condition). It is misguided to use antibiotics to try to prolong gestation in this situation; all it will succeed in doing is delaying the manifestations of severe chorio-amnionitis by which time both the mother and baby may be very sick. Tocolytics are contraindicated in PPROM, for fear of preventing delivery in the situation of chorio-amnionitis.

When should delivery occur in PPROM? Most obstetricians would aim to manage these women conservatively until 34–36 weeks, and then decide on the mode of delivery depending upon obstetric

🔑 Key Points

- PPROM with breech presentation or in multiple gestation is especially risky (cord prolapse, risk of feet/legs/arms prolapsing through the cervix)
- Very little amniotic fluid at an early gestation carries a very poor prognosis
- Severe, overwhelming chorio-amnionitis may develop suddenly and endanger the wellbeing and lives of the mother and baby
- Severe oligohydramnios is associated with limb deformities and pulmonary hypoplasia

factors. Factors in favour of earlier delivery include maternal group B streptococcal vaginal colonization, and breech presentation. If women with PPROM are managed on an outpatient basis, they must be reviewed at least weekly by an obstetrician when a full blood count, and usually ultrasound scan will be carried out. They must take their temperature daily and be told explicitly to return to the obstetric unit should their temperature rise above 37.5°C, their heart rate rise to >100 or if they have flu-like symptoms. Overwhelming sepsis may occur and may be fatal if the early signs are missed.

Polyhydramnios

Polyhydramnios is the term given to an excess of amniotic fluid, i.e, AFI > 95th centile for gestation on ultrasound estimation. It may present as severe abdominal swelling and discomfort. On examination, the abdomen will appear distended out of proportion to the woman's gestation (increased symphysis–fundal height [SFH]). Furthermore, the abdomen may be tense, tender and the fetal poles will be hard to palpate. The condition may be caused by maternal, placental or fetal conditions:

- Maternal
  - diabetes
- Placental
  - chorioangioma
  - AV fistula
- Fetal
  - multiple gestation (in monochorionic twins it may be twin-to-twin transfusion syndrome)
  - idiopathic

– oesophageal atresia/tracheo-oesophageal fistula
– duodenal atresia
– neuromuscular fetal condition (preventing swallowing)
– anencephaly

The management of polyhydramnios is directed towards establishing the cause (hence determining fetal prognosis), relieving the discomfort of the mother (if necessary by amniodrainage), and assessing the risk of preterm labour due to uterine over-distension. The latter may require assessment of cervical length by ultrasound. If prior to 24 weeks following amniotic fluid drainage the cervical length is less than 25 mm, consideration might be given to cervical suture insertion.

Polyhydramnios due to maternal diabetes needs urgent investigation as it often suggests high maternal blood glucose levels. In this context, polyhydramnios should correct itself when the mother's glycaemic control is optimized.

Twin-to-twin transfusion syndrome is a rare cause of acute polyhydramnios in the recipient sac of monochorionic twins. It is associated with oligohydramnios and a small baby in the other sac. The condition may be rapidly fatal for both twins; amnio-drainage and removal by laser of the placental vascular connections are two therapeutic modalities employed in dealing with this condition. This is further discussed in Chapter 13.

Abdominal pain in pregnancy

Abdominal pain is exceptionally common in pregnancy; the problem is in distinguishing pathological from 'physiological' pains. Most experienced obstetricians will remember women with ill-defined symptoms and signs where a diagnosis of acute appendicitis, pyelonephritis or lobar pneumonia has been missed for crucial hours or days. This is not to excuse mis-diagnosis, but with so many possibilities to exclude a balance must be struck between over-investigation and complacency.

The causes listed in Table 14.1 are not exhaustive, but cover over 95 per cent of possible diagnoses. The crucial point to make is that certain conditions are potentially so dangerous or debilitating (pneumonia, pulmonary embolus, renal stones, intestinal obstruction, pancreatitis) that obstetricians may have to perform X-rays and arrange invasive assessments to make a diagnosis. To avoid this, and risk not making an early diagnosis, means that the woman may not be treated appropriately for possibly very serious conditions.

Venous thromboembolism

Pulmonary embolus (PE) is the major cause of direct maternal death in the UK, and is responsible for approximately 16 fatalities per year. Pregnancy is a hyper-coagulable state because of an alteration in thrombotic and fibrinolytic system. There is an increase in clotting factors VIII, IX, X and fibrinogen levels, and a reduction in protein S and antithrombin III concentrations. The net result of these changes is possibly nature's way of reducing the likelihood of haemorrhage following delivery.

These physiological changes predispose a woman to thromboembolism (the obstruction of a blood vessel by a blood clot), and any underlying preponderance to thrombosis may be unmasked in pregnancy. High levels of circulating oestrogen are associated with changes in clotting factors; the situation is in some ways analogous to that of women developing a deep vein thrombosis (DVT) while using the oral contraceptive pill. The additional factor that makes pregnancy a particular risk is venous

Risk factors for DVT/PE

Pre-existing
- maternal age (>35 years)
- thrombophilia
- obesity (>80 kg)
- previous thromboembolism
- severe varicose veins
- smoking
- malignancy

Specific to pregnancy
- multiple gestation
- pre-eclampsia
- grand multiparity
- Caesarean Section, especially if emergency
- damage to the pelvic veins
- sepsis
- prolonged bedrest

Table 14.1 – Abdominal pain in pregnancy: causes and clinical assessment

	Specific history	Key investigation
Extrauterine, non-pathological		
Ligament stretching (inguinal/round)		
Rib pain/costo-chondritis 'wind'		
Constipation		
Heartburn	• Relieved with food	
Extrauterine, pathological		
UTI	• Frequency, dysuria, haematuria, hesitancy	• MSU, microscopy culture and sensitivities
Pyelonephritis	• As above, plus feverish	• Blood culture, renal ultrasound
Renal stones	• As above, but intermittent, spasmodic pains	• Urine microscopy (haematuria, precipitated crystals), renal ultrasound, limited IVU
Cholecystitis	• Nausea, temperature, vomiting	• LFTs, ultrasound upper abdomen
Pancreatitis	• Alcoholism, gallstones, autoimmune disease	• Serum amylase, abdominal ultrasound, may require CT/MRI
Appendicitis	• Often non-specific right-sided pain and tenderness	• Temperature, white cell count, abdominal ultrasound
Intestinal obstruction	• Bilious vomiting	• U+Es, abdominal X-ray
HELLP syndrome	• Headache, blurred vision, bruising, bleeding gums	• BP, urinalysis, LFTs, FBC, clotting, liver, ultrasound
Fulminating pre-eclampsia	• Headache, visual disturbance, oedema	• As for HELLP syndrome
Uterine/feto-placental		
Preterm labour	• Intermittent pains; low backache; show	• CTG for uterine activity
Placental abruption	• Sudden severe abdominal pain,	• CTG, FBC, clotting, senior
	• Vaginal bleeding, reduced FM	• Obstetric input immediately
Fibroids (torsion, red degeneration)	• Intermittent severe pain, nausea, vomiting	
Ovarian cysts (torsion, rupture)	• As above	
Painful Braxton-Hicks contractions		
Medical conditions		
Diabetes	• Weight loss, polydipsia, polyuria	• Urinalysis (ketones, glucose), U+E, glucose
Pneumonia (especially lower lobe)	• Cough, temperature, chest pain	• Examination, chest X-ray
Pulmonary embolus	• Short of breath, haemoptysis, insp. dyspnoea (possibly calf pain)	• ECG, chest X-ray, blood gases, then ventilation perfusion scan, spiral CT or pulmonary angiograph
Sickle cell crisis	• Ill-defined abdominal pain, temperature	• Sickle status, % sickle Hb
Malaria	• Recent travel in endemic area (within 1 year)	• Urinalysis (protein, blood), thick film for parasites

stasis in the lower limbs due to the weight of the gravid uterus placing pressure on the inferior vena cava; this is compounded by immobility.

Pregnancy itself increases the risk of DVT by five times; Caesarean Section by 10 times. The risk of DVT after Caesarean Section is probably around 1 per cent.

Thrombophilia

Some women are predisposed to thrombosis through changes in the coagulation/fibrinolytic system. These factors may be inherited or acquired. Inherited thrombophilias include protein C, protein S and antithrombin (AT) III deficiency. New thrombophilias are now being discovered at an alarming rate. One of the most common of these is resistance to activated protein C (APCR) caused by the Leiden mutation in the factor V gene. The preponderance of this and other thrombophilias varies widely depending on ethnicity. For instance APCR is commonest in Scandinavian countries but is present in <5 per cent of other European populations.

Acquired thrombophilia is most commonly associated with the antiphospholipid syndrome (APS). APS is the combination of lupus anticoagulant with or without anti-cardiolipin antibodies, with a history of recurrent miscarriage and or thrombosis. APS may (or more commonly may not) be associated with other auto-antibody disorders such as systemic lupus erythematosus (SLE).

It is crucial that women with a history of thrombotic events are screened for thrombophilia, even if this is first done in pregnancy (when protein S and AT III levels fall physiologically anyway and may complicate result interpretation). The presence of thrombophilia, with a history of thrombotic episode(s), means that prophylaxis should be considered for pregnancy.

Deep vein thrombosis (DVT)

The commonest symptoms are of pain in the calf, with varying degrees of redness or swelling. A pregnant woman's legs are frequently swollen in pregnancy, therefore unilateral symptoms should ring alarm bells. Signs are few, except that the calf will frequently be tender to gentle touch. It is mandatory to ask about symptoms of PE (see later) as a woman with PE might present initially with a DVT. In any woman with suspicion of DVT, heparin or a low-molecular weight heparin should be given in treatment doses until the diagnosis is confirmed or refuted. A firm diagnosis by one of the methods below is mandatory.

The two methods of diagnosing a DVT are venography, or Doppler ultrasound. Venography is invasive, requiring the injection of contrast medium and the use of X-rays. It does, however, allow excellent visualization of veins both below and above the knee.

Colour Doppler ultrasound is now the preferred first-line method of investigating suspected DVT. It is now more widely available, allowing non-invasive assessment of the deep veins between the knee and the iliac veins. Calf veins are often poorly visualized, however it is known that a thrombus confined purely to the calf veins with no extension is very unlikely to give rise to a PE. The main advantage of colour Doppler is in allowing a dynamic assessment of the femoral and iliac veins.

Pulmonary embolus

Pulmonary embolus (PE) is crucial to recognize, as missing the diagnosis could have fatal implications. The classic presentation of inspiratory chest pain and breathlessness, with a pleural 'rub', hypoxia and S1QT3 changes on electrocardiograph (ECG) is rarely seen. The most common presentation is of mild breathlessness, or inspiratory chest pain, in a woman who is not cyanosed but may be slightly tachycardic (>90/min) with a mild pyrexia (37.5°C). The presence of these signs, together with risk factors for PE, makes immediate full anticoagulation and confirmation of the diagnosis (preferably within 24 hours) not merely advisable, but essential. A positive diagnosis of PE has major implications regarding long-term anticoagulation.

Anticoagulants

Heparin prolongs the activated partial thromboplastin time (APTT, otherwise known as kaolin cephalin time, KCT). The activity of low-molecular weight heparin derivatives is assessed by factor X assay. Both are given intramuscularly or intravenously. They do

---

'Labour ward' management of a non-moribund 'walk in' woman with suspected PE

History (ask about risk factors)

Examine (pulse, BP, temperature, examine calves, percuss and auscultate lung fields)

Investigate: arterial blood gases, chest X-ray, ECG, oxygen saturation monitor, baseline coagulation screen and blood count

Don't forget to ask about the pregnancy and monitor the fetus (pre-eclampsia or chorio-amnionitis might predispose to PE)

If PE is suspected...

Give oxygen

Heparinize immediately (full anticoagulant dosage IV; 36,000 iu/24 hours with a bolus dose)

Call for senior help (anaesthetic/medical/cardiothoracic)

Definitive diagnosis: ventilation/perfusion scan or pulmonary angiography

Further management: life-threatening PE may warrant thrombolytic drugs or surgery. This is rarely the case, however.

---

not cross the placenta, are not teratogenic and the effect can be stopped within hours by witholding further doses. They are regarded as relatively safe; maternal thrombocytopaenia is a rare idiosyncratic reaction and osteoporosis is a risk if treatment is prolonged (>6 months).

Warfarin is given orally and prolongs the prothrombin time (PT). Warfarin crosses the placenta and can cause limb and facial defects in the first trimester, and fetal intracerebral haemorrhage in the second and third trimesters. Its use is largely confined to women at highest risk of thromboembolism requiring full anticoagulation; if it is used exposure should be limited to the second and third trimesters.

Prophylaxis and treatment issues

These are controversial and the examples below are given as a guide.

- Low dose daily aspirin may be used in those women judged 'at risk' but who are not sufficiently 'high risk' to warrant prophylactic subcutaneous heparin (for example, previous DVT below the knee).
- Women with risk factors for DVT (for example, a woman aged 43, weighing 105 kg) should receive subcutaneous heparin prophylaxis and elasticated stockings if admitted to hospital or undergoing a surgical procedure such as Caesarean Section.
- Those with a previous history of thromboembolism in pregnancy or whilst taking the combined oral contraceptive pill may require

prophylactic subcutaneous heparin throughout the pregnancy.

- Some women require full anticoagulation throughout pregnancy, for instance those with artificial heart valves, women having had a PE in this pregnancy and women with antiphospholipid syndrome having had recurrent DVTs.

Antepartum haemorrhage

This is defined as vaginal bleeding from 24 weeks to delivery of the baby. The causes are placental, or local. Placental causes are obviously the most worrying, as potentially the mother's and/or fetus' life is in danger. These include placental abruption, placenta praevia and vasa praevia. Local causes include cervicitis, cervical 'erosion', cervical carcinoma, vaginal trauma or vaginal infection.

Antepartum haemorrhage must always be taken seriously, and any woman presenting with a history of fresh vaginal bleeding must be investigated promptly and properly. The key question is whether the bleeding is placental, and is compromising the mother and/or fetus, or whether it has a less significant cause. Normally, it will be obvious from looking at the woman whether the situation is in extremis or not. A pale, tachycardic woman looking anxious with a painful firm abdomen, underwear soaked in fresh blood and reduced fetal movements needs emergency assessment and management for a possible placental abruption. A woman having had a small postcoital bleed with no systemic signs or symptoms represents a different end of the spectrum.

History

- How much bleeding?
- Triggering factors (for example, postcoital bleed).
- Associated with pain or contractions?
- Is the baby moving?
- Last cervical smear (date/normal or abnormal)?

Examination

- Pulse, blood pressure.
- Is uterus soft or tender and firm?
- Fetal heart auscultation/CTG.
- Speculum vaginal examination, with particular importance placed on visualizing the cervix (having established that placenta is not a praevia, preferably using a portable ultrasound machine).

Investigations

- Depending on degree of bleeding, FBC, clotting and if suspected praevia/abruption cross-match 6 units of blood.
- Ultrasound (fetal size, presentation, amniotic fluid, placental position and morphology).

Placental abruption

The premature separation of the placenta is termed abruption. The bleeding is maternal and/or fetal and abruption is acutely dangerous for both mother and fetus (Figs 14.2 and 14.3). See Chapter 11.

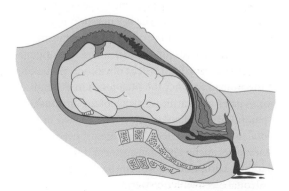

Figure 14.2 Placental abruption with revealed haemorrhage.

Vasa praevia

- An aberrant feto-placental vessel running in the membrane
- Risk factors: placenta praevia; multiple pregnancy
- Associated with velamentous (eccentric) cord insertion 'unwinding' the cord vessels to expose them; bilobed or succenturiate lobe of placenta
- Rupture of vasa may occur in labour or with PPROM. Can cause acute fetal exsanguination and death. Tachycardic/bradycardic CTG; small amount of bright red vaginal bleeding (differentiate fetal from maternal blood by Kleihauer test)
- Treatment of ruptured vasa is delivery, usually immediate Caesarean Section

Placenta praevia

A placenta covering or encroaching on the cervical os may be associated with bleeding, either provoked or spontaneous. The bleeding is from the maternal not fetal circulation and is more likely to compromise the mother than the fetus (Fig. 14.4).

Further management

If there is minimal bleeding and the cause is clearly local vaginal bleeding, then symptomatic management

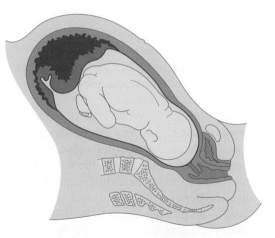

Figure 14.3 Placental abruption with concealed haemorrhage.

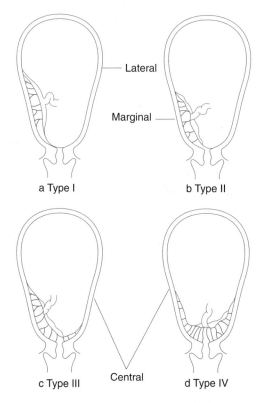

Figure 14.4 Classification of degrees of placenta praevia. a = lateral, b = marginal, c and d both central.

🔑 Key Points

- Placenta praevia is most dangerous for the mother
- Placental abruption is more dangerous for the fetus than mother
- Ruptured vasa praevia is very dangerous for the fetus

may be given (for example, antifungal preparations for candidiasis), as long as there is reasonable certainty that cervical carcinoma is excluded by smear history and direct visualization of the cervix.

Placental causes of bleeding are a major concern. A large gauge intravenous cannula is sited and FBC, clotting, cross-match must be sent and appropriate fetal and maternal monitoring instituted. If there is major fetal or maternal compromise, decisions may have to be made about immediate delivery for fetal or maternal indication irrespective of gestation; an attempt at maternal steroid injection should still be given. If this is the situation, and bleeding is continuing, refer to Chapter 20 for emergency management. If bleeding settles, then the woman must be admitted for 48 hours as the risk of re-bleeding is high within this time frame. Rhesus status is important: if the mother is rhesus negative, send a Kleihauer test (to determine whether any, or how much fetal blood has leaked into the maternal circulation) and administer anti-D.

Breech presentation, oblique and transverse lie at term

Breech presentation occurs in 40 per cent of babies at 26 weeks, 20 per cent at 30 weeks and 3 per cent at term. Similarly oblique and transverse positions are not uncommon antenatally. They only become a problem if the baby (or first presenting baby in a multiple gestation) is not cephalic by 37 weeks. There are three types of breech; the commonest is extended (frank) breech (Fig. 14.5). Less common is a flexed (complete) breech (Fig. 14.6) and least common is footling breech; in this case a foot presents at the cervix. Cord and foot prolapse are risks in this situation.

The predisposing factors for abnormal lie or breech presentation include:

Uterine
- Fibroids
- Congenital abnormalities, e.g. susceptible uterus
- Uterine surgery
- Oligohydramnios
- Polyhydramnios

Fetal
- Multiple gestation
- Abnormality, e.g. anencephaly
- Neuromuscular condition

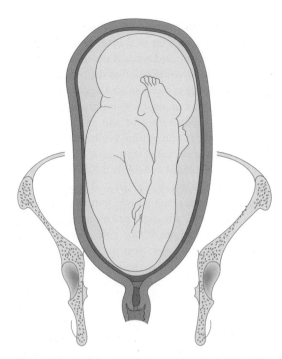

Figure 14.5 Frank breech (also known as extended breech) presentation with extension of the legs.

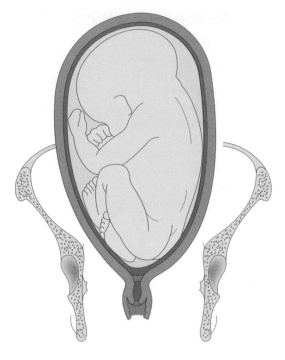

Figure 14.6 Breech presentation with flexion of the legs.

Abnormal presentation or unstable lie at term

Any woman presenting at term with a transverse or oblique lie is at potential risk of cord prolapse following spontaneous rupture of the membranes, and prolapse of the hand, shoulder or foot once in labour. In most cases, the woman is multiparous with lax uterus and abdominal wall musculature and gentle version of the baby's head in clinic or on the ward will restore the presentation to cephalic. If this does not occur, or the lie is unstable (alternating between transverse, oblique and longitudinal), then it is important to think of possible uterine or fetal causes of this (see box opposite, as for breech presentation).

The diagnosis of transverse or oblique lie might be suspected by abdominal inspection; the abdomen often appears asymmetrical. The symphysis-fundal height may be less than expected, and on palpation the fetal head or buttocks may be in the iliac fossa. Palpation over the pelvic brim will reveal an 'empty' pelvis.

It goes without saying that a woman in labour with the baby's lie anything other than longitudinal will not be able to deliver vaginally; this is one situation where if Caesarean Section is not performed then both the mother and baby are at considerable risk of morbidity and mortality. The only exception to this is for exceptionally preterm or small babies, where vaginal delivery may occur irrespective of lie or presentation.

A woman with an unstable lie at term should be admitted to the antenatal ward. The normal plan would be to deliver by emergency Caesarean Section if the presentation is not cephalic in early labour or if spontaneous rupture of the membranes occurs. In a multiparous woman, an unstable lie will often correct itself in early labour (as long as the membranes are intact).

Assessment of women with breech presentation

There are no reliable data over the perinatal mortality associated with breech versus cephalic delivery at term. Most obstetricians suspect that vaginal delivery is probably safer for the mother and less safe for the baby, and vice versa for Caesarean Section. So, when a primiparous woman at 38 weeks with a breech baby asks you in clinic, 'Shall I have a Caesarean, doctor?'

Factors for vaginal breech delivery

Adverse factors against vaginal breech delivery include:
- Large or small baby (ultrasound estimated weight >3.5 or <2.5 kg)
- Small pelvis on pelvimetry or very flat sacrum
- Primigravid
- Previous caesarean section
- Poor obstetric history
- Long history of subfertility/assisted conception
- Advanced maternal age
- Extended neck

Positive factors in favour of a vaginal breech delivery
- Normal size baby (2.5–3.5 kg)
- Good pelvimetry
- Flexed neck
- Multiparous
- Breech deeply engaged
- Positive mental attitude of woman and partner
- Obstetric unit with staff familiar with breech delivery

your answer will have to be carefully considered. Before planning the mode of delivery, it is advisable to estimate the fetal weight and attitude from ultrasound, and some obstetricians still advocate pelvimetry (either erect lateral, or computerized tomographic) to determine pelvic shape. Then, take into account the factors shown in the symptoms box above.

Your counselling should not be directive, and the ultimate decision rests with the woman. It is your duty to present her with the options, not to scare her with horror stories of head entrapment at delivery. On the other hand, the woman should know that a vaginal breech delivery is probably more risky for her

🔍 Key Points in breech presentation

- ECV should be offered at 36–37 weeks in carefully selected women
- Most women with breech presentations end up with caesarean section (80 per cent)
- A vaginal breech delivery must be carefully planned
- Preterm breeches (<34 weeks) are probably better delivered by caesarean
- Ensure that experienced, senior obstetric staff are present at a breech delivery

baby and perinatal mortality is probably higher in vaginal breech babies. The fear of obstetric litigation should not force obstetricians to deter women from vaginal breech delivery. A well-planned, well-conducted vaginal breech delivery can be very satisfying for the woman, her partner and the staff involved.

External cephalic version

The most common situation arises when a woman, with an otherwise uncomplicated pregnancy, presents in the antenatal clinic at 36 weeks' gestation with a breech baby. If there are no contraindications (see box below), an external cephalic version (ECV) may be performed at 36–37 weeks. The procedure is mildly uncomfortable, and is usually carried out by a senior obstetrician at or near delivery facilities. The woman lies comfortably, and under ultrasound guidance, the baby is gently manipulated into the cephalic position. ECV is much more difficult in women who are overweight or have fibroids, and deep engagement of the breech makes any manipulation more difficult. A fetal heart rate trace must be performed before and after the procedure. If the procedure fails, or becomes difficult, it is abandoned. It is hoped that approximately two-thirds of babies can be turned to cephalic using this method (Fig. 14.7).

ECV is a relatively straightforward and safe

Contraindications and risks of ECV

Contraindications to ECV:
- Placenta praevia
- Oligo- or polyhydramnios
- History of antepartum haemorrhage
- Previous Caesarean or myomectomy scar on the uterus
- Multiple gestation
- Pre-eclampsia or hypertension
- Plan to deliver by Caesarean Section anyway

Risks of ECV include:
- Placental abruption
- Premature rupture of the membranes
- Cord accident
- Transplacental haemorrhage (remember anti-D administration to rhesus-negative women)
- Fetal bradycardia

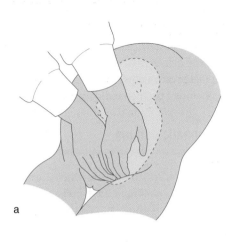

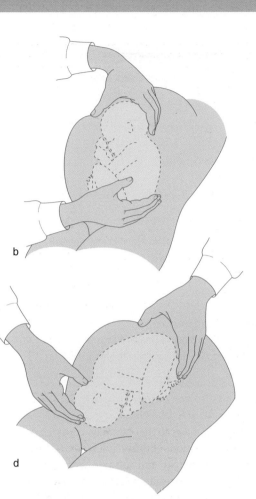

Figure 14.7 External cephalic version. (a) The breech is disengaged from the pelvic inlet; (b) version is usually performed in the direction which increases flexion of the fetus and makes it do a forward somersault (c); on completion of version the head is often not engaged for a time (d). The fetal heart rate should be checked after the external version has been completed.

technique and has been shown to reduce the number of Caesarean Sections due to breech presentation. There is a strong argument in favour of an ECV in most delivery units, especially those where primigravid women are normally delivered by Caesarean Section. The technique is easier to perform in multiparous women where the uterus is already relatively lax. ECV is occasionally performed with tocolytics such as ritodrine, salbutamol, nifedipine or GTN.

Substance abuse in pregnancy

Drug dependence

Addiction to hard drugs is unfortunately becoming more common throughout the western world. It is crucial to have a high index of suspicion about drug abuse if there are subtle or not so subtle signs. The picture of an 'addict' depends upon her degree of compensation and ability to adapt and may range from the very top to the lowest socio-economic groups. The classic dishevelled, thin, malnourished woman with venous access scars visible up her arm represents the very severest end of the spectrum.

Problems frequently encountered in drug addicts (Table 14.2):

- Social problems: housing, crime, other children in care or abused.
- Co-existent addictions: alcohol and smoking.
- Malnutrition: especially iron, vitamins B and C.
- Risk of viral infections, e.g. HIV or Hepatitis B.
- Fetal and neonatal risks.

Table 14.2 – Effects of some drugs of abuse on the fetus and neonate

	Fetal effects	Neonatal effects
Opiates	Preterm labour SGA Anaemia Multiple gestation	Neonatal withdrawal syndrome Higher risk sudden infant death syndrome Higher perinatal mortality
Cocaine and derivatives	Placental abruption Preterm delivery SGA	Increased cerebral infarction risk
Cannabis	Preterm delivery Theoretical risk of chromosome damage	

Management only becomes more complex once drug addiction is identified. The aims of management are to stabilize the mother's drug-taking habits, ensure contact with social/care workers and psychiatric/drug liaison services as appropriate. It is important not to try to reduce opiate dose too rapidly in pregnancy as this can easily precipitate acute withdrawal in both mother and fetus; the principle is to administer the lowest effective dose of methadone liquid in three divided doses every day.

Screening for infections such as hepatitis B and HIV should be performed for the former and considered for the latter if risk factors (bisexual partner, origin in a high prevalence area, IV drug abuse) are present. In many cases, multidisciplinary case conferences should be held to make arrangements and decisions for when the baby is delivered.

Alcohol

There is much doubt over what a 'safe' dose of alcohol is during pregnancy. What is likely is that intake of <100 g per week (approximately two drinks per day, e.g. two medium glasses of wine or one pint of beer) is not associated with any adverse effects. Doses greater than this have been related to IUGR. Massive doses, in excess of 17 drinks per day, have been associated with fetal alcohol syndrome (see box opposite).

If alcohol abuse is suspected, it may be necessary to involve social workers and arrange for formal

Fetal alcohol syndrome

- Narrow palpebral fissures
- Depressed bridge, short nose
- Widely spaced eyes
- Mental retardation
- Club foot
- IUGR
- Cardiac defects

psychiatric/addiction assessment. It is extremely difficult to 'test' for alcohol abuse as even markers such as mean corpuscular volume and gamma GT are not reliable in pregnancy. Malnutrition is very likely in heavy alcohol abuse and requires in addition to a change in basic diet, B vitamin supplements and iron; the problem is that the majority of such patients not only don't take their medicines but also default antenatal appointments.

Smoking and pregnancy

Smoking is not advisable in pregnancy. Although smokers have a lower incidence of pre-eclampsia than non-smokers, overall perinatal mortality is increased, babies are smaller at delivery, there is a higher risk of antepartum haemorrhage and there is some evidence of a link between antenatal maternal smoking and later development of leukaemia in childhood. It is estimated that a baby will weigh less than its target weight by a multiple of 15 g times the average number of cigarettes a woman smokes per day; smoking less than five cigarettes per day has a barely discernible obstetric effect. Smoking acutely reduces placental perfusion; this probably contributes to the IUGR.

Post-term pregnancy

Term, by definition, is 37–42 weeks' gestation. A very small proportion (<5 per cent) of pregnancies would proceed beyond 42 weeks if left alone. It should be said at the outset that the definition of post-term pregnancy for a woman depends on her accurate dates, and preferably a first trimester ultrasound estimation of crown–rump length.

Post-term pregnancy is a problem because at this gestation, the baby is at its maximum size, and the placenta is becoming more calcified, less efficient and more prone to failure. There are no known tests that can predict fetal outcome post-term; an ultrasound scan may give temporary reassurance if the amniotic fluid and fetal growth are normal; similarly a CTG

should be performed at and after 42 weeks. Some women wish to wait for their labour to start naturally, and in these cases, it is usually reasonable to wait a day or two over 42 weeks as long as appropriate surveillance is carried out and the woman is aware of the increased risk of stillbirth or neonatal death.

Immediate induction of labour or delivery post-dates should take place if:
- there is reduced amniotic fluid on scan;
- fetal growth is reduced;
- there are reduced fetal movements;
- the CTG is not perfect;
- the mother is hypertensive or suffers a significant medical condition.

So, when counselling the parents regarding waiting for labour to start naturally after 42 weeks, it is important that the woman is aware that no test can guarantee the safety of her baby, and that perinatal mortality is increased (at least two-fold) beyond 42 weeks. A labour induced post-term is more likely to require Caesarean Section; this may partly be due to the reluctance of the uterus to contract properly, and the possible compromise of the baby leading to abnormal CTG.

CASE HISTORY

Ms W

38 years old, second ongoing pregnancy

Severe nausea and vomiting earlier in pregnancy requiring hospital admission

Now 22 weeks' gestation, presents to casualty with severe retrosternal pain on lying down

Finds it difficult to eat and drink: 'stomach is burning'

Occasionally brings up blood-stained vomitus

Losing weight

What is the most likely diagnosis?

The symptoms sound like heartburn, however, this is simply the description of a symptom and it is quite possible that her hyperemesis earlier in the pregnancy was associated with gastro-oesophageal reflux, gastro-oesophagitis or even ulceration.

How would you manage Ms W?

You must concentrate on making a diagnosis, and alleviating her symptoms allowing her to eat and drink. Severe upper GI symptoms causing weight loss may

warrant upper GI endoscopy; at the very least a gastroenterologist should be consulted. At the same time, remember that the following conditions can all present with vomiting and even weight loss in pregnancy, so the appropriate investigations should be carried out:

- urinary tract infections (send mid-stream urine sample to the laboratory)
- multiple gestation or triploidy/partial molar pregnancy (perform ultrasound if not done already)
- liver disease (send liver function tests)

The most likely diagnosis is mild reflux with heartburn so provide a liquid antacid preparation to be taken three times daily and possibly and H2 blocker. Advise her to eat frequent small meals and to avoid spicy foods, smoking, caffeine and alcohol. Depending on her hydration and nutritional status, you may need to admit her to the antenatal ward, commence IV rehydration and give protein 'build-up' drinks.

Rhesus iso-immunization

Blood group is defined in two ways. Firstly, there is the ABO group allowing four different permutations of blood group (O, A, B, AB). Secondly, there is the rhesus system, which consists of C, D and E antigens. The importance of these blood group systems is that a mismatch between the fetus and mother can mean that when fetal red cells pass across to the maternal circulation, as they do to a greater or lesser extent during pregnancy, sensitization of the maternal immune system to these fetal 'foreign' red blood cells may occur.

ABO blood group iso-immunization may occur when the mother is blood group O and the baby is blood group A or B. Anti-A and anti-B antibodies are present in the maternal circulation naturally, hence do not require prior sensitization in order to be produced. This means that ABO incompatibility may occur in a first pregnancy. In this situation, anti-A or anti-B antibodies may pass to the fetal circulation, causing fetal haemolysis and anaemia. ABO incompatibility causes mild haemolytic disease of the baby, but may sometimes explain unexpected jaundice in an otherwise healthy term infant.

The rhesus system is more commonly associated with severe haemolytic disease. Of all the antibodies (C, D and E), the D antigen is associated most commonly with severe haemolytic fetal disease, however, this can only occur if the mother is D rhesus-negative and the baby is D rhesus-positive. Both anti-C and anti-E antibodies may also be associated with haemolytic disease requiring intrauterine fetal blood transfusion, but are much less commonly implicated.

Rare antibodies such as those listed below may unusually be associated with haemolytic disease.

The aetiology of rhesus disease

Rhesus disease does not affect a first pregnancy. It requires that the mother has had exposure to D rhesus-positive fetal cells in a previous pregnancy and then developed an immune response that has lain dormant until a following pregnancy of a D rhesus-positive baby. In the subsequent pregnancy, when maternal resensitization occurs (rhesus-positive red cells pass from the baby to the maternal circulation) (Fig. 14.8), IgG antibodies cross from the mother to the fetal circulation. If these antibodies are present in sufficient quantities fetal haemolysis may occur leading to such severe anaemia that the fetus may die unless a transfusion is performed. It is for this reason that rhesus-negative women have frequent antibody checks in pregnancy; an increasing titre of atypical antibodies may suggest an impending problem. It is important to note, however, that although the amount of D antibodies must be over a certain threshold limit (see later on), absolute measure of the antibodies does not correlate well with the degree of fetal anaemia. It is for this reason that invasive and non-invasive assessments of the fetus are indicated in risk situations to determine whether the fetus is becoming anaemic.

However the other two rhesus antigens (C and E) may also be associated with haemolytic disease of the fetus or neonate; these are inherited in exactly the same way as is D.

The problem of iso-immunization occurs when fetal cells have caused a maternal antibody response, and IgG antibodies are produced which cross the placenta and destroy fetal red cells, leading to fetal anaemia. Once a mother is sensitized to a fetal red cell antigen, the sensitization cannot be lost and the response will magnify with successive exposure, for instance in subsequent pregnancies.

The genetics of rhesus disease (Fig. 14.9):
- rhesus-negative mother, rhesus-negative father (homozygote);
- rhesus-negative mother, rhesus-positive father (heterozygote)
- rhesus-negative mother, rhesus-positive father (homozygote).

Antibodies associated with haemolytic disease

- ABO
- Rhesus (C, D, E)
- Kell
- Duffy
- c (known as 'little c')
- S

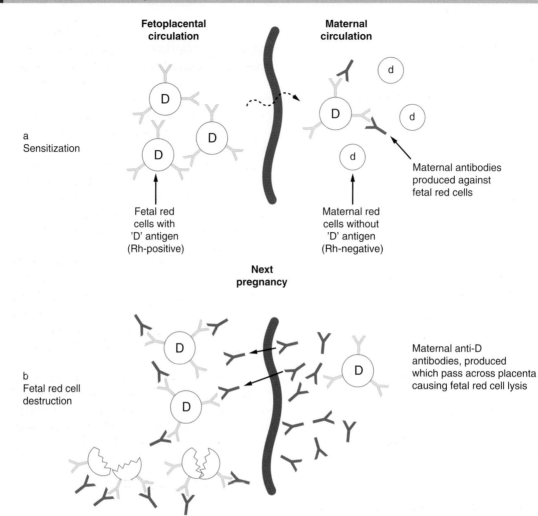

a
Sensitization

Fetal red
cells with
'D' antigen
(Rh-positive)

Maternal red
cells without
'D' antigen
(Rh-negative)

Maternal antibodies
produced against
fetal red cells

Next pregnancy

b
Fetal red cell
destruction

Maternal anti-D
antibodies, produced
which pass across placenta
causing fetal red cell lysis

Figure 14.8 The mechanism of Rhesus sensitization and fetal red cell destruction.

Prevalence of the disease

The presence of D rhesus negativity is 15 per cent in the Caucasian population, but lower in all other ethnic groups. It is very uncommon in Orientals. Rhesus disease is commonest in countries where anti-D prophylaxis is not widespread such as the Middle East and Russia.

Preventing rhesus iso-immunization

The process of iso-immunization can be 'nipped in the bud' by the intramuscular administration of anti-D immunoglobulins to a mother preferably within 72 hours of exposure to fetal red cells. Anti-D

Signs

Features of fetal anaemia
Note: clinical and ultrasound features of fetal anaemia do not usually become evident unless fetal haemoglobin is >5g/dL less than the mean for gestation. Usually features are not obvious unless the fetal haemoglobin is <6g/dL
- Polyhydramnios
- Enlarged fetal heart
- Ascites and pericardial effusions
- Hyperdynamic fetal circulation (can be detected by Doppler ultrasound by measuring increased velocities in the middle cerebral artery or aorta)
- Reduced fetal movements
- Abnormal CTG with reduced variability, eventually a 'sinusoidal' trace

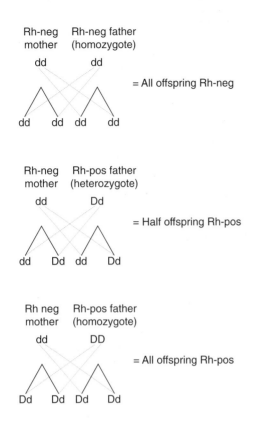

Figure 14.9 Parental genotype determinants of Rhesus group.

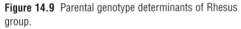

Potential sensitizing events for rhesus disease

- Miscarriage
- Termination of pregnancy
- Antepartum haemorrhage
- Invasive prenatal testing (chorion villus sampling, amniocentesis and cordocentesis)
- Delivery

In the first trimester of pregnancy, because the volume of fetal blood is so small, it is unlikely that sensitization would occur and a 'standard' dose of anti-D (the exact dose varies from country to country) is given; this will more than cover even the largest fetomaternal transfusion. In the second and third trimesters, fetal blood volume is greater and because there is a possibility of a fetomaternal transfusion of several millilitres, a larger dose is given and a Kleihauer test performed. A Kleihauer is a test of maternal blood to determine the proportion of fetal cells present (relying on their ability to resist denaturation by alcohol or acid); it will allow a calculation of the amount of extra anti-D immunoglobulin required should a large transfusion have occurred.

In many countries, rhesus-negative women are given anti-D at 28 and/or 34 weeks routinely. This is based on the finding that a small number of rhesus-negative women become sensitized during pregnancy despite the administration of anti-D at delivery and without a clinically obvious sensitizing event. The likelihood is that a small fetomaternal haemorrhage occurs without any obvious clinical signs, therefore prophylactic anti-D would reduce the risk of iso-immunization from this event.

The spectrum of the disease

(Mildest)…
- Normal delivery at term; mild jaundice requiring phototherapy
- Preterm delivery of an anaemic fetus requiring exchange transfusion
- Delivery of a fetus at 34 weeks following fortnightly blood transfusions from 26 weeks' gestation
- Stillbirth or neonatal death due to rhesus (earlier gestation = worse prognosis)
…(Severest)

The management of rhesus

This depends on the clinical scenario.
- The woman is D rhesus-negative, as is her partner. In this situation, there is no risk that the baby will be D rhesus-positive (assuming that her partner is the father of the baby). There is therefore no chance of rhesus disease.
- The woman is D rhesus-negative, and the partner

immunoglobulins 'mop up' any circulating rhesus positive cells before an immune response is excited in the mother. The practical implications of this are that after any potential sensitizing event (see symptoms box), anti-D immunoglobulin must be given intramuscularly as soon as possible afterwards. It is normal practice to administer anti-D after any of these events; the exact dose is determined by the gestation at which sensitization has occurred and the size of the fetomaternal haemorrhage.

is rhesus-positive. She has no (or a very low titre of) D rhesus antibodies and it is either her first pregnancy or she has not had a pregnancy previously affected by D rhesus disease.

Monitor atypical antibody levels at booking, 24 and 36 weeks. An increase in antibody titre to >10 iu/mL requires review in a fetal medicine centre so that early signs of fetal anaemia can be detected by ultrasound and, if appropriate, invasive assessment performed.

- The woman is D rhesus-negative and she has been sensitized to the D rhesus antigen, manifesting itself in an adverse pregnancy outcome. Once a woman is sensitized to the D rhesus antigen, no amount of anti-D will ever turn back the clock. In this situation there is therefore no role whatsoever for anti-D.

   Depending on her history (see 'the spectrum of the disease'), close surveillance is necessary. Begin by monitoring atypical antibodies every 2–4 weeks from booking. If the antibodies are at a low level (<10–15 iu/mL) then the baby is unlikely to become infected. If the antibodies rise by >15 iu/mL, and/or there are features of fetal anaemia, a fetal medicine opinion must be sought urgently as the baby may be very anaemic.

   If a previous pregnancy resulted in a stillbirth or neonatal death, fetal blood sampling by cordocentesis may be performed at 10 weeks before the onset of previous clinical disease. For example, if in a previous pregnancy a stillbirth occurred at 34 weeks due to previously unrecognized rhesus disease, then in the next pregnancy fetal blood sampling should be performed from 24 weeks for estimation of fetal haemoglobin and possible intrauterine transfusion of blood into the umbilical vein. In some units, the bilirubin concentration of amniotic fluid is determined optically to give an indirect measure of fetal haemolysis; this avoids the risks to the baby from cordocentesis should the baby not require transfusion. The most severely affected fetuses may require repeat transfusions

Blood transfused to the fetus must be

- Concentrated (Hb normally 22–24 g/dL)
- Cytomegalovirus-negative
- Rhesus-negative
- Irradiated (to reduce the risk of graft versus host disease)

every 7–10 days; after 34 weeks the risks of cordocentesis (fetal bradycardia, cord tamponade or haemorrhage, fetal death; see Chapter 12) outweigh the risk of prematurity and delivery of the baby is normally undertaken. Prior to 24 weeks, intra-peritoneal transfusion may be performed.

Blood transfusion

Blood may be given to the baby by a needle introduced through the mother's abdomen. Blood is given either intravascularly (into the umbilical vein or heart), or intraperitoneally. The first method is preferable, as blood enters the fetal circulation directly and severely anaemic fetuses may be saved. Intraperitoneal transfusion is reserved for cases of technical difficulty, or if the gestation is less than 22 weeks. If blood is taken from the fetus, the haemoglobin, fetal blood group and karyotype are usually checked. Clearly, if the baby is D rhesus-negative, it will not develop D rhesus disease.

At delivery

If the baby is known to be anaemic or has had multiple transfusions, a neonatologist must be present at delivery should exchange transfusion be required. Blood must therefore always be ready for the delivery. All babies born to rhesus-negative women should have cord blood taken at delivery for a blood count, blood group and indirect Coomb's test.

🔧 Key Points

Key points in D Rh disease

- Rh disease gets worse with successive pregnancies
- If the father of the fetus is Rh-negative, the fetus cannot be Rh-positive
- If the father of the fetus is Rh-positive, he may be a heterozygote (50 per cent likelihood that the baby is D Rh-positive) or a homozygote (100 per cent likelihood)
- Anti-D is given only as prophylaxis and is useless once sensitization has occurred
- Prenatal diagnosis for karyotype, or attempts at determining fetal blood group by invasive testing (e.g. chorion villus sampling) may make the antibody levels higher in women who are already sensitized

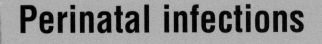

Chapter 15

Perinatal infections

OVERVIEW

Infection presents a major challenge to the obstetrician both in developed and developing countries. The extremely high rates of maternal mortality due to puerperal sepsis during the nineteenth and early twentieth centuries were mainly due to transmission of infection within the hospital. Group A streptococcus was the commonest pathogen. Semmelweis, working in mid-nineteenth century Vienna, was the first to demonstrate the value of aseptic technique and handwashing between patients. With improved infection control measures and the availability of IV antibiotics, maternal death from sepsis in hospital is now rare. Unfortunately, neonatal death still occurs from infections, such as group B streptococcal meningitis, septicaemia and viral infections, such as herpes encephalitis.

     Altered maternal physiology during pregnancy places the mother at additional risk of certain infections. Decreased smooth muscle tone leads to increased vulnerability to pyelonephritis developing as a complication of cystitis. Subtle shifts in immunity due to T-helper cells may lead to increased susceptibility to intracellular infections such as tuberculosis, chicken pox (varicella zoster infection), listeria and *Chlamydia psittaci*.

Infections associated with congenital infection

The infections that cause congenital abnormality have been traditionally summarized by the acronym TORCH (Toxoplasmosis, Rubella, cytomegalovirus, herpes). It is clear that many other infections may adversely affect a fetus or neonate and these have been resummarized as STORCH[5], (Table 15.1). However, pregnancy loss may occur in the first trimester in association with any acute infections in the mother, e.g. influenza.

Syphilis

Syphilis is a sexually transmitted infection caused by the sphirochete *Treponema pallidum*. It is common in many developing countries where up to 10 per cent of pregnant women may have positive serological tests. There has been an explosive epidemic in Russia and Eastern Europe during the 1990s but in Western Europe and the USA the incidence has fallen progressively over the course of the second half of the twentieth century.

     Primary syphilis presents as a painless genital ulcer

Table 15.1 – STORCH[5] Specific infections that adversely effect a fetus, neonate or pregnant woman

S   Syphilis
T   Toxoplasmosis
O   Other
     Bacterial vaginosis
     Trichomoniasis vaginalis
     Group B streptococcus
     Escherichia coli
     Ureaplasma urealyticum
     Haemophilus influenzae
     Varicella
     Listeria monocytogenes
R   Rubella
C   Cytomegalovirus
H[5]   Herpes
     HIV
     Hepatitis B
     Human papillomavirus
     Human parvovirus

(Fig. 15.1) three to six weeks after the infection is acquired, with local lymphadenopathy. In women the ulcer is most often on the cervix and may therefore pass unnoticed. At this stage the infection is highly contagious. Secondary manifestations of syphilis occur six weeks to six months after infection, often just as the primary chancre is regressing, and present as a non-itchy maculopapular rash affecting the palms of the hands and soles of the feet. Lesions affecting the mucous membranes are warty growths called condylamata lata. Other manifestations include alopecia, uveitis, and sensorineural deafness. If no specific treatment is administered the lesions regress after 2–4 weeks but the infected patient may suffer relapses during the following two years when lesions may reappear. At this stage the infection is called early latent, as it may be transmitted during relapses. Subsequently late infection ensues and syphilis cannot be transmitted sexually. Ultimately 20 per cent of untreated patients will develop symptomatic cardiovascular tertiary syphilis and 5–10 per cent will develop symptomatic neurosyphilis.

Up to 70 per cent (the highest risk) of fetuses become infected if the mother has primary or secondary syphilis during pregnancy. With later stages of syphilis the risk is smaller, being approximately 14

per cent, five years after the mother has acquired infection. The spectrum of congenital syphilis varies from a severe fetal infection causing intrauterine death, to a neonate with symptomatic disease (early congenital syphilis), a child who subsequently develops the stigmata of congenital syphilis (late congenital syphilis) to a child who is asymptomatically infected. The key features are summarized in Table 15.2.

Any woman presenting during pregnancy with small genital ulcers should be screened for syphilis and herpes. A dark ground examination should be performed to look for *T. pallidum* and blood taken for serology. A fluorescent treponemal antibody absorption (FTA) test is the first serological test to become positive in early syphilis. The *Treponemal pallidum* haemagglutination assay (TPHA) and FTA are specific tests for treponemal antibody, confirming exposure to infection at some stage of life; these remain positive even after treatment. The Veneral Diseases Research Laboratory test (VDRL) is measured quantitatively; a high titre of 1:64 or greater is found in secondary or early latent syphilis. After treatment the VDRL titre falls progressively and will be unreactive in most individuals after two years.

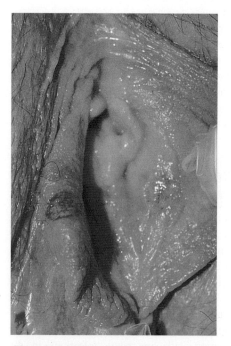

Figure 15.1 Primary syphilis. There is one painless ulcer on each side of the labia minora. (Courtesy of Dr Raymond Maw, Royal Victoria Hospital, Belfast.)

Table 15.2 – Features of congenital syphilis

Severe intrauterine infection leading to miscarriage
Early congenital syphilis:
      Maculopapular rash
      hepatitis splenomegaly
      mucus patches, lymphadenopathy
      bone abnormalities, anaemia
      active neurosyphilis
Late congenital syphilis
      Stigmata: Hutchinson's triad —
            interstitial keratitis,
            sensorineural deafness
            Hutchinson's teeth
            Clutton's joints
      Active disease: general paresis of the insane
            (GPI), gummata

The majority of pregnant women with syphilis are detected during routine screening at their booking visit. Biological false-positive VDRL tests may occur in women with systemic lupus erythematosus (SLE) or the anti-phospholipid syndrome, usually at a titre of 1:8 or less. Thus, if the VDRL is positive, but FTA and TPHA are negative an auto-antibody screen should be performed and lupus antibody sought. People originating from tropical countries may have one of the tropical treponematoses that are not sexually transmitted or transmissible to a fetus, such as Pinta and Yaws.

Treatment
Penicillin is the treatment of choice for syphilis. For early syphilis (primary, secondary or early latent) prescribe protein penicillin 1.2 MU daily, intramuscularly, for 12 days. Later stages of syphilis require 21 days of treatment. A Jarisch-Herxheimer reaction may occur with treatment as a result of release of pro-inflammatory cytokines in response to dying organisms. This presents as a worsening of symptoms, and fever for 12–24 hours after starting treatment and may be associated with uterine contractions and the onset of preterm labour. Some clinicians therefore advocate admitting women to initiate treatment with IV penicillin (1.2 MU per day in divided doses).

Women who are allergic to penicillin represent a problem. Tetracycline is the usual second line treatment but is contraindicated in pregnancy.

Erythromycin is less reliable and resistance has been reported; it is best administered IV. It is essential that current and recent sex partners of women with syphilis are screened themselves. Older children may also need to be screened.

Toxoplasmosis

Toxoplasma gondii is a protozoan parasite that may be acquired from exposure to cat faeces, or from eating uncooked meat. The prevalence varies widely according to eating habits. In France more than 70 per cent of pregnant women have been infected and acquired immunity before pregnancy, whilst in the UK only 10–20 per cent of women are immune. Despite this it is estimated that approximately 1 in 140 pregnant women in France acquire the infection during pregnancy compared to 1 in 400 in the UK. Primary infection often passes asymptomatically. It may cause a glandular fever-like illness with atypical lymphocytes seen on a blood film, but rarely it causes fulminating pneumonitis or fatal encephalomyelitis. Eye infections, presenting as chorioretinitis can occur from either congenital or acquired infection. In AIDS, as immunity deteriorates, previously quiescent toxoplasma may recur, causing multiple brain abscesses.

Most infections, however, are asymptomatic. Infection during the first trimester of pregnancy is most likely to cause severe fetal damage, but only 10–25 per cent of infections are transmitted to the fetus. In the third trimester 75–90 per cent of infections are transmitted but the risk of fetal damage decreases from 65 per cent in the first trimester to almost zero for those infected near to the time of delivery. Severely infected infants may have the classic tetrad of hydrocephalus or microcephaly, chorioretinitis, convulsions and cerebral calcifications. In such cases extensive neurological damage occurs and the neonate may die. The majority of infected infants are asymptomatic at birth but develop sequelae several years later.

Only 10 or so severely affected babies are diagnosed per year in the UK. Routine screening in pregnancy is therefore not undertaken. A variety of serological tests are available. The Sabin-Feldman dye test is performed in reference laboratories. Enzyme-linked immunosorbant assays (ELISA) are available and immunoglobin (Ig) M antibody can also be measured. The most definitive test is demonstration of the parasite in lymph node tissue or cerebral spinal fluid (CSF). It can be isolated by inoculation into mice. A high titre of antibody on the dye test (1 to 500 or higher) is suggestive but not diagnostic of current infection as titres may fall for several years. Similarly IgM antibody may persist for several months in adults. A presumptive clinical diagnosis can be made for congenital infection if the full clinical features are present and the infant has an elevated toxoplasma antibody titre. If the titre remains high for at least six months the diagnosis becomes definite. The presence of IgM antibody in cord blood is suggestive, but can occur from a placental leak and repeat testing should be performed. A negative IgM test does not exclude congenital toxoplasmosis.

Treatment

A combination of sulphadiazine and pyrimethamine is used in symptomatic adults. Pyrimethamine, however, is potentially teratogenic and should not be used during the first trimester. Spiramycin, a macrolide antibiotic is less toxic and is devoid of teratogenic effects. A three-week course of 2–3 gm per day is administered during pregnancy. Whilst this reduces the incidence of transplacental infection, it has not been shown definitively to reduce the incidence of clinical congenital disease. In France, where many more women acquire infection during pregnancy, women are screened antenatally, but again the benefits of such a programme appear to be limited. Congenital toxoplasmosis should always be treated with pyrimethamine and sulphonamide.

Prevention

Pregnant women should be informed of the mode of spread of toxoplasmosis from meat and cat faeces. They should avoid eating rare steaks or hamburgers and take care when handling raw meat in the kitchen. Handwashing with soap and water is essential. Pregnant women should avoid handling cats and particularly cat litter. Children's sandpits should be covered to prevent cats from defaecating in them.

Cytomegalovirus

Cytomegalovirus (CMV) is a herpes virus and therefore has the ability to establish latency. In the UK approximately 40 per cent of women are susceptible when they become pregnant. It is spread through the respiratory and genitourinary tracts and high levels of virus may be present in the urine. Primary infection often produces no symptoms or mild non-specific symptoms. The incidence of infection in pregnancy is therefore not known precisely but is estimated to be as high as 1 in 200 pregnancies, of which around 40 per cent will result in fetal infection. It is possible that infection later in pregnancy is more likely to result in fetal morbidity. Ninety per cent of infected infants are asymptomatic. Thus of an estimated 1,000 infected babies born per year in the UK, approximately 100 are damaged by the virus.

The principle features are microcephaly, blindness and deafness. Other manifestations include pneumonitis, chorioretinitis, cerebral calcification and developmental delay. Because the primary infection in the mother is usually asymptomatic the diagnosis is rarely made before birth. Probably about another 100 children are born each year with sensorineural hearing loss as the only sign of congenital CMV infection.

After infection the virus is excreted for weeks or months by adults and by infants for years. It persists in the lymphocytes throughout life and can therefore be transmitted by blood transfusion or transplantation. Reactivation occurs intermittently with shedding in the genital, urinary or respiratory tract. In temperate countries infection is usually transmitted by close contact, kissing or sexual contact; approximately 1–2 per cent of the population become infected each year. In tropical countries, most infections take place in childhood and 60–70 per cent of individuals are infected within six months of birth. The remainder are mostly infected by the age of five and therefore there are few susceptible pregnant women. Clinical features in infected infants include hepato-splenomegaly, jaundice and purpura.

Diagnosis

A definitive diagnosis of congenital infection can be made by isolating the virus in cell culture from throat swabs, urine, blood or CSF in the first three weeks of life. Infants may secrete the virus for a prolonged period and therefore isolation in the postnatal period does not confirm recent infection. Serological diagnosis is made by demonstrating a rising titre of IgG antibody or specific CMV IgM antibody. Specific IgM antibodies persist for a few weeks to a few months and specific IgA antibodies from a few months to a year. The diagnosis may be made *in utero* by amniocentesis and polymerase chain reaction (PCR), as the virus is concentrated in the urine. The congenital manifestations need to be differentiated from other congenital infections such as toxoplasmosis, rubella, herpes simplex and syphilis.

Treatment

Specific antiviral agents are available for CMV such as ganciclovir and foscarnet. These are not used in pregnancy, and have to be given by IV infusion. These agents are used in immunosuppressed individuals with AIDS or after transplantation but are not indicated for infected infants with congenital defects. Assistance with rehabilitation for congenital abnormalities may be required.

Rubella

This togavirus causes a usually insignificant infection in adults or adolescents but can cause devastating congenital infection. In most countries between 70–90 per cent of young adults are immune to rubella. In some parts of Asia only 50 per cent are immune. In temperate climates acquired disease is most common in the spring and early summer with an increase in local incidence every 3–5 years.

The incubation period is 2–3 weeks and clinical manifestations include mild fever, sore throat, enlarged cervical glands and a rash that may be discreet or give a general pink flush to the trunk. Painful joints are common in adults and symptoms persist for 3–7 days. However, infection in children often passes unnoticed. Any symptoms suggestive of rubella during pregnancy should lead to investigation. Similar clinical pictures (except those of congenital infection) are produced by many other viral infections.

Gregg's triad of cardiovascular defects, eye defects and deafness summarizes congenital infection. In addition, hepatitis, thrombocytopenia, bone involvement, microcephaly, behavioural change and mental retardation have been reported. Abortions and stillbirths can occur as can preterm birth. The diagnosis should be suspected in any small-for-gestational-age baby with congenital abnormalities. The congenital syndrome occurs most commonly in early pregnancy; the incidence is 50 per cent following infection in the first month, dropping to 10 per

cent if infection occurs in the fourth month of pregnancy. The virus can be isolated from over 90 per cent of embryos of infected pregnancies and it appears that approximately half the cases are able to clear the infection as only 50 per cent of proven maternal infections result in infants with persistent IgG or IgM antibodies.

Diagnosis is based on serological tests. At booking, maternal antibody levels are measured and if the antibody titre is low (< than 15 IU/mL) a booster vaccination should be given after delivery. A very high IgG antibody titre is suggestive of recent infection but specific IgM is only detectable for 4–6 weeks in most cases. Non-immune women should be advised to stay away from known cases of rubella, as there is no specific treatment available. Congenital rubella can be diagnosed by detecting the virus and secretions from the throat, urine and faeces. It can also be found in CSF, blood, eyes and ears. Excretion diminishes slowly and has ceased by the age of six months in 70 per cent of cases. Presence of IgG antibody after six months of age is confirmatory. Rubella-specific IgM may be found for 3–9 months.

Many children are so handicapped by deafness or blindness that they are unable to attend normal schools. If rubella is diagnosed during the first trimester, the risk of congenital infection is so high that many women elect to have a termination of pregnancy. In the past, adolescent girls were vaccinated against rubella and in the last decade vaccination has been incorporated in infancy within the measles, mumps, rubella (MMR) vaccine. Following scares related to the measles vaccine uptake has recently dropped below 90 per cent in the UK meaning that a cohort of women susceptible to rubella will continue to present in pregnancy. However, a vaccination programme has led to a significant reduction in the incidence of congenital rubella to two per year for the UK.

Varicella zoster

Varicella zoster virus is another herpes virus. It is transmitted easily from adults with chicken pox or shingles (herpes zoster) and 90 per cent of adults in the UK are immune to chicken pox. Shingles is a reactivation that can occur during pregnancy but does not pose any threat to the fetus. Transmission occurs through droplet spread, with an incubation period of about two weeks. In children the illness is often mild and there may be only a handful of lesions. In adults there is usually a prodrome with headache, general aches and pains and malaise. Clusters of vesicles emerge at different stages, usually most are densely grouped centrally. If there is any doubt the diagnosis can be confirmed by electron microscopy and culture of vesicle fluid. Once the infection clears latent infection of both sensory and motor nerve cells is established. This infection can reactivate with dissemination of the virus into a dermatome causing the eruption recognized as shingles. Pregnant women are more vulnerable to chicken pox and may develop pneumonitis, which can be fatal (to which smokers are particularly prone). Early administration of IV acyclovir may ameliorate the severity but intensive care support may be needed.

Varicella zoster can affect the fetus in two ways. If infection occurs prior to 20 weeks' gestation there is a small risk, approximately 1 per cent, of a congenital varicella syndrome. This consists of hypoplastic limbs, scarring and central nervous system anomalies. If a pregnant woman is exposed to chicken pox or shingles she should be tested for varicella zoster antibody. If she is not immune, varicella zoster immune globulin (VZIG) should be administered. The possible role of antiviral agents has not yet been evaluated.

Neonatal chicken pox can occur if the mother presents with infection from two days before to five days after delivery, as the fetus is exposed to virus in the absence of maternal antibody. Neonatal varicella may be very severe although early reports of a mortality rate of up to 30 per cent were over-estimated. VZIG should be administered to the neonate immediately if the mother develops chicken pox. If chicken pox develops during the first month of life, IV acyclovir should be administered.

The diagnosis of chicken pox is usually clinical but can be confirmed by electron microscopy or culture of scrapings taken from vesicles. Serological tests are negative during the acute presentation but the absence of antibody confirms that mother is susceptible to infection. Chicken pox should be differentiated from other acute viral exanthems. Small pox has now been eradicated. Eczema herpeticum might be mistaken for chicken pox.

Other infections associated with pregnancy loss and preterm birth

Parvovirus B19

Infection with human parvovirus has been recognized to cause acute aplastic crises in individuals with reduced red cell survival, such as those with sickle cell anaemia. In children it causes the viral exanthem known as 'fifth disease', erythema infectiosum or slapped cheek syndrome.

The infection is asymptomatic in 25 per cent of adults and >50 per cent of children. It may be associated with only mild symptoms of malaise or present with a macular rash and it can be associated with severe arthralgia. In approximately 15 per cent of infections occurring during pregnancy the fetus becomes chronically infected. This leads to persistent anaemia *in utero*, which may develop into non-immune hydrops fetalis. This can resolve spontaneously or may require intrauterine blood transfusion.

The diagnosis of parvovirus infection is confirmed by demonstrating virus-specific IgM in maternal serum or demonstrating seroconversion with a specimen that previously proved negative. It should be sought in mothers who have the clinical features, or when hydrops fetalis develops. There is no specific treatment for parvovirus infection but the baby should be monitored carefully with repeat ultrasound examinations. The virus is not teratogenic.

Listeria monocytogenes

This bacterium has been isolated from more than 50 species of domestic and wild animals including birds, fish, insects and crustaceans. It is found in sewage, water and mud and can grow in refrigerated food including meat, eggs and dairy products, particularly soft cheeses. Asymptomatic carriage in man as well as animals is common with up to 29 per cent of healthy people having detectable organism in the faeces. Such carriage is often transient. Cooking destroys it and therefore the risk of infection is greatest with uncooked food. Most infections are probably subclinical but pregnant women are more vulnerable to the infection. In the UK the incidence of *Listeria* infection is approximately 1 in 37,000 births.

In adults the anginose type of listeriosis may be confused with glandular fever and in pregnancy, an episode of malaise, headache, fever, backache, conjunctivitis and diarrhoea associated with abdominal or loin pain may occur. In 40 per cent of cases fever is not marked at any time and the disease presents as a mild, flu-like illness. In animals, recurrent or persistent genital *Listeria* infection causes habitual abortion and it may do the same in humans.

Listeria infection of the newborn occurs in two forms: the early onset type from *in utero* infection that manifests as septicaemia within two days of birth. Usually the infant is born premature with signs of respiratory distress and there may be a rash. The late form presents predominantly as meningoencephalitis after the 5th day. Approximately 30 per cent of babies with early onset disease are stillborn. In France, *Listeria monocytogenes* ranks third, after *E. coli* and group B streptococcus as a cause of neonatal sepsis. The organism has a predilection for infecting the CNS in the newborn and also in immunosuppressed adults. There may be only a low-grade fever and focal neurological signs may develop.

Diagnosis in the neonate requires a high index of suspicion. Specimens from affected sites including throat, liver, CSF, vagina, placenta, urine, faeces, blood can be used for culture. Isolation is enhanced by cold passage at 4°C. Serological diagnosis is unsatisfactory, although finding a rising titre of *Listeria*-specific IgM can be helpful.

The organism is susceptible to penicillins, macrolides and tetracyclines and ampicillin is the treatment of choice. Without recognition of the diagnosis the mortality for infantile Listeriosis is as high as 90 per cent and the prognosis is worse in preterm babies. Early diagnosis and prompt treatment has reduced this figure to only 50 per cent.

Malaria

Malaria is prevalent throughout the tropics and is a major cause of mortality in both children and adults. Major polymorphisms such as thalassaemia and sickle cell trait provide a selection advantage in these areas because affected individuals are more resistant to severe manifestations of malaria. *Plasmodium falciparum* causes the most severe type of malaria, which can present with hepatic and cerebral forms of infection. It is transmitted between human hosts by the female *Anopheles* mosquito. Attempts to eradicate this intermediate host during the 1960s and 70s with spraying of toxins such as dichlorodiphenyltrichloroethane (DDT) have now been abandoned. *P. falciparum* has been able to develop resistance to most antimicrobials, creating a need for new agents to be developed. The other strains of malaria (*P. ovale* and *P. vivax*) seldom cause fatal disease and have not so far developed chloroquine resistance but cause considerable morbidity. The development of the parasite in the mosquito only occurs at warm temperatures, therefore, infection is rarely transmitted at altitudes above 2,200 metres.

The principal feature of malaria is episodes of temperatures associated with rigors as the temperature rises followed by sweating as the temperature falls. There is headache, nausea and vomiting and with *P. falciparum* malaria the pyrexia may be continuous. The incubation period is approximately two weeks. In severe infections 20 per cent or more of the red cells may be infected and haemolysis occurs leading to anaemia. This may result in haemoglobinuria (blackwater fever), associated with acute renal failure. Hyponatraemia and disseminated intravascular coagulation may also occur. Cerebral malaria presents with disturbances in consciousness due to obstruction of cerebral capillaries by infected red cells that have reduced deformability. Pregnant women are at increased risk of severe manifestations of malaria; infection may trigger a miscarriage or premature labour. Even non-*falciparum* malaria has been associated with intrauterine growth restriction. Congenital malaria has been described.

The diagnosis should be suspected in anybody who has been to the tropics and presents with a febrile illness. A history of taking prophylaxis does not exclude the diagnosis, as no prophylaxis is 100 per cent effective. A blood film should be requested and stained for malaria parasites. Repeated blood films should be taken during episodes of fever if the initial test is negative. As well as anaemia there may be thrombocytopenia and elevation of liver enzymes. Fever in the tropics or in those recently returned may be caused by many other infections including typhoid, food poisoning organisms, and viral infections such as dengue fever.

Malaria is usually treated with quinine sulphate, initially administered IV. Individuals with *P. falciparum* malaria should be admitted to hospital and monitored closely as sudden deterioration requiring intensive care may occur. Non-*falciparum* malaria establishes chronic infection of the liver. If the individual is not returning to an endemic area acute treatment should be followed by a course of fansidar to eradicate infection. Individuals living in endemic areas acquire immunity to malaria but this is lost within a few months of moving away, therefore anyone travelling from the UK to an endemic area should consider taking prophylaxis. A combination of chloroquine and proguanil taken weekly provides protection against non-*falciparum* malaria and *falciparum* in some areas. Malaria resistant to many antimicrobials is present in sub-Sahara and Africa and South East Asia where even mefloquine resistance has been reported. The choice of prophylactic agent should therefore be made after consulting current recommendations giving details of resistance patterns. Chloroquine is probably the least toxic prophylactic agent for pregnant women and those travelling to areas of chloroquine resistance must balance the risk of malaria against the potential toxicity of prophylactic agents. It is safest to avoid travel to such areas when pregnant but if the mother cannot be persuaded to delay travel the potential risks and benefits of chemoprophylaxis must be discussed.

Chlamydia psittaci

This organism causes epidemic abortion in ewes. In humans it causes an atypical pneumonia. Exposure to lambing ewes, and the products of conception can lead to infection in pregnant women. This results in intrauterine infection and abortion. It has occurred most commonly in vets and farm workers and all pregnant women should be advised to avoid sheep during the lambing season.

Urinary tract infection (see page 201)

Bacterial vaginosis

Bacterial vaginosis (BV) is the commonest cause of vaginal discharge in women of childbearing age. The principle symptom is an offensive fishy-smelling vaginal discharge that is often more apparent during menstruation or following unprotected intercourse. In some populations its prevalence is greater than 50 per cent although in the UK it is found in 10–15 per cent of women. It is thought to represent a disturbance of the vaginal ecosystem in which the usually dominant lactobacilli are overwhelmed by an overgrowth of predominantly anaerobic organisms including *Gardnerella vaginalis*, *Bacteroides spp.*, *Mycoplasma hominis* and *Mobiluncus spp.* Some of these organisms produce polyamines and trimethylamine, which are responsible for the fishy smell. There is also a rise in the vaginal pH from the normal level, below 4.5, to levels as high as 6 or 7. It is not a sexually transmitted infection and there is no benefit from treating male partners.

BV is not usually associated with vaginal soreness. However, it may co-exist with either candidiasis or trichomoniasis, both of which cause irritation and soreness. On examination a white or yellow thin homogenous discharge is seen. Examination of a 'wet mount' of vaginal fluid microscopically shows the presence of many small bacteria. These adhere to the epithelial cells giving them a fuzzy border, the so-called 'clue cell'. Similar features are seen on a Gram-stained smear. Vaginal pH can be measured simply by placing a small amount of vaginal fluid onto pH paper. The fourth criterion is the potassium hydroxide test where a sample of vaginal fluid is mixed with potassium hydroxide on a microscope slide. A strong fishy smell is produced if the woman has BV. The condition may also be recognized on Papanicolaou-stained cervical smears. Culture of vaginal fluid is not useful for making the diagnosis as the organisms can be found in more than 50 per cent of normal women.

Trichomoniasis or candida can both co-exist along with BV and the discharges they produce can look similar to those of BV. Microscopy and culture of vaginal fluid can confirm both of these alternatives. Discharge due to cervicitis is usually more mucoid or mucopurulent and there should be signs of clinical cervicitis on examination. Many observational studies have confirmed that women with BV have an increased risk of second trimester loss and preterm birth: indeed it may be the most important cause of idiopathic preterm birth. It is associated with chorioamnionitis that can progress to deciduitis or amniotic fluid infection. Fetal pneumonitis and ultimately fetal death may follow this from sepsis.

Chorio-amnionitis is associated with elevated levels of pro-inflammatory cytokines such as TNF-Alpha, Il6 and Il12. These can stimulate the metabolism of arachidonic acid to prostaglandins, which are the final pathway for cervical ripening and the onset of labour. At present, studies are evaluating the use of antibiotics to treat women in pregnancy with BV. Studies of selected women at high risk of preterm birth have shown a benefit from treatment with metronidazole. However, it is less clear whether women without high-risk factors for preterm birth should be screened and treated. Symptomatic women should of course be treated.

Standard treatment for BV in the UK is metronidazole 400 mg twice a day for five days. This produces resolution within a few days but relapse can occur and as many as 30 per cent of women have BV again within one month. Alternative treatments include intravaginal 0.75 per cent metronidazole gel, 2 per cent clindamycin cream and oral clindamycin 300 mg twice a day for 5 days. Physicians have been wary of prescribing metronidazole during pregnancy because of reputed teratogenicity. Several meta-analyses have reviewed pregnancies where it was prescribed and have shown no excess of birth defects. If a woman requires treatment it is sensible to discuss the potential risks and weigh them against the benefits. Both oral and intravaginal clindamycin have been associated with pseudomembranous colitis, a potentially fatal condition. Women who develop diarrhoea following such treatment, particularly with blood, should cease treatment and seek medical advice.

Infections affecting the neonate at birth

Herpes simplex virus

Herpes simplex is a virus well adapted to its human host. Primary infection usually presents within seven days of exposure and may be accompanied by widespread lesions around the mouth and oro-pharynx and, in the case of oral herpes around the vulva, vagina and cervix. If inoculation occurs on skin, such as occupational exposure for a health care worker, a herpetic whitlow may result. In many populations more than 70–80 per cent are exposed to oral herpes, herpes simplex virus type 1 (HSV1), during childhood. This gives some degree of cross-protection against herpes simplex virus type 2 (HSV2), traditionally the causative agent of genital herpes, and primary infection may be mild. With less exposure to childhood infections in Western societies fewer young adults have been exposed to HSV1 and at present 50 per cent of cases of genital herpes are now due to this strain of virus. Primary infection may therefore follow oro-genital contact. Seroprevalence studies suggest that 15–70 per cent of the population have antibodies to HSV1 and approximately 20 per cent to HSV2.

Primary genital herpes presents with soreness and irritation of the affected part (Fig. 15.2). It may, however, pass completely unnoticed or be manifest with a widespread eruption of painful ulcers preceded by vesicles. Severe dysuria and peripheral nerve involvement may lead to urinary retention in women requiring admission for analgesia and a temporary suprapubic catheter. In pregnancy with altered T-helper cell immunity, recurrent herpes may be more severe than usual and mimic primary herpes. In primary herpes the lesions heal during the course of 2–3 weeks. Recurrences (Fig. 15.3) usually last 3–7 days and are more localized, in a similar manner to an oral cold sore.

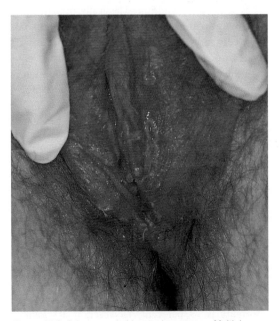

Figure 15.2 Primary genital herpes in a woman. Multiple ulcers are seen with a wide distribution, and confluent in some areas. In pregnancy, recurrent herpes can resemble a primary episode. (Courtesy of Dr Richard Lau, St. George's Hospital, London.)

On examination vesicles and ulcers are seen. The cervix may be severely inflamed and haemorrhagic. Cases of severe herpes mimicking pelvic inflammatory disease (PID) have been described particularly in postnatal HIV-infected women.

More than half the men and women infected with genital herpes are unaware of its presence. Close and careful questioning may reveal a history of transient almost trivial sores occurring sporadically usually in the same site. HSV2 is more likely to cause symptomatic recurrences than HSV1. The frequency of recurrences varies from person to person and a small minority will have more than six recurrences often per year; some are incapacitated due to neurological symptoms such as pains going down the legs.

The initial diagnosis is clinical but should always be confirmed by taking a swab from a vesicle or ulcer for culture or electron microscopy. Specific viral transport medium is essential. Serological tests have not been useful, as assays have not been able to distinguish between antibodies to HSV1 and HSV2.

Herpes simplex needs to be differentiated from other causes of genital ulcers. These include infections such as syphilis and tropical genital ulcer disease (see below). Genital ulcers can occur in association with systemic diseases such as sarcoidosis or SLE. Behçet's syndrome classically presents with oral and genital ulceration and may be accompanied by uveitis and CNS manifestations. The diagnosis is made by exclusion.

In the non-pregnant woman a first presentation of herpes should be treated with a five-day course of acyclovir 200 mg five times a day. This will stop further lesions developing and allow those that are present to heal. In many cases it will be a recurrent rather than a true primary infection that is being treated, but it is not possible to differentiate reliably unless there was a history of herpes infection. There is insufficient data to confirm that acyclovir is safe during pregnancy. However, to date there is no excess of birth defects associated with its use. Topical acyclovir cream is not effective in the treatment of genital herpes.

Herpes is important to diagnose in pregnancy because a devastating neonatal infection can occur with involvement of skin, liver and CNS. Neonatal mortality is 75 per cent. However, if acyclovir is administered rapidly, this can be reduced to 40 per cent. This syndrome is more common in the USA than the UK with a rate of 1 in 5000 live births

compared to 1 in 33,000. The vast majority of these cases are associated with a primary herpes infection in the mother in the weeks prior to delivery. The baby then has no protective antibody and is vulnerable to disseminated infection, or localized herpes encephalitis. If primary herpes presents around the time of delivery the case should be discussed with the paediatrician. Caesarean section will provide protection to the infant as long as the membranes have not ruptured for more than four hours. Genital swabs should be cultured from the mother and throat swabs from the baby and IV acyclovir should be administered to the neonate. Women known to have recurrent herpes have also been offered caesarean section if a recurrence occurs at the time of delivery. It has been found that the risk of infection to the neonate from a maternal recurrence of herpes is very small and many units have now abandoned caesarean section for this indication. The potential role of acyclovir administration for the last 2–4 weeks of pregnancy in women with recurrent herpes has not been fully evaluated because neonatal herpes in such cases is so rare.

Infection during the first trimester may cause miscarriage. A congenital syndrome has also been described, associated with micro-ophthalmia, chorioretinitis and microcephaly.

Group B Streptococcus

This organism is a commensal in the gut and genital tract and found in 20–40 per cent of women. It may

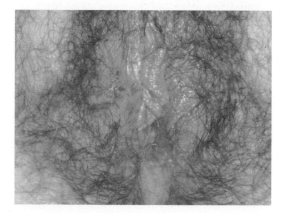

Figure 15.3 Recurrent genital herpes in a woman. (Courtesy of Dr. Colm O'Mahony, Countess of Chester Hospital.)

cause severe neonatal infection leading to neonatal death and can cause upper genital tract infection progressing to septicaemia and occasionally maternal death.

Carriage of the organism is asymptomatic. It colonizes the vagina from the gut and then ascends into the uterus. It can be detected on culture of vaginal swabs, but colonization of the vagina can occur at any stage of pregnancy. Attempts have been made to screen for infection in early pregnancy and eradicate the organism with penicillin, however recolonization frequently occurs and this approach has not been shown to reduce the incidence of neonatal infection. The current recommendation is therefore that the organism should be sought by culture of vaginal swabs in complicated pregnancies or those with a prior preterm birth. If the organism is present penicillin should be administered IV at the time of delivery. The infants most at risk are premature, those where deliveries undergo prolonged rupture of membranes, are growth restricted or have birth asphyxia. Early disease presents as overwhelming septicaemia and pneumonia. Occasionally an infant colonized in the perinatal period may develop secondary disease between 1 and 4 weeks of age, presenting as meningitis. Hospitals in which there is a high incidence of neonatal infection have developed protocols to screen mothers whose pregnancies are considered high-risk, and to treat them at about 28 weeks' gestation with penicillin, if the organism is detected on a vaginal swab. The case for such screening is weaker in units with a low prevalence of neonatal infection.

Chlamydia trachomatis

Chlamydia trachomatis is an obligate intracellular parasite. Genital infection with serotypes D–K is the commonest bacterial sexually transmitted infection in developed countries. It is also very common in developing countries. In many tropical countries trachoma, caused by serotypes A–C, is endemic and transmission is thought to occur amongst household contacts; it leads to blindness in the most severe cases. *Chlamydia trachomatis* is important in pregnancy because it causes neonatal eye infection (ophthalmia neonatorum) and neonatal pneumonitis.

Estimates of the prevalence of genital *Chlamydia trachomatis* infection vary between 2 per cent and 10 per cent of women in the UK. The organism is detected much more commonly in young sexually active women and women under the age of 25. The spectrum of disease varies from chronic asymptomatic infection to cervicitis, endometritis, salpingitis (PID) and intraperitoneal spread leading to perihepatitis (Fitz-Hugh Curtis). In men it causes non-gonococcal urethritis which may present with urethral discharge and dysuria. Many male partners of women with *Chlamydia trachomatis* however, are asymptomatic.

PID is uncommon during pregnancy and many pregnant women carrying *Chlamydia trachomatis* are only diagnosed after the neonate develops clinical disease. Where screening is undertaken, in communities with a high prevalence of *Chlamydia trachomatis*, asymptomatic infection will be detected. An infected cervix is friable and bleeds easily on contact, with an associated purulent discharge from the cervical os, termed 'mucopurulent cervicitis'. The changes induced by pregnancy may be similar so that the specificity of such findings is lower than in the non-pregnant woman. Tubal damage associated with previous chlamydial infection is an important predisposing factor for ectopic pregnancy.

Approximately 50 per cent of babies born to women with chlamydial infection develop ophthalmia neonatorum. This usually presents about a week after birth with a red sticky eye, which may be bilateral. Chloramphenicol drops, which are commonly prescribed, will only produce partial resolution. A swab for *Chlamydia trachomatis* should be taken from the baby's eye. The organism can also be sought in nasopharyngeal aspirates. Diagnosis of chlamydial infection is made by detecting the organism. ELISA tests are easily used to screen large numbers of samples but unfortunately the sensitivity is only 60 per cent. For this reason culture, DNA detection based tests or direct immunofluorescence must be used. Tests that rely on amplification of DNA provide greater sensitivity and specificity and will be used increasingly as routine. The organism can be detected with such tests in endocervical swabs, first pass urine samples, and even self-administered vaginal swabs. The most important differential diagnosis for cervicitis is gonorrhoea, which is described below.

The treatment of choice for *Chlamydia trachomatis* is tetracycline, usually doxycycline. However, tetracycline should be avoided in the second and third

CASE HISTORY

A 21-year-old primigravida is admitted in labour at 26 weeks' gestation with a twin pregnancy. The membranes ruptured spontaneously two hours earlier. An emergency Caesarean Section is performed. The first child is stillborn, and the second survives for only 12 hours in the neonatal intensive care unit. At postmortem the first child had a Gardnerella pneumonitis. The mother develops pyrexia of 39°C and is commenced on IV co-amoxiclav. Cultures of blood and urine are sterile. A vaginal swab grows mixed anaerobes. The fever settles and she is discharged from hospital five days later.

Six months later she presents with amenorrhoea of seven weeks, and right-sided pelvic pain. An ectopic pregnancy is confirmed and removed laparoscopically.

At this point she is screened for sexually transmitted infections and found to have chlamydial cervicitis. Her partner is also infected. Both are treated with doxycycline 100 mg twice daily for two weeks. After a further six months she falls pregnant again with a singleton fetus. A screen for

BV, chlamydia, gonorrhoea and trichomonas is negative. She has an uneventful pregnancy, delivering a healthy boy at 38 weeks' gestation.

Discussion points

- Infection is a major factor in the aetiology of idiopathic preterm birth. BV is associated with chorio-amnionitis, fetal sepsis and postpartum endometritis. Gardnerella pneumonitis is suggestive of BV in the mother.
- Preterm birth is commoner in twin pregnancies than in singleton pregnancies.
- *Chlamydia trachomatis* is an important cause of ectopic pregnancy. It should be sought in women with an ectopic pregnancy and their sex partners must also be screened and treated before intercourse is resumed.
- Forty per cent of women with a prior preterm birth have preterm delivery in the next pregnancy. It is possible that by eradicating infections the risk of preterm birth is reduced.

trimester of pregnancy because it binds to developing bones and teeth in the fetus, causing brown staining of the teeth and dysplastic bones. Erythromycin 500 mg twice a day for two weeks is therefore prescribed. This causes nausea, and the pharmacokinetics are not reliable in pregnancy so a test of cure two weeks after completing treatment is obligatory. It is essential that male partners are screened and treated before sexual intercourse is resumed. Azithromycin as a single one-gram dose is licensed for the treatment of *Chlamydia trachomatis* and may be useful if the woman is unable to tolerate erythromycin. Although penicillins are not considered adequate treatment to eradicate *Chlamydia trachomatis*, a recent study has shown that co-amoxiclav is effective in preventing neonatal infection and may be used if macrolides are contraindicated. Definitive treatment with a tetracycline should be administered after delivery and breastfeeding. Neonates with ophthalmia neonatorum should be treated with tetracycline eye ointment. Because there is a risk of subsequent chlamydial pneumonitis they should also be treated with a two-week course of erythromycin syrup.

Many women with *Chlamydia trachomatis* have subclinical endometritis, which may predispose to early pregnancy loss, chorio-amnionitis and preterm birth, and clinical postpartum endometritis. It has been associated with failure of implantation in women undergoing IVF. Such women and their partners should therefore be screened.

Gonorrhoea

Neisseria gonorrhoeae is a sexually transmissible agent causing cervicitis, urethritis, endometritis, salpingitis (PID) and perihepatitis in women. In men it causes urethritis and epididymitis and in both men and women it causes proctitis and pharyngitis. It is common worldwide although the incidence has decreased in developed countries since the Second World War. Infection in both sexes is frequently asymptomatic.

Like chlamydia, gonorrhoea is commonest in young sexually active women with the incidence declining over the age of 25. Its importance in obstetrics is due to a neonatal eye infection that if untreated can progress to blindness due to corneal scarring. The introduction of silver nitrate drops as prophylaxis produced a dramatic decline in the incidence of this complication.

The diagnosis of gonorrhoea is established by microscopy and culture. Gram-stained microscopy of cervical urethral and rectal swabs is performed, although the sensitivity of Gram stain is only 50 per cent compared to culture in women. The organism prefers a high CO_2 environment and is cultured on selective media such as blood agar. Even with optimal conditions, however, a single set of cultures has a sensitivity of only 60–70 per cent for detecting infection. If clinical suspicion is high a second set of cultures should be taken. It is routine practice to perform two sets of cultures as a test of cure following treatment. DNA detection based tests are now available and these offer superior sensitivity to culture, however at present they do not allow the opportunity for antibiotic resistance testing for which culture remains necessary.

Neisseria gonorrhoeae has demonstrated a great ability to acquire resistance to antibiotics. It readily exchanges plasmids with other bacterial species and plasmid-mediated resistance to penicillin and tetracycline appear rapidly under selection pressure with such antibiotics. In many developing countries the price of antibiotics is prohibitive for most individuals, so that suboptimal doses are used. This encourages the development of resistant strains, which are then exported worldwide. Chromosomal mutation has also produced moderate levels of penicillin resistance and is responsible for resistance to quinolones. Quinolones are contraindicated in pregnancy and therefore in a penicillin-allergic woman, or a woman with penicillin-resistant infection a cephalosporin, such as cefotaxime 2 gm in a single IM dose, should be administered. Table 15.3 details antibiotics and their use in pregnancy.

Neonates may present with ophthalmia neonatorum due to gonorrhoea a few days after birth. If *Neisseria gonorrhoeae* is cultured, topical and systemic treatment should be administered according to antibiotic sensitivities. In a similar way to *Chlamydia trachomatis*, gonorrhoea is associated with chorioamnionitis and preterm birth.

Trichomoniasis

Trichomoniasis vaginalis causes severe vulvovaginitis in susceptible women. It is generally sexually transmitted although infection may persist asymtomati-

cally for many months in women and in some men. In men it may cause urethritis but is frequently asymptomatic. Transient infection can be transmitted to female infants who will present with purulent vaginal discharge.

The incidence of trichomoniasis has fallen in the last decade in developed countries. It remains highly prevalent in many developing countries where as many as 20–30 per cent of pregnant women carry the infection. It presents with a purulent vaginal discharge and may be associated with severe inflammation causing soreness and itching with a tide mark extending on to the thighs. The diagnosis is made by detecting the organism on wet mount microscopy, with a sensitivity of approximately 50–60 per cent.

Newborn girls have stratified squamous epithelium in the vagina, similar to that of an adult due to the influence of high levels of maternal oestrogen *in utero*. They are therefore susceptible to infection and may develop asymptomatic discharge. As the influence of maternal oestrogen wanes over the first few weeks of life such infection usually resolves spontaneously and specific treatment is rarely necessary.

Trichomoniasis frequently co-exists with disturbed vaginal flora that develops into BV. The only established treatments for trichomoniasis are metronidazole or tinidazole but these have been considered to

Table 15.3 – Commonly used antibiotics in pregnancy

Thought to be safe
    Penicillins e.g. amoxycillin
    Cephalosporins e.g. cefotaxime
    Erythromycin
    Nitrofurantoin in first and second trimesters

Probably safe but limited experience
    Co-amoxiclav
    Azithromycin

Significant caution required
    Quinolones, e.g. ciprofloxacin
    Folate reductase inhibitors e.g. cotrimoxazole

Contraindicated
    Tetracyclines

carry a risk of teratogenecity. Recent reviews have concluded that there is extremely limited animal data to support such a claim although there is some evidence of mutagenesis. Retrospective studies of women who have taken metronidazole during pregnancy have shown no excess of fetal abnormalities and it is therefore reasonable to treat symptomatic women with a five-day course of metronidazole 400 mg twice a day. It is sensible, however, to discuss the potential risks of any treatment with the mother so that she can make an informed decision. Clotrimazole has some activity against trichomoniasis and application of intravaginal clotrimazole pessaries may control symptoms until the end of the first trimester if a woman is particularly concerned about systemic treatment.

Other infections

Ureaplasma urealyticum is an organism in the Mycoplasma family, which is a common commensal organism in the vagina. It has been detected in the membranes of women delivering preterm and has also been associated with neonatal pneumonitis. Its importance in inducing preterm birth and neonatal lung disease is not yet established and further research is continuing. *Mycoplasma genitalium* is a recently described organism that appears to cause a spectrum of disease similar to *Chlamydia trachomatis* with cervicitis, PID and non-gonococcal urethritis. It has not yet been studied extensively in pregnancy.

Infections affecting the mother

Vaginal candidiasis

Over three-quarters of women have at least one episode of vaginal candidiasis during their lifetime. A few women get frequent recurrences. The organism is carried in the gut, under the nails, in the vagina and on the skin. The yeast *Candida albicans* is implicated in more than 80 per cent of cases. *Candida glabrata*, *C. krusei* and *C. tropicalis* account for most of the rest. Sexual acquisition is rarely important although the physical trauma of intercourse may be

sufficient to trigger an attack in a predisposed individual. Candida is an opportunist, growing under favourable conditions. Symptomatic episodes are common in pregnancy. Its growth is favoured by the high levels of oestrogen, increased availability of sugars, and subtle alterations in immunity.

The classical presentation is itching and soreness of the vagina and vulva with a curdy white discharge that may smell yeasty but not unpleasant. Not all candida presents in the same way, in some cases there may be itching and redness with a thin, watery discharge.

The pH of vaginal fluid is usually normal, between 3.5 and 4.5. The diagnosis can be confirmed by microscopy and culture of the vaginal fluid. Asymptomatic women from whom candida is grown on culture do not require treatment.

Recurrent candida, or resistance to treatment is relatively uncommon. If this appears to be the case, it is important to consider other diagnoses, particularly herpes simplex that causes localized ulceration and soreness, and dermatological conditions such as eczema and lichen sclerosis.

In general it is better to use a topical treatment rather than systemic. This minimizes the risk of systemic side effects, and exposure of the fetus. Vaginal creams and pessaries can be prescribed at a variety of doses and duration of treatment. For uncomplicated candida, a single dose treatment, such as clotrimazole 500 mg, is adequate. If oral therapy has to be used, a single 150 mg tablet of fluconazole is usually effective, but its activity is limited to *Candida albicans* strains and its role in pregnancy is not yet defined.

Genital warts

Warts are caused by human papillomavirus (HPV) infections. More than 100 strains have so far been identified and certain strains are generally transmitted sexually, producing genital warts on the mucosa of the genital tract. Most symptomatic infections develop within eight months of starting a sexual relationship with a new partner but the incubation period may be a few years in some cases. It is thought that cell-mediated immunity is important for suppressing wart virus infections. With the alterations in maternal immunity that occur during pregnancy a previously asymptomatic infection may start to produce genital warts or established infections may become more florid (Fig. 15.4). Topical application of podophyllin or podophyllotoxin is often used as first line treatments but these are contraindicated in pregnancy. The risk of fetal damage from administration of a small amount of such chemicals to genital warts in a woman who does not realise she is pregnant is so low that it is not an indication for termination of pregnancy, unless applied to a very large area, >10 cm^2. Surgical methods such as cryotherapy or excision are therefore the only treatments available for pregnant women. Even so, the warts may not fully resolve until the woman has delivered. Male partners should be advised to attend a genitourinary medicine clinic for screening and treatment of any warts that they may have and condoms should be used during sexual intercourse. In an established relationship it is likely that wart virus transmission has already occurred and therefore it is no longer necessary to give such advice unless a new relationship has started. HPV types 6 and 11 are the ones found most often in symptomatic lesions. These have a low association with malignant change in the cervix. The oncogenic strains 16 and 18 may be found alongside the other types, but do not often produce typical lesions on their own.

Any baby born to a mother harbouring wart virus will be exposed to such virus during delivery. It appears, however, that few neonates acquire infection from their mothers. Rarely, infants may present with laryngeal warts due to a genital strain of wart virus, but transmission appears to occur from less than 1 per cent of infected mothers. It is unlikely that maternal transmission leads to established infection in the genital tract of boys or girls.

Tropical genital ulcer disease

In many tropical areas infections causing genital ulcers are common. Herpes simplex remains an important cause of genital ulcers worldwide but lymphogranuloma venereum caused by the LGV strains of *Chlamydia trachomatis,* Donovanosis caused by *Calymmatobacterium donovanii* and chancroid caused by *Haemophilus ducreyii* are common. Specific diagnostic tests are expensive and such infections are usually managed according to protocols for syndromic management. The precise antibiotics prescribed depend on local availability and sensitivity

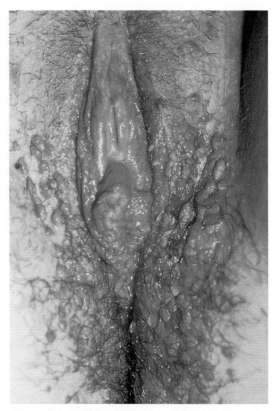

Figure 15.4 Multiple genital warts in a pregnant woman. Warts often increase in size and number during pregnancy. (Courtesy of Dr Richard Lau, St. George's Hospital, London.)

patterns established in reference laboratories. In some areas of sub-Saharan Africa up to 30 per cent of pregnant women are infected with HIV therefore, altered immunity may lead to atypical presentation of any of these infections making diagnosis and treatment more difficult.

Other infections

With the altered immune state of pregnancy chronic infections requiring cell-mediated immunity may flare up. These include wart virus infections as discussed above. With the increasing incidence of tuberculosis worldwide and recent increases in the UK and the USA, increasing numbers of pregnant women may present with severe manifestations of disease such as miliary tuberculosis. Pregnancy produces a transient fall in the CD4 lymphocyte count of HIV-infected women. This will be discussed more fully

Table 15.4 – Infection screening during pregnancy (universal in UK, or some parts of the UK)

Infection	Test	Action
Syphilis	VDRL/ TPHA	Refer to specialist if reactive. If no history of prior treatment, will need parenteral penicillin for 12 days
Rubella	IgG	If negative, advise to avoid contact: vaccinate after delivery
Hepatitis B	surface antigen test	Immunoglobulin and vaccination for neonates. Check maternal liver function tests, and refer to hepatitis clinic
HIV	HIV antibody	Discuss ways to reduce risk of vertical transmission. Manage with multidisciplinary team
UTI	urinalysis/M,C&S	Prescribe antibiotics and check again after treatment

May be indicated in some cases/routine in some countries
Group B Streptococcus
Herpes simplex
Toxoplasmosis
Bacterial vaginosis
Chlamydia trachomatis
Gonorrhoea
Hepatitis C

below. Most of the UK now has an effective screening programme, these are listed in Table 15.4.

Other vertically transmissible viral infections

Human T-cell leukaemia virus-1

Human T-cell leukaemia virus (HTLV-1) is a retrovirus which establishes life-long infection in infected individuals. The majority of such individuals remain asymptomatic but a small proportion may develop T-cell leukaemia in adult life. It also causes tropical spastic paraparesis, which presents with demyelination of the spinal cord causing spastic weakness in the legs. Its prevalence is greatest in Japan, the Caribbean, the Indian sub-continent and parts of Africa. It is transmitted sexually or through breast milk, therefore if infection is identified the mother should be advised not to breastfeed. There is no specific treatment but barrier methods of contraception should be advised if the sex partner is uninfected.

Hepatitis A

This is caused by an RNA virus, which is spread through the oral-faecal route. Approximately 50 per cent of the UK population have antibodies from childhood infection but the prevalence is falling. The majority of individuals in developing countries acquire infection during childhood. It is usually a benign illness but occasionally fulminating hepatitis has been described in pregnant women but it has not been associated with congenital abnormalities. Individuals are most infectious before they develop jaundice. Some degree of protection may be provided through vaccination or administration of human immune globulin during the incubation period.

Hepatitis B

Hepatitis B is a more severe infection that may be followed by chronic carriage and disease ending in cirrhosis. It is transmitted sexually, through blood products and through vertical transmission from an infected mother. A majority of acute infections are not clinically recognized as only 20 per cent of individuals develop jaundice. The earlier in life the infection occurs the more likely the person is to become a carrier; 80 per cent of infants infected perinatally become carriers. Infection is particularly common in China and South East Asia but prevalent in most tropical countries.

Pregnant women are screened for hepatitis B at booking. During acute infection hepatitis B surface antigen (HBsAg) and e antigen (HbeAg) are detectable in serum. Hepatitis B core antibody appears after approximately six weeks and remains detectable thereafter as a marker of exposure. As immunity develops anti-e antibody develops and the e antigen becomes undetectable. With clearance of the virus, surface antigen disappears and surface antibody is detectable. When HBeAg is present the individual is highly infectious. Only a small proportion of individuals who are sAg-positive but eAg-negative have replicating virus and are infectious. Thus to screen for chronic infection anticore antibody is sought. If this is positive the other markers are tested to establish the degree of infectivity.

A proportion of individuals do not clear the acute infection and go on to develop chronic hepatitis. Treatment is available with interferon under the guidance of a liver specialist and antiviral drugs with specific activity against hepatitis B are being introduced at present. Vertical transmission can be prevented by vaccination of neonates born to mothers with hepatitis B. Hepatitis B immune globulin is given at birth additionally if the mother is eAg-positive. Countries with a higher prevalence of hepatitis B infection than the UK have a policy of universal vaccination of all infants.

Hepatitis C

This is another RNA virus that causes chronic hepatitis. Again acute infection often passes asymptomatically but more than 50 per cent of infected individuals have active hepatitis which will progress to cirrhosis and possibly hepatocellular carcinoma. The prevalence varies widely across the world with the highest incidence in Egypt, possibly associated with the use of contaminated needles for mass treatment for schistosomiasis. In the UK infection is highly prevalent in those with a history of IV drug use. It may be transmitted sexually but transmission is not very efficient with only 1–2 per cent of long-term partners becoming infected. Vertical transmission again occurs uncommonly although the risk is increased in those co-infected with HIV.

Hepatitis D

This is a defective virus that can only replicate in the presence of hepatitis B. Individuals who have this super infection are more likely to develop severe hepatitis.

Hepatitis E

This virus is spread through the oral–faecal route and causes acute hepatitis. It can, like hepatitis A, be fulminating in pregnant women, with up to 20 per cent mortality. It is found mainly in tropical countries, where epidemics have occurred after natural disasters allowed contamination of water with sewage. It is not thought to cause chronic hepatitis.

HIV infection

HIV infection is a major challenge for the obstetric team. There is a need to reduce the risk of vertical transmission to the fetus, and to maintain optimal health of the mother. This, however, usually involves the use of interventions such as drugs of known or unknown fetal toxicity, performing caesarean section and advice not to breastfeed. It is best managed through a multidisciplinary team incorporating obstetricians, midwives, paediatricians and HIV specialists.

Acquired immunodeficiency syndrome (AIDS) was first described in San Francisco in 1983. It is caused by infection with human immunodeficiency virus (HIV). More than 20 million individuals are now infected worldwide and in countries with a high prevalence it is the leading cause of death in young adults. It is a particularly devastating disease because of the stigma of sexual transmission, the risk of vertical transmission to children, and the likelihood that other family members are infected. Even if a child is not infected, the death of one or both parents threatens their development and survival in many parts of the world. At present, HIV is increasing in prevalence in most parts of the world. In sub-Saharan Africa there are several cities in which as many as a third of pregnant women are infected. The epidemic in South East Asia is a few years behind that of Africa. By contrast in London the prevalence in pregnant women is less than 1 per cent, and considerably lower in most other parts of the UK. A resurgence in tuberculosis has occurred hand-in-hand with the AIDS epidemic.

The onset of immunodeficiency can be manifest in any organ system so that a high index of suspicion is required to recognize the way in which other disease processes are altered.

Natural history and principles of treatment of HIV infection

Twenty per cent of those infected with HIV experience an acute seroconversion illness a few weeks after acquisition. Clinical features include: fever, generalized lymphadenopathy, a macular erythematous rash, pharyngitis and conjunctivitis. A steady decline in immune function over the first few years may be manifest by non-life-threatening opportunistic conditions, such as recurrent oral and vaginal candidiasis, single dermatome herpes zoster (shingles), frequent and prolonged episodes of oral or genital herpes, persistent warts and genital ulcers (Fig. 15.5). Furry white patches on the sides of the tongue, termed oral hairy leukoplakia (OHL), may come and go. It is pathognomic of immunodeficiency. Persistent generalized lymphadenopathy may be present. Skin problems include seborrhoeic dermatitis, folliculitis, dry skin, tinea pedis and a high frequency of allergic reactions.

Without antiretroviral treatment the average time for the development of AIDS is 10 years. Essentially AIDS is defined by the onset of life-threatening opportunistic infections, or malignancies associated with immunodeficiency. The commonest presentations are listed in Table 15.5. There are two strategies used in treatment. Combinations of antiretroviral drugs are prescribed. The acronym HAART has been adopted, for Highly Active AntiRetroviral Therapy. Combinations may include two or more nucleoside analogues reverse transcriptase inhibitors, such as zidovudine or didinasine, a non-nucleoside reverse transcriptase inhibitor such as nevirapine, or one or more protease inhibitors such as nelfinavir. If successful the immune system improves after a few months. These drugs, particularly some of the

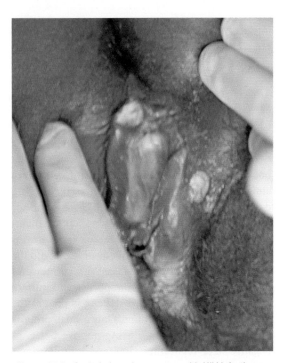

Figure 15.5 Genital ulcers in a woman with HIV infection. These persistent painful ulcers were due to herpes simplex. Persistence for more than one month is AIDS defining. In the tropics the differential diagnosis includes chancroid and Donovanosis.

protease inhibitors, have many potential interactions with other drugs through effects on the cytochrome P-450 enzymes. This includes increasing the rate of breakdown of both natural oestrogens and synthetic oestrogens used in oral contraceptive pills.

If immunodeficiency has already occurred treatment and prevention of opportunistic infections is needed. This may include cotrimoxazole to prevent *Pneumocystis carinii* pneumonia (PCP) and in severely immunosuppresed individuals with CD4 counts <0.05/L, azithromycin to prevent disseminated *Mycobacterium avium* intracellulare complex (MAC) infection, and ganciclovir to prevent cytomegalovirus (CMV) infection. Regular administration of antifungal agents may be necessary to control oral and vaginal candidiasis.

Virology

HIV is a retrovirus, with its genetic code in a single strand of RNA. Reverse transcriptase is carried

Table 15.5 – Common AIDS-presenting illnesses

Pulmonary
    Pneumocystis carinii pneumonia
    Tuberculosis – pulmonary or extra-pulmonary

Neurological
    Cerebral toxoplasmosis
    Cryptococcal meningitis
    AIDS dementia

Gastrointestinal
    Diarrhoea and wasting syndrome which may
      be due to infection with Cryptosporidium,
      Microsporidium, Isospora
    Oesophageal candidiasis

Ophthalmic
    Cytomegalovirus retinitis

Malignancy
    Kaposi's sarcoma
    Non-Hodgkin's lymphoma

Systemic
    Mycobacterium avium intracellulare complex
      (MAC) infection

within the core to enable pro-viral DNA to be produced in an infected cell. The outer membrane protein, gp-120 binds to CD4 receptors, which are present on T-helper lymphocytes, macrophages, dendritic cells and microglia. Co-receptors, such as the CCR-5 chemokine receptor are also used to enhance viral entry. Approximately 1 per cent of Caucasians has a homozygous mutation in the receptor, which is associated with resistance to acquiring infection. Another viral protein, p24, surrounds the RNA and enzymes present within the core of the virus, which enters the cytoplasm of an infected cell. Once pro-viral DNA has been integrated into the host, genome viral peptides are transcribed. Specific viral protease enzymes cleave these, before the daughter virus particles are assembled.

Current antiretroviral drugs target reverse transcriptase or viral proteases. The aim of therapy is to reduce the level of virus in the plasma to zero with a combination of antiretroviral agents. If total suppression of viral replication is not achieved, resistant strains of virus will inevitably arise within the patient over the course of a few months. This is because reverse transcription is inherently inaccurate, leading to a high rate of mutation. With each cycle of replication of virus, which takes 48 hours, single point mutations arise, which will confer reduced sensitivity to antiviral agents. If therapy is effective the CD4 lymphocyte count rises progressively, and at least partial immune restoration occurs. Unfortunately HIV infects long-lived memory cells from which virus can rapidly reseed the body on cessation of therapy. Eradication, and thus cure, is unlikely even after several years of treatment.

Diagnosis

HIV infection is diagnosed by finding antibodies to gp-120. During seroconversion p24 antigen is detectable in the serum before antibodies are produced. We monitor the disease by measuring the level of CD4 lymphocytes in peripheral blood. A normal level is >0.5/L. There is a 10 per cent risk of AIDS developing within one year when the CD4 lymphocyte count drops to 0.2/L. This is the level at which primary prophylaxis against PCP is recommended. Using PCR technology we can also measure the concentration of viral RNA in the plasma. A high level, >100,000 particles/mL predicts rapid disease development, whilst a low level, <10,000 HIV viral load copies/mL is associated with a low risk of disease progression.

Because the consequences of receiving a diagnosis of HIV are serious a test should only be performed with informed consent from the patient. She may wish to discuss it with a partner, for whom the test may have major implications. To avoid the serious consequences of incorrect labelling or other human errors occurring it is good practice to confirm correct labelling of the sample and request form with another health care worker.

If you suspect an individual has HIV look for HOL, generalized lymphadenopathy and skin rashes. Kaposi's sarcoma may be evident with multiple red or purple tumours anywhere on the body. There is often lymphopenia or thrombocytopenia on a full blood count. Polyclonal IgG production produces a raised total protein level.

Transmission

In most developing countries HIV is principally spread through vaginal intercourse, with approximately equal numbers of men and women infected. In developed countries the majority of infections have been acquired through homosexual sex or IV drug use, although the incidence of heterosexual transmission is increasing. Genital infections are risk factors for HIV transmission and acquisition, including genital ulcer disease, chlamydia and gonorrhoea. BV may also be a risk factor, and is very common in some African countries, with a prevalence of 50 per cent or greater. Good control of sexually transmitted infections should reduce the incidence of HIV infection.

Vertical transmission

Vertical transmission occurs in 25–40 per cent of pregnancies, if no interventions are used to reduce the risk. It is thought that a minority of infections occur during gestation. These babies can present with AIDS in the neonatal period. The majority of infections occur during parturition. Breastfeeding accounts for transmission in up to 15 per cent of pregnancies, corresponding to 37 per cent of

Key Points

HIV and pregnancy

As a minimum the following information needs to be discussed before a test is performed:

- The antibody test may take three months to become reactive after exposure
- If there has been a recent high-risk exposure the test should be repeated three months and six months after the event
- A confirmatory sample should always be taken if the first test is reactive
- Without specific treatment the average time to develop AIDS is 10 years. It is possible to remain healthy even 15 years after initial infection
- In countries with adequate health-care resources the prognosis is greatly improved by treatment
- In pregnancy the risk of vertical transmission is about 1 in 4 if no interventions are undertaken
- A combination of antiretroviral medication, Caesarean Section and avoidance of breastfeeding reduce the risk to <3 per cent.
- Who, if anyone, does the individual plan to tell about the test and its result?

CASE HISTORY

A 25-year-old primigravida attends a booking clinic at 18 weeks' gestation. She has a history of IV drug use. After discussion with the midwife she agrees to be screened for hepatitis viruses and HIV. She tests positive for syphilis; TPHA and FTA both reactive, VDRL negative. She also has evidence of past infection with hepatitis B; core antibody positive, surface antigen and e antigen negative. She is hepatitis C and HIV antibody positive.

She gives a history of treatment for syphilis five years earlier, with a 14-day course of penicillin injections. The HIV and hepatitis C tests are confirmed on a second sample. Her CD4 lymphocyte count is 0.35 cells/L, and HIV viral load 15,000 copies/mL. She has vaginal candidiasis.

She is seen by the multidisciplinary HIV team and agrees to a three-pronged approach to reduce the risk of vertical transmission: taking zidovudine 250 mg twice daily starting at 28 weeks' gestation, an elective Caesarean Section at 38 weeks' gestation and not to breastfeed.

The pregnancy progresses uneventfully, and the child has negative HIV PCR tests at three months, six months and nine months of age, confirming that HIV has not been transmitted. He is also hepatitis C negative.

Discussion points

- Tests for HIV and hepatitis B and C should be encouraged in all women with a history of IV drug use. Pre-test discussion is essential, and positive results should be confirmed on a second sample.
- If the history of prior syphilis treatment is confirmed she does not need further treatment. Her serological test results are compatible with treated infection.
- There are no interventions to reduce vertical transmission of hepatitis C, which is more common in mothers co-infected with HIV.
- With the measures to prevent HIV vertical transmission the risk of infection for the fetus is less than 3 per cent.
- The CD4 and viral load results suggest a low risk of developing AIDS in the next three years for the mother. She does not require aggressive triple therapy for HIV, or prophylaxis against opportunistic infections at this stage.
- In developing countries the risks of gastroenteritis from bottle feeding have to be balanced against the risk of infection through breast milk. With prolonged breastfeeding, >1 year, 15–20 per cent of infants might acquire infection through this route.

infected infants. Transmission by this route may occur even after several months. The risk of vertical transmission is increased if there is a high HIV viral load or a preterm delivery. The role of genital infections in vertical transmission is still being assessed. Many children infected with HIV will survive into adolescence.

Three interventions have been shown to reduce the risk of vertical transmission of HIV.

- Avoiding breastfeeding.
- Elective Caesarean Section.
- Antiviral medication prescribed during the latter half of pregnancy, and to the neonate for six weeks.

If all three interventions are undertaken the risk of transmission is probably less than 3 per cent. Zidovudine monotherapy has been studied most extensively in this context in randomized controlled trials. Since maternal HIV plasma viral load is predictive of vertical transmission it is likely that combination therapies will be more effective. This approach has to be balanced against unknown potential toxicities for the neonate.

References for further reading

Barton S, Hay P. (eds) *Handbook of Genitourinary Medicine.* London: Arnold, 1999.

Chapter 16

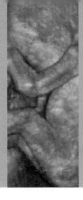

Medical diseases complicating pregnancy

OVERVIEW

Pregnancy is a normal event in life and as the majority of the population does not have medical disorders, most women will remain medically fit and well for the duration of their pregnancy. There are few medical disorders that are associated with sterility although some may reduce a woman's fertility. Thus potentially any woman of fertile age, irrespective of any pre-existing medical disorder may fall pregnant. For any medical condition in pregnancy there is always a spectrum of disease from the very mild forms, which are unlikely to have a sinister effect on the pregnancy, to the most severe, which in some circumstances may be associated with significant maternal mortality.

In an age of increasing medical subspecialization an obstetrician will often work in partnership with a specialist physician, for example a cardiologist or endocrinologist, with a particular interest in pregnancy. Other members of a team, including specialist nursing staff, dieticians and physiotherapists, will often provide support. This multidisciplinary approach is vital in helping to ensure that the levels of care afforded to the non-pregnant population are provided for pregnant women. In the ideal world the assessment of a woman's medical condition and the implications for future pregnancies would be discussed and a plan of care detailed before the woman fell pregnant. Pre-conception counselling of this type does occur, but usually after the first pregnancy has ended in failure. For example, women with insulin-dependent diabetes should only fall pregnant when their diabetic control is very tight;

failure to do so is associated with a significantly increased risk of pregnancy failure and fetal abnormality. Counselling prior to the pregnancy allows women, particularly those with congenital heart disease, to come to terms with the possible risks they may be taking by falling pregnant and the level of care they will require.

HEART DISEASE

Heart disease is a rare, but potentially serious medical condition that complicates approximately 1 per cent of all pregnancies. The prevalence and incidence of all heart disease in pregnancy may vary from one community to another, principally because the incidence of rheumatic heart disease is more commonly found in less affluent societies. In the UK 50 years ago rheumatic heart disease accounted for 90 per cent of all heart disease in pregnancy, but since the widespread use of antibiotics in streptococcal infection this figure has fallen to less than 50 per cent. Rheumatic heart disease nonetheless remains an important cause of heart disease especially in ethnic minorities. In contrast with the advances in paediatric cardiac surgery that have been pioneered since the mid 1960s more women with congenital heart disease are now surviving and reaching child-bearing age. Congenital heart disease now accounts for approximately 50 per cent of women with heart disease in pregnancy in the UK.

Irrespective of the underlying condition pregnancy imposes a significant burden on the heart due to the normal physiological changes that occur. Both blood volume and cardiac output increase by 40 per cent. The increase in cardiac output is achieved by an increase both in stroke volume and a rise in heart rate of 12–15 beats per minute. These changes are discussed in more detail in Chapter 5.

Maternal risks

Although maternal mortality is seen with all forms of heart disease, it is most likely in conditions that restrict an increase in pulmonary blood flow, typically pulmonary hypertension and mitral stenosis. In these circumstances an obstruction exists either within the pulmonary vessels or at the mitral valve. This situation is at its worst in Eisenmenger's syndrome, where the mortality is 25–50 per cent. In other complex cardiac lesions, such as Fallot's tetralogy, the risk of maternal mortality is much lower, 5 per cent in some series, because there is less resistance at the pulmonary valve. In less severe forms of cardiac disease, including rheumatic heart disease, the maternal mortality may be as low as 1 per cent. Other cardiac complications associated with pregnancy include infection, cardiac arrhythmia and the development of a cardiomyopathy. Infective endocarditis is very rare since the routine use of antibiotics in such women.

Fetal risks

The fetal outcome in cases of maternal rheumatic heart disease is usually very good, although there is

an increased incidence of growth restriction and preterm delivery; these are more common in pregnancies complicated by congenital heart disease, especially if the cardiac disease results in a restriction of maternal cardiac output. The outcome is especially poor in cases of cyanotic heart disease and the total fetal loss rate may be as high as 40 per cent. Uncorrected coarctation of the aorta is associated with fetal growth restriction in over 10 per cent of cases due to reduced placental perfusion.

The aetiology of congenital heart disease is multifactorial and is present to some degree in 8 per 1000 live born babies. If a parent is affected the risk is increased to 5 per cent. Therefore all pregnant women with congenital heart disease should be referred for expert fetal cardiology during the antenatal period.

Pre-pregnancy management

Most women with heart disease will be aware of their condition prior to falling pregnant. Ideally such women should be fully assessed before embarking on a pregnancy and the maternal and fetal risks carefully explained. A cardiologist should be involved in this assessment, which should include maternal echocardiography. Any concurrent medical problems should be aggressively treated and medical therapy optimized. If there is a possibility that the heart disease will require surgical correction it is recommended that this should be undertaken before a pregnancy if at all possible. Key points in pre-pregnancy counselling are shown in the box below.

Key Points

Issues in pre-pregnancy counselling of women with heart disease
- Risk of maternal death
- Possible reduction of maternal life expectancy
- Risk of fetus developing congenital heart disease
- Risk of preterm labour and fetal growth restriction
- Need for frequent hospital attendance and possible admission
- Intensive maternal and fetal monitoring during labour

Antenatal management

All pregnant patients with heart disease should be managed in a joint obstetric and cardiac clinic, by experienced physicians and obstetricians. Continuity of care makes the detection of subtle changes in maternal wellbeing more likely. This is important because many of the signs of heart failure are common symptoms in normal pregnancy, such as breathlessness, tachycardia, ankle swelling and an ejection systolic heart murmur. In trying to distinguish between these 'normal' symptoms and impending cardiac failure it is important to ask the patient if she has noted any breathlessness, particularly at night, any change in her heart rate or rhythm, any increased tiredness or a reduction in exercise tolerance. Physical examination should include the points listed in the box opposite. In the majority of cases patients will remain well during the antenatal period and outpatient management is usually possible, although patients should be advised to have a low threshold for reducing their normal physical activities. Risk factors for the development of heart failure include:

- respiratory or urinary infections;
- anaemia;
- obesity;
- multiple gestation;
- hypertension;
- arrhythmias;
- pain-related stress.

Any signs of deteriorating cardiac status should be carefully investigated and treated. Hospital admission for bedrest will reduce the workload of the heart. Admission should not be a blanket policy, but rather it should be assessed on an individual basis.

The use of anticoagulants during pregnancy is a complicated issue because warfarin is teratogenic, especially if used in the first trimester. However anticoagulation may be essential in patients with congenital heart disease who have pulmonary hypertension, artificial valve replacements and those in atrial fibrillation. In the first trimester therefore warfarin is usually stopped and heparin used. Until recently subcutaneous heparin was not considered to be sufficient prophylaxis and therefore intravenous heparin was required. The new low molecular weight heparins may be able to provide sufficiently good anticoagulation to avoid IV preparations. In the second trimester, warfarin may be restarted until 37 weeks' gestation, when heparin should be reintroduced until the patient delivers. Should labour commence whilst the patient is still using warfarin, vitamin K should be given to reduce the bleeding tendency.

🔍 Key Points

Essential points of examination in pregnant women with heart disease

- Pulse rate and rhythm
- Blood pressure
- Jugular venous pressure
- Presence of basal crepitations
- Ankle and sacral oedema
- Symphysis–fundal height measurement

Treatment of heart failure in pregnancy

The development of heart failure in pregnancy is a very ominous sign. The principles of treatment are the same as in the non-pregnant individual. The patient will require admission and the diagnosis confirmed by clinical examination to confirm signs of heart failure and investigation, principally echocardiography. Drug therapy may include digoxin either in cases of heart failure and certainly if atrial fibrillation is present. Although there is some evidence that diuretic therapy is associated with fetal growth restriction, in the acute situation with the development of pulmonary oedema, diuretic therapy is indicated. Oxygen and morphine may also be required. Dysrhythmias also require urgent correction and drug therapy including selective beta-adrenergic blockade may have to be used. The indications for the use of these drugs is unaltered by pregnancy although some studies have reported an increased incidence of growth restriction. In all cases assessment of the fetal wellbeing is essential and would include fetal ultrasound to assess fetal growth and regular cardiotocography (CTG). If there is evidence of fetal compromise premature delivery may have to be considered. Similarly in cases of intractable cardiac failure the risks to the mother of continuing the pregnancy and the risks to the fetus of premature delivery must be carefully balanced.

Management of labour and delivery

In nearly all cases the aim of management is to await the onset of spontaneous natural labour as this will minimize the risk of intervention and maximize the prospects for a normal delivery (see box below). Induction of labour should only be considered for the normal obstetric indications. Epidural anaesthesia is recommended, as this will certainly reduce the pain-related stress, but is not without significant risk to both the mother and baby in some cardiac conditions, principally because of the complication of maternal hypotension. In these circumstances epidurals should be the responsibility of a senior anaesthetist to minimize the procedure-related risks. Prophylactic antibiotics should be given to reduce the risk of bacterial endocarditis. Depending on the severity of the condition other forms of monitoring may be appropriate during labour including oxygen saturation and continuous arterial blood pressure monitoring.

Additional points in management

Management of labour in women with heart disease
- Avoid induction of labour if possible
- Use prophylactic antibiotics
- Careful fluid balance
- Avoid supine position
- Epidural anaesthesia by senior anaesthetist
- Short second stage
- Syntocinon for delivery of placenta

Assuming normal progress in labour, the second stage is deliberately kept short and if normal delivery does not occur readily an elective forceps or ventouse delivery is undertaken to reduce maternal effort. Caesarean Section should only be performed for the normal obstetric indications. Liberal use of caesarean delivery will be associated with an increased risk of haemorrhage and infection, conditions that are likely to be much less well tolerated in cases of cardiac disease. Ergometrine is associated occasionally with intense vasoconstriction, hypertension and heart failure and therefore the management of the third stage is helped by using syntocinon only.

Specific heart conditions occurring during pregnancy

Mitral stenosis is the commonest acquired cardiac lesion accounting for 90 per cent of rheumatic valvular problems. It is the leading cause of death in the developing world. The stenosis produces a left atrial obstruction with a consequent elevated left atrial and pulmonary wedge pressure (Fig. 16.1). Eventually pulmonary oedema and atrial fibrillation may occur. There is a fixed cardiac output with limited ability to adapt to the increased demands placed on the heart during pregnancy by a raised intravascular volume and heart rate. The most useful investigation is echocardiography, which is able to assess the mitral valve area. Echocardiography performed early in pregnancy will act as a baseline against which subsequent investigations may be compared if there is a deterioration in the patient's symptoms. Significant problems may be anticipated if the valvular area falls below the normal 8 cm^2 to 4 cm^2. A valve with an area of 2 cm^2 or less will require surgical valvotomy and although ideally this would be undertaken before the pregnancy, it may be performed during pregnancy.

Eisenmenger's syndrome is associated with a very high maternal mortality, up to 50 per cent. Initially there is a left to right shunt across a ventricular-sep-

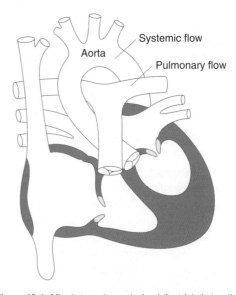

Figure 16.1 Mitral stenosis producing left atrial obstruction.

tal defect with consequent pulmonary hypertension. Eventually the shunt may reverse and cyanosis occurs (Fig. 16.2). The major risk in pregnancy is during labour and delivery when there may be sudden changes in systemic vascular resistance leading to syncope. Because of the very high maternal mortality the option of terminating the pregnancy should be carefully discussed with the mother. In mothers who decide to continue with their pregnancy, miscarriage and fetal growth restriction are more common.

Coarctation of the aorta and Marfan's syndrome

Although coarctation may be detected in childhood, in less severe cases it may not present until the second and third decades when hypertension develops. The principal risk is of dissection of the aorta associated with the increased cardiac output of pregnancy and a possible increase in medial vessel degeneration. In addition, endocarditis, intracranial haemorrhage and death have been reported. There is a 2 per cent risk that the fetus will also develop coarctation. The risk of maternal death is approximately 15 per cent and the option of termination should be discussed. Antenatally the development of hypertension is the most serious sign and an epidural during labour is recommended.

Marfan's syndrome is a connective tissue abnormality that may lead to mitral valve prolapse and aortic regurgitation or dissection. Pregnancy increases the risk of cardiac compromise and has been associated with maternal mortality of up to 50 per cent depending on the severity of the lesions.

Echocardiography is the principal investigation as it is able to determine the size of the aortic root and the degree of regurgitation.

HYPERTENSIVE DISORDERS

Hypertensive disease may complicate 5–7 per cent of all pregnancies. Although the diagnosis of hypertension may be made on blood pressure measurements alone, the complex aetiology of hypertension in pregnancy has led to considerable confusion both in its definition and its management.

Hypertension is defined as changes of blood pressure recorded on at least two occasions at least six hours apart of either:

- diastolic blood pressure greater than 90 mmHg, or
- systolic blood pressure greater than 140 mmHg, or
- a rise in diastolic blood pressure of at least 15 mmHg, or
- a rise in systolic blood pressure of at least 30 mmHg.

Significant proteinuria is defined as 300 mg/L or more in a 24-hour urine sample. Although reagent strips give an indication as to the degree of proteinuria, accurate quantification relies on a 24-hour collection. Other causes of proteinuria include renal disease, vaginal discharge or contamination and urinary tract infection. Oedema is a non-specific generalized accumulation of fluid, but which affects more

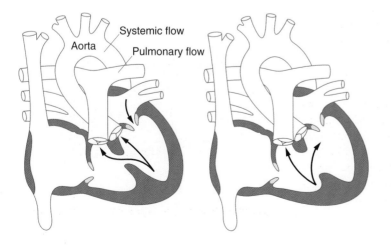

Aorta
Systemic flow
Pulmonary flow

Figure 16.2 Eisenmenger's syndrome, initial left to right shunting is reversed with consequent cyanosis.

than 50 per cent of the pregnant population and is therefore non-discriminatory. Pre-eclampsia and eclampsia (see Chapter 11) will typically relate to elevations in blood pressure after the 20th week of pregnancy. It is for this reason that it is useful to have a pre-pregnancy or early pregnancy recording of blood pressure with which to compare subsequent changes in blood pressure.

Chronic hypertension preceding pregnancy

Essential hypertension is the underlying cause in 90 per cent of cases. A complete list of causes is shown in the box below. Before a diagnosis of essential hypertension is made, these other possibilities need to be excluded. Irrespective of the underlying cause the principal concern for the obstetrician is that the patient may develop superimposed pregnancy-induced hypertension. This may occur in up to one-third of women with pre-existing hypertension and is more likely in women with renal disease. Those at increased risk of developing superimposed pregnancy-induced hypertension are listed in the box (opposite) and the incidence of superimposed problems in this group is 50 per cent. The maternal risks include eclampsia, abruption, heart failure and intracerebral haemorrhage. Abruption is rare, but in severe hypertensive disease the risk is in the order of 10 per cent. Fetal morbidity and mortality are closely related to the degree of severity and the gestational age at delivery. Placental insufficiency may lead to growth restriction and abruption is often associated with a poor outcome.

Causes of chronic hypertension

- Essential hypertension
- Renal disease
  - glomerulonephritis
  - polycystic disease
  - diabetic nephropathy
  - renal artery stenosis
- Collagen vascular disease
  - systemic lupus erythematosus (SLE)
  - scleroderma
- Coarctation of the aorta
- Phaeochromocytoma

Risk factors for developing superimposed pregnancy-induced hypertension

- Renal disease
- Maternal age >40 years
- Diabetes
- Connective tissue disease e.g. SLE
- Coarctation of the aorta
- Blood pressure >160/100 mmHg in early pregnancy

Management

If the blood pressure is elevated for the first time in pregnancy, appropriate investigations should be performed to exclude renal, cardiac and autoimmune disease. In mild cases (blood pressure less than 150/100 mmHg) there is no immediate indication to treat, however the pregnancy will require careful monitoring to detect any further possible rise in blood pressure. Women who are using anti-hypertensive medication before the onset of pregnancy can often be advised to stop in anticipation of a slight fall in blood pressure during the second trimester. Some anti-hypertensives such as the angiotensin-converting enzyme inhibitors should definitely be avoided because of the risk of fetal damage. The development of proteinuria is a sinister feature. Fetal growth restriction should be watched for and serial ultrasound examination is appropriate.

In more severe hypertension women will often need to be admitted for bedrest and intensive monitoring. If the blood pressure is consistently noted to be in excess of 150/100 mmHg antihypertensive medication will need to be introduced to reduce the risk of intracerebral haemorrhage or heart failure.

Investigation of hypertension

- Creatinine, electrolytes, urate
- Liver function tests
- 24-hour urinary protein/creatinine clearance
- Renal scan
- Auto-antibody screen
- Complement studies
- Cardiac investigations including ECG and echocardiography

Care should be taken not to excessively lower the blood pressure as this may adversely affect the fetus by reducing placental blood flow. The preferred anti-hypertensive medication is methyldopa, which is generally well tolerated. Other commonly used drugs include labetalol and hydralazine, although the latter is more often used intravenously in the acute situation. The aim of antihypertensive medication is to maintain the blood pressure below 160 mmHg systolic and 100–110 mmHg diastolic.

The obstetric management is similar to that for pregnancy-induced hypertension. The critical feature is the timing of delivery to maximize the chances of fetal survival if premature delivery is considered and to prevent serious maternal complications that may arise if delivery is postponed too long. Each case must be individually assessed but in general it is reasonable to attempt vaginal delivery by induction of labour if the maternal blood pressure is reasonably controlled. If delivery is contemplated before 34 weeks' gestation the mother should be given steriods to increase fetal lung maturation. Continuous fetal monitoring is advocated in labour as the fetus will often be growth restricted. There should be a low threshold for Caesarean Section. If there is evidence of rapidly deteriorating maternal or fetal wellbeing then Caesarean Section is appropriate. Magnesium sulphate may be administered if the patient shows signs of fulminating pre-eclampsia.

Postnatally the maternal blood pressure will often resume its pre-pregnancy level, but careful observation is required in the first 48 hours because of a persisting risk of eclampsia. Breastfeeding is encouraged and although some antihypertensive medication may enter the breast milk, it is not significant.

ENDOCRINE DISORDERS

Diabetes

Significant hormonal changes affect carbohydrate metabolism during pregnancy. In particular there is an increase in human placental lactogen and cortisol, both of which are insulin antagonists and therefore relative insulin resistance develops in the mother. These changes are most marked during the third trimester. To balance these changes during normal pregnancy the maternal pancreas secretes increased amounts of insulin to maintain carbohydrate metabolism. Typically in pregnancy this will result in a fall in the fasting level of glucose. In contrast, following a carbohydrate challenge the levels of glucose are higher than normal. Glucose crosses the placenta by means of a facilitated diffusion process and the fetal blood glucose level closely follows the maternal level. Fetal glucose levels will normally be maintained within narrow limits if the maternal levels are also well controlled.

Diabetes may complicate a pregnancy either because the woman has pre-existing insulin-dependent diabetes before her pregnancy begins or she may develop an impaired glucose tolerance during the course of her pregnancy. Approximately 1–2 per cent of women will develop gestational diabetes during pregnancy. Certain groups of women are more likely to develop diabetes at some time during their life and are labelled as potential diabetics. The risk factors that are important for the obstetrician to note are listed below.

Risk factors for the development of diabetes in pregnancy

- Obesity (body mass index 30)
- Family history
- Previous baby >4.5 kg
- Previous unexplained stillbirth
- Previous congenital abnormality

Definition of diabetes

The WHO has defined diabetes mellitus as either a raised fasting blood glucose level of >7.8 mmol/L or a level of >11.1 mmol/L 1–2 hours following a 75 gram glucose load. The significance of impaired glucose tolerance has been much debated, but many now feel that it is unlikely to have any untoward effect on pregnancy outcome unless the WHO criteria are reached. The importance of good glycaemic control during pregnancy is reinforced by the direct relationship between blood glucose levels and the incidence of fetal and maternal complications. For this reason diabetic women who plan to become pregnant should ensure that their diabetes is optimally controlled to reduce the risk of obstetric complications. Patients should be advised of the risks of pregnancy, their own insulin regime, diet and exercise. Careful self-monitoring of glucose levels by patients is a critical aspect of diabetic care. This helps to highlight excessive swings in blood sugar levels. Patients will often have to change from a twice-daily insulin regime to a four times daily insulin regime. Insulin-dependent diabetics are likely to require increased insulin doses during pregnancy.

Fetal and neonatal complications of diabetic pregnancy

There is an increased risk of miscarriage in early pregnancy and congenital fetal abnormality. Good diabetic control, particularly prior to conception reduces these risks substantially. Measurement of glycosylated haemoglobin gives a retrospective assessment of diabetic control; high levels in early pregnancy are associated with neural tube defects, congenital heart disease and other spinal anomalies including a rare condition called caudal regression syndrome. Congenital abnormality is the most important cause of mortality and morbidity in diabetic pregnancies and is seen 2–4 times more often than in normal pregnancies. Malformations at present account for 40 per cent of the perinatal mortality associated with diabetic pregnancies. The mechanism that gives rise to these abnormalities is not fully understood, but it is thought that hypoglycaemia in the critical stages of organogenesis may be the underlying cause and this has certainly been demonstrated in animal models. Apart from structural malformations fetal macrosomia is a major problem which is associated with traumatic birth,

shoulder dystocia and therefore possible hypoxic damage (Fig. 16.3). Accelerated growth patterns are typically seen in the late second and third trimesters and are associated with poorly controlled diabetes (Fig. 16.4). Until recently sudden, unexplained, late stillbirths occurred in 10–30 per cent of diabetic pregnancies but are much less common now that diabetic control has improved. However, it remains a risk in patients whose diabetes is poorly controlled, that have vascular disease and in pregnancies complicated by macrosomia or polyhydramnios. The mechanism of such losses is not understood although several possible mechanisms may contribute to chronic hypoxia.

Maternal mortality and morbidity in diabetic pregnancy

There has been a marked reduction in maternal mortality in diabetic pregnancies and this is now a very rare event. Those at most risk are women with pre-existing coronary artery disease. In general the maternal morbidity is related to the severity of diabetic-related disease preceding the pregnancy. Women with co-existing renal nephropathy are at particular risk of developing pre-eclampsia and studies suggest that although the renal condition may worsen during pregnancy, this is rarely permanent and tends to improve following delivery. In contrast patients with diabetic retinopathy are at risk of progression of the disease and they should be kept under careful surveillance. Other complications include an increased incidence of infection, severe hyper- or hypoglycaemia, and the complications that may arise from the increased operative delivery rate, including thromboembolic disease (see box below).

Maternal complications of diabetic pregnancy

- Nephropathy
- Retinopathy
- Coronary artery disease
- Hyperglycaemia/hypoglycaemia
- Pre-eclampsia
- Infection
- Thromboembolic disease

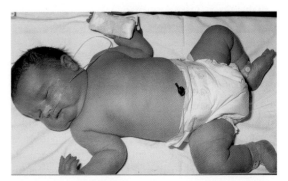

Figure 16.3 5.1 kg macrosomic infant of a diabetic mother.

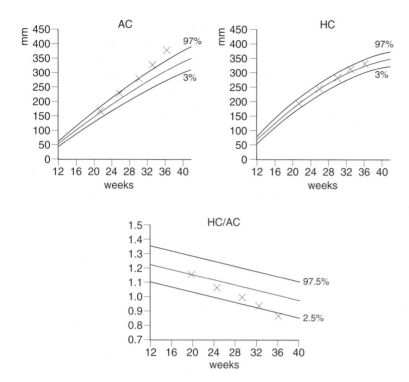

Figure 16.4 Growth patterns of the fetal head circumference (HC) and abdominal circumference (AC) and the HC/AC ratio in the fetus of a poorly-controlled insulin-dependent diabetic mother. The increased growth mainly affects the abdominal organs hence the accelerated growth rate of the AC.

Neonatal complications

Neonatal morbidity has fallen dramatically over the last three decades, with the improvement of glycaemic control antenatally, but it remains significant and is related to the degree of antenatal control. Diabetic babies will usually be cared for on the special care baby unit for the first 24–48 hours of life to monitor for possible complications, especially hypoglycaemia. The causes of neonatal morbidity include:

- Congenital abnormalities
  - Cardiac
  - Neural tube defects
- Macrosomia
  - Birth asphyxia
  - Traumatic birth injury e.g. brachial nerve injury
- Respiratory distress syndrome
- Hypoglycaemia
- Hypomagnesemia
- Polycythaemia
- Hyperbilirubinaemia

The gestational age connected incidence of respiratory distress syndrome is six times that of normal infants.

It has been suggested that this is a consequence of diminished surfactant production as a result of fetal hyperinsulinaemia. Hypoglycaemia particularly in the first 24 hours following delivery is now anticipated because the fetus continues to excrete large amounts of insulin in the immediate neonatal period. Mothers should be encouraged to breastfeed straight away, but careful monitoring of the baby's blood sugar should be undertaken and if necessary a glucose infusion commenced. Less common abnormalities include disturbances of hypocalcaemia and magnesium deficiency, in extreme cases leading to apnoeic episodes and fits. Polycythaemia is often found and may need correction by a partial exchange transfusion. Finally, jaundice caused by hyperbilirubinaemia may result from the neonatal polycythaemia.

Screening for diabetes in pregnancy

No single screening test has been shown to be perfect. Urinary glucose has been shown to be an unreliable method of detecting potential diabetes and most screening tests now rely on blood glucose estimation. A full glucose tolerance test would be the ideal method, but this would be too expensive and time-consuming. Recognizing that blood glucose measurement was more useful, Lind advocated a random blood sugar test. If the value was greater than 5.8 mmol/L more than two hours after a meal or greater than 6.2 mmol/L within two hours of a meal he suggested that a full glucose tolerance test should be performed. Unfortunately the sensitivity of this test is only about 60 per cent although this can be improved if the test is repeated at 28 weeks' gestation.

The sensitivity of a single glucose measurement can be increased to 80 per cent if the measurement is taken one hour following a 50 g glucose meal, sometimes called a mini glucose tolerance test, which can conveniently be provided by a bottle of Lucozade. This method of screening is now widely used and if the glucose level is greater than 7.7 mmol/L a full glucose tolerance test is arranged.

Antenatal management

Diabetic pregnant women should be managed in a joint clinic with an obstetrician and physician. Women with pre-existing diabetes should be referred directly to this clinic at booking and those in whom a diagnosis is made at a later stage should also be referred. The principal of treatment is to maintain the blood sugar level with a mean 24-hour profile of less than 5 mmol/L. This will usually require three or four daily doses of insulin. Some diabetics may be controlled using a continuous infusion pump, typically in an established diabetic. All diabetic women should be instructed in self-monitoring with their own glucose meters. The long-term control may be checked using glycosylated haemoglobin measurements. Input from a dietician is also important and frequently a nurse specialist will act as an adviser to adjust the dose of insulin, should glucose levels become erratic.

The obstetric management is aimed initially at ensuring that the appropriate screening tests are performed including detailed ultrasound assessment and fetal echocardiography. Serial growth scans are recommended to help detect possible fetal macrosomia, although this is rarely a problem before the third trimester. As well as assessing the fetal size, ultrasound may also alert the team to developing polyhydramnios. Concern for the fetal wellbeing should lead to increased surveillance with biophysical profile scores, Doppler ultrasound and CTG. In principal, provided the pregnancy has gone well, management would attempt to achieve a vaginal delivery between 38–40 weeks' gestation. The development of macrosomia or maternal complications such as pre-eclampsia together with the failed rate of induction means that the Caesarean Section rate amongst diabetic women may be as high as 50 per cent.

The management of preterm labour or polyhydramnios is particularly difficult in diabetic pregnancies. Tocolytics such as ritodrine or salbutamol, are themselves diabetogenic and will tend to elevate blood glucose levels. In addition the administration of intramuscular steroids to improve fetal lung aspiration, will also destabilize diabetic control. Under these circumstances an IV insulin and glucose infusion should be used to ensure normoglycaemia.

Management in labour

During either induced or spontaneous labour normoglycaemia should be maintained using a sliding scale of insulin administration. Blood glucose levels should be tested at two-hourly intervals. Continuous fetal monitoring is advised and fetal scalp blood sampling should be undertaken in the presence of an abnormal CTG. Following delivery the insulin requirements of established diabetics will rapidly fall and return to pre-pregnancy levels. Women who for the first time became diabetic during a pregnancy

Key Points

Diabetes in pregnancy

- In gestational diabetes the incidence of large babies (macrosomia) can be reduced with good blood glucose control
- Gestational diabetes has a very high recurrence rate in subsequent pregnancies
- The highest risk of congenital abnormalities are cleft palate, sacral agenesis and cardiac defects
- Reduced fetal movements at or near term in diabetics with a CTG that is not perfect should lead to delivery as a priority (especially if there are abnormal ultrasound findings, as is the case with Mrs K)

Mrs A K

Aged 38, Asian, 3rd pregnancy

2 previous pregnancies complicated by gestational diabetes: both caesarean sections at term; weighed 3.9 and 4.2 kg

Body mass index = 8

Mrs K booked for a hospital delivery at 12 weeks. An ultrasound showed a singleton pregnancy with a normal nuchal scan giving a risk of Down's of 1:1400. An anomaly scan and fetal echocardiography at 20 weeks was normal.

In her previous pregnancy, Mrs K had required insulin in a four times daily regimen from 20 weeks' gestation. Unfortunately she was poorly motivated to check her BMs and modify her diet (regularly eating cream cakes and chocolate). In this pregnancy, insulin was started at 14 weeks (Hba1c prior to commencing insulin was 8.6) with short-acting insulin before meals and long-acting at night. Despite advice from dieticians and weekly diabetic clinic attendance, blood glucose control was poor and serial ultrasound (Fig. 16.4) showed fetal growth accelerating beyond the 95th centile from 32 weeks onwards. At 36 weeks and 3 days, Mrs K noticed reduced fetal movements. An ultrasound scan showed polyhydramnios (amniotic fluid index 26 cm) and an estimated fetal weight of 4.6 kg. CTG was reactive but variability was reduced (<5 beats/min).

A semi-elective Caesarean Section was performed the following day; a 5.1 kg female infant (Usha) was delivered in good health. Usha was hypoglycaemic after delivery and required four days' care on the neonatal unit while blood sugar levels stabilized and feeding became established. Luckily, Usha suffered no respiratory complications.

may stop their insulin and a full glucose tolerance test is repeated some six weeks following delivery.

Contraceptive advice

Particular care must be given in the postnatal period regarding the use of appropriate contraception. Barrier methods may be the best option although they do have a slightly higher failure rate. An IUCD is associated with a failure rate and also infection, which is, of course, not to be desired in a diabetic. The combined contraceptive pill increases the risk of vascular complications whilst the progesterone-only pill is associated with irregular bleeding and a higher failure rate, unless used meticulously.

Thyroid disorders

Pregnancy has a significant impact on the normal maternal thyroid physiology. During pregnancy the production of thyroid-binding globulin by the liver doubles as a result of oestrogenic stimulation. As a consequence there is an increased amount of total thyroxine (T4) and tri-iodothyronine (T3), but importantly there is no significant change in the amount of circulating free thyroid hormone (FT4 and FT3). The renal clearance of iodine increases in pregnancy.

Maternal hyperthyroidism

Hyperthyroidism in the mother occurs in 1 in every 500 pregnancies. In the majority of cases the condition has been diagnosed before pregnancy and 90 per cent of cases are secondary to Graves' disease. This autoimmune disorder is associated with the presence of circulating thyroid stimulating antibodies. Rarer causes of hyperthyroidism include:

- toxic nodules;
- Hashimoto's thyroiditis;
- multiple nodule goitre;
- trophoblastic disease (extremely rare).

Clinically the diagnosis may be difficult to make in pregnancy because mild maternal tachycardia, weight loss, heart murmurs and heat intolerance are all symptoms in early pregnancy. If there is a past history or clinical suspicion of thyroid disease, thyroid function tests should be performed in pregnancy. Hyperthyroidism is confirmed by high levels of FT4 and FT3 together with reduced levels of thyroid-stimulating hormone (TSH). Uncontrolled maternal hyperthyroidism is associated with maternal cardiac arrhythmias including atrial fibrillation, diarrhoea, vomiting, abdominal pains and psychosis. If the underlying aetiology is autoimmune disease the thyroid-stimulating antibodies may cross the placenta and cause a fetal goitre. The main complications for the fetus include fetal growth restriction, stillbirth, fetal tachycardia and premature delivery.

Following the diagnosis of hyperthyroidism the treatment during pregnancy should be drug therapy aiming to maintain maternal FT3 and FT4 levels in the high/normal range. Radioactive iodine is contraindicated because it completely obliterates the fetal thyroid gland. Treatment is usually medical with carbimazole although occasionally beta-blockers and surgical treatment will be undertaken. The lowest dose of carbimazole must be used as high doses cross the placenta and may cause fetal hypothyroidism. Careful monitoring of maternal thyroid function is therefore essential under these circumstances.

Maternal hypothyroidism

The commonest worldwide cause for this is iodine deficiency, but this is rarely seen in the UK. Maternal iodine deficiency is associated with the development of cretinism in the newborn as a result of congenital hypothyroidism. The commonest reason for maternal hypothyroidism in the UK is usually over-treated hyperthyroidism. Women treated with radioactive iodine will frequently be using thyroxine supplements and the dose should be checked in early pregnancy to ensure appropriate levels of FT4 and FT3 are available. If a patient is diagnosed as having hypothyroidism they should receive full thyroid replacement during pregnancy. Thyroid function tests should be performed serially. In the postnatal period there is a relationship between thyroid dysfunction and postnatal depression, which may occur 6–12 months following delivery. Although this is often a self-limiting condition, 20 per cent of patients who are hypothyroidic during pregnancy will remain so postnatally.

Pituitary disorders

Hyperprolactinaemia is an important cause of infertility and amenorrhoea. It is most often due to a benign pituitary microadenoma. It may also be due to drugs that act as dopamine antagonists, such as methyldopa and the phenothiazines. The diagnosis is confirmed with a combination of measurement of the prolactin level and computerized tomography scanning of the pituitary fossa. In 80 per cent of cases it may be treated with the dopamine agonist bromocriptine which causes the tumour to diminish in size. Larger tumours may require surgery or radiotherapy, which is best undertaken before pregnancy. Bromocriptine is usually stopped once pregnancy is diagnosed. It is rare for microadenomas to increase in size, but it is important to monitor the patient's visual fields during pregnancy. If there is evidence of tumour growth during pregnancy bromocriptine should be recommenced. In patients with larger tumours it is best to continue with the bromocriptine because of the risk of the tumour enlarging under oestrogenic stimulation. There is no evidence that bromocriptine is teratogenic.

Adrenal disorders

Cushing's syndrome

All adrenal disease is rare in pregnancy. Cushing's syndrome is characterized by increased glucocorticoid production usually because of hypersecretion of adrenocorticotrophic hormone from a pituitary tumour. Most women with Cushing's syndrome are infertile and in the few reported cases of pregnancy a high incidence of preterm delivery and stillbirth is described. Diagnosis may be difficult because many of the symptoms mimic normal pregnancy changes such as striae, weight gain, weakness and hypertension. Glucose intolerance may be seen. If suspected, cortisol levels should be assayed and adrenal imaging with computerized tomography or magnetic resonance imaging should be used.

Addison's syndrome

Addisons's disease (adrenal insufficiency) is usually an autoimmune process. The clinical picture is of exhaustion, nausea, hypotension, hypoglycaemia and weight loss. The diagnosis is difficult to make in pregnancy because the cortisol levels, instead of being characteristically decreased, may be in the low-normal range due to the physiological increase in cortisol-binding globulin in pregnancy. Occasionally the disease may present as a crisis and treatment consists of glucocorticoid and fluid replacement. In adequately treated patients the pregnancy usually continues normally.

Phaeochromocytoma

Phaeochromocytoma is a rare catecholamine-producing tumour. The tumours arise from the adrenal medulla in 90 per cent of cases. Its importance in pregnancy is that it may present as a hypertensive crisis and the symptoms may be very similar to severe pregnancy-induced hypertension. A characteristic feature is paroxysmal hypertension, whilst the other symptoms of headaches, palpitations, blurred vision, anxiety and convulsions may occur in severe pregnancy-induced hypertension. The diagnosis is confirmed by measurement of catecholamines and their metabolites in a 24-hour urine collection. Levels of metanephrine and vanillylmandelic acid are present. Treatment is by alpha-blockade with phentolamine. Caesarean Section is the preferred mode of delivery as it minimizes the likelihood of sudden increases in catecholamines associated with vaginal delivery.

RESPIRATORY DISORDERS

Asthma

Asthma is reversible bronchial airway obstruction, a common complaint that may complicate up to 2 per cent of pregnancies. In most cases the disease is well controlled with conventional inhalation drugs. Pregnancy itself does not seem to increase the frequency or severity of asthma. Problems may occur in patients whose asthma is poorly controlled and this is usually due to a lack of compliance with their medication or resulting from a failure of physicians to recognize the severity of the problem. In such cases there is an increased incidence of fetal growth restriction. Care should be aimed at optimizing medical treatment to prevent asthmatic attacks and the use of aggressive treatment should these attacks occur. Patient inhalation techniques should be carefully reviewed and regular respiratory peak flow assessment is the best way of monitoring the severity of the condition. Drug therapy includes the use of the inhaled beta$_2$–agonist salbutamol and inhaled glucocorticoids such as betamethasone. In severe exacerbations hospital admission may be needed to provide nebulized treatment with bronchodilators, IV antibiotics and steroids.

In cases of suspected growth restriction serial ultrasound scans should be undertaken to document fetal growth. Labour is rarely a problem for asthmatics and epidural is the preferred analgesia. General anaesthesia should be avoided if possible as it increases the risk of bronchospasm and chest infection. Ergometrine should not be used because it may cause intense bronchospasm and similarly in the postnatal period non-steroid anti-inflammatory drugs, often used for pain relief should also be avoided.

Sarcoid

Sarcoid is a non-caseating granulomatosis that may affect any organ, but principally affects the lung and skin. It is a rare condition to diagnose in pregnancy, although erythema nodosum, which is not uncommon, may be the first clue. Pregnancy does not influence the natural history of the condition. A few patients may develop severe progressive lung problems with pulmonary fibrosis, hypoxemia and pulmonary hypertension and these complications are associated with a poor prognosis. If the diagnosis is considered or diagnosed prenatally patients are best jointly managed with a chest physician. Treatment is with steroid therapy. If there is progressive lung involvement anaesthetic input should be obtained prior to labour.

Cystic fibrosis

This is an autosomal recessive condition. The life expectancy of affected patients is increasing all the time and although many patients are subfertile, many more women are now surviving to an age where pregnancy is possible. It is a multisystem disorder, principally affecting the lungs and liver. Malabsorption is often a major problem and patients are typically underweight.

It is important to check the cystic fibrosis carrier status of the patient's partner and the couple should be offered genetic counselling as to the risks of the fetus having cystic fibrosis or being a carrier. The principal risks to the fetus are of growth restriction and preterm delivery, the latter usually being iatrogenic if there is evidence of deteriorating maternal respiratory function. Fetal growth and wellbeing are monitored by serial ultrasound scans. Maternal wellbeing should be jointly managed between the obstetrician and an expert respiratory physician. Most patients will have a daily physiotherapy regime and during exacerbations will require prolonged antibiotic therapy and hospital admission.

Many pregnancies will require preterm delivery because of significant intrauterine growth restriction or worsening maternal respiratory function despite optimal medical treatment. If delivery is contemplated before 34 weeks' gestation, steroid therapy should be given to improve fetal lung maturation. Ideally a vaginal delivery should be aimed for and an epidural analgesia offered. A short second stage will reduce the possibility of maternal exhaustion.

HAEMATOLOGICAL ABNORMALITIES

The WHO defines anaemia as a haemoglobin concentration of less than 11.0g/dL. During pregnancy, although the red cell mass increases the plasma volume expansion is relatively greater and therefore the haemoglobin concentration falls. Anaemia in pregnancy is most commonly due to a lack of haemoglobin production because of low levels of essential precursors such as iron and folate. Less commonly it may be secondary to chronic blood loss or haemolysis.

Microcytic anaemia

Iron demand in pregnancy increases from 2 mg to 4 mg daily. A healthy diet contains 10 mg. The diagnosis of iron deficiency is made by noting a fall in the mean corpuscular volume (MCV) below 85 fl, assuming that the electrophoresis is normal. Low levels of serum iron and ferritin help to confirm the diagnosis. Treatment is with iron supplementation and a single 60 mg tablet daily should suffice, however if this is poorly tolerated by the patient, different iron preparations are available including liquid formulae. Other means of increasing haemoglobin concentration have their drawbacks: intramuscular iron is painful, IV iron may cause allergic reactions and blood transfusions carry the small risk of infection in addition to the problems of transfusion reactions.

Macrocytic anaemia

Folate deficiency is rarely seen, but is suggested by an increased MCV. It is not often seen in the UK as many foods have folate supplements added. Folate requirements are increased in pregnancy as all tissues require it for the manufacture of DNA. The normal values of folate concentrations fall in pregnancy due to the haemodilutional effect of plasma expansion. All women considering pregnancy should be encouraged to use folate supplementation as it has been shown to reduce the incidence of neural tube defects. Additional supplements are required in women on anticonvulsant medication, in particular phenytoin.

Worldwide, the commonest cause of a raised MCV however is an increased alcohol consumption. Vitamin B12 deficiency (pernicious anaemia) is another cause of macrocytic anaemia, but is unlikely to occur in pregnancy as severe cases are associated with infertility.

Haemolytic anaemia

Sickle cell syndromes

These are autosomally inherited diseases. Abnormal haemoglobin (HbS) contains β-globin chains with an amino acid substitution that results in it precipitating when in its reduced state. The red blood cells become sickle-shaped and occlude small blood vessels and this is known as sickling.

Sickle cell disease (HbSS)

Sickle cell disease is a severe condition and in pregnancy women are at high risk of complications. Pregnancy is associated with an increased incidence of sickle cell crises that may result in episodes of severe pain, typically affecting the bones or chest. These crises may be precipitated by hypoxia, stress, infection and haemorrhage. Mothers are at increased risk of miscarriage, pre-eclampsia, chest and urinary tract infections and premature labour. The fetal loss rate is higher as is the incidence of growth restriction. Ideally the potential problems of pregnancy should be discussed with the patient before pregnancy.

Sickle cell trait (HbAS)

Sickle cell carriers have a 1:4 risk of having a baby with sickle cell disease if their partner also has sickle cell trait. Carriers of the trait are usually fit and well, but are at increased risk of urinary tract infection. Very rarely they may suffer from crises.

Sickle cell haemoglobin C disease (HbSC)

Although this condition may cause only mild degrees of anaemia, it is associated with very severe crises that are more common throughout pregnancy.

Antenatal management

All women should be screened at booking to detect haemoglobinopathies. If a woman is found to be heterozygote for a haemoglobinopathy her partner should also be tested. Prenatal diagnosis can be offered to couples at risk of having an affected baby. No specific treatment exists to prevent sickle cell crises, however episodes of hypoxia, dehydration and infection should be avoided by aggressive treatment with adequate analgesia, antibiotics, oxygen and rehydration. Ideally a haemoglobin concentration of at least 10.0 g/dL with 60 per cent normal HbA will minimize the risk of crises. In some cases blood transfusion or exchange transfusion may be used to increase the percentage of circulating normal haemoglobin A, however blood transfusion is not without risk and this form of management is less commonly used today.

A vaginal delivery should be aimed for and epidural anaesthesia advised to reduce the stress of labour. Care should also be taken to avoid dehydration, infection or hypoxia during the labour. Continuous fetal monitoring is recommended. In the postnatal period patients with sickle cell disease remain at increased risk of suffering a crisis as this is a stressful time for any mother. Contraception should be carefully discussed and the combined contraceptive or progesterone-only pill may both be safely used.

Thalassaemia

The thalassaemia syndromes are the commonest genetic blood disorders. The defect is a reduced production of normal haemoglobin. The syndromes are divided into the alpha and beta types, depending on which globin chain is affected. In alpha thalassaemia minor there is a deletion of one of the two normal alpha genes required for haemoglobin production. Although the affected individual is chronically anaemic this condition rarely produces obstetric complications except in cases of severe blood loss. It is important to screen the patient's partner for thalassaemia and consider prenatal diagnosis if he is also affected as there is a 1:4 chance of the fetus having alpha thalassaemia major.

In alpha thalassaemia major there are no functional alpha chains, no normal haemoglobin is synthesized and the condition is incompatible with life. Fetuses develop marked hydrops and the pregnancies are complicated by polyhydramnios and preterm delivery. If affected the baby will only survive a few hours following delivery. These pregnancies are also complicated by severe pre-eclampsia thought to be related to the enlarged and hydropic placenta. There is no treatment, but individuals can be offered the option of antenatal diagnosis in subsequent pregnancies.

The beta thalassaemias are due to defects in the normal production of the beta chains. Normal haemoglobin contains mostly HbA1 with a small percentage of HbA2. If the gene for HbA1 is missing the individual has beta thalassaemia minor. These abnormalities are more commonly found in people from the East Mediterranean, but may also occur sporadically in other communities. Consequently all pregnant women should be offered electrophoresis as part of the antenatal screening process. Beta thalassaemia is not a problem antenatally although women will tend to be mildly anaemic and have a low MCV. Iron and folate supplements should be given and their partners should also be screened. If, however, both partners have beta thalassaemia minor there is a 1:4 chance the fetus could have no gene for the production of HbA1 and this is termed beta thalassaemia major. The fetus produces HbF *in utero* and this is not a problem, however in postnatal life normal HbA1 cannot be produced and severe anaemia develops requiring serial blood transfusion. Eventually this leads to the problems of iron overload and death.

Thrombocytopenia

Thrombocytopenia is a reduction in platelet number below 150 x 10^9/L. There are many causes and these are classified in the box above.

Incidental thrombocytopenia

Incidental thrombocytopenia is a surprisingly common condition and may be present to some degree in 7–8 per cent of the pregnant population. Mild falls in platelet counts to between 100–150 x 10^9/L are only very rarely associated with a poor maternal outcome as bleeding is rarely a complication unless the count is 50 x 10^9/L or less. Similarly neonatal thrombocytopenia is only seen in 4 per cent of these cases and is not related to the degree of maternal thrombocytopenia. The majority of neonates will have platelet counts in excess of 50 x 10^9/L. The diagnosis of incidental thrombocytopenia is a diagnosis of exclusion and can only be made when the autoimmune and other causes have been excluded.

Autoimmune thrombocytopenia purpura

This condition may present acutely typically in children after a viral illness. In adults the presentation is more chronic. The incidence in pregnancy is 1:5000. Auto-antibodies are produced against platelet surface antigens leading to their destruction by the reticulo-endothelial system. In pregnancy these antibodies may cross the placenta and destroy the fetal platelets, however there is no relationship between the degree of maternal and fetal thrombocytopenia.

In pregnancy the condition may present with bruising or be suspected for the first time following a routine blood count. The count is typically 30–80 x 10^9/L and it is rare for it to fall to extremely low levels. Other conditions should be considered including SLE. Serial platelet counts are measured and provided the count remains above 80 x 10^9/L no bleeding complications are likely and normal epidural anaesthesia may be used. If the count falls below 80 x 10^9/L, the

Classification of thrombocytopenia

- Incidental thrombocytopenia of pregnancy
- Increased consumption
- Autoimmune thrombocytopenia
- Activated clotting mechanism
  - Pre-eclampsia
  - HELLP syndrome
  - Disseminated intravascular coagulation
- Platelet thrombus formation e.g. thrombocytopenic purpura
- Hypersplenism
- Decreased platelet production
- Malignant marrow infiltration

anaesthetist should be informed and other forms of pain relief for the labour, including possibly an infusion pump, should be used.

If the platelet count falls below 50 x 10^9/L treatment should be considered. Until recently corticosteriods were the mainstay of therapy and act by changing immune function and improving capillary fragility. However high doses are often required to improve the platelet count and their long-term use is associated with weight gain, hypertension, diabetes and osteoporosis. Although more expensive, the use of IV IgG immunoglobulin has been a major advance in the treatment of autoimmune thrombocytopenia. The precise mechanism of its action is not known, but it is thought that the administration of human IgG prolongs the clearance time of IgG-coated platelets by the reticulo-endothelial system. Administration will usually consist of an IV infusion over five days and the platelet response is rapid. Clinicians need to consider the cost of this treatment and therefore it is usually reserved until after 36 weeks' gestation. The resulting increase in platelets will normally allow delivery in the next 2–3 weeks with adequate platelet cover and therefore the option of an epidural in labour can be considered. A final treatment is splenectomy, but this is very rarely undertaken in pregnancy as it has a high fetal and maternal loss rate.

Thrombophilia

Please see Chapter 14.

Table 16.1 – Congenital malformations associated with anti-epileptic medication

	Na Valproate	Carbamazepine	Phenytoin
Neural tube defect	++	+	
Facial cleft		+	+
Developmental delay		+	+
Nail hypoplasia		+	+
Growth restriction			+

NEUROLOGICAL ABNORMALITIES

Epilepsy

Epilepsy is a relatively common disorder occurring in 0.15–1 per cent of women of child-bearing age. Pregnancy has no consistent effect on epilepsy and although several studies have shown an increase in the frequency of fits, others have shown no difference or a decrease in their frequency. In the majority of cases women will have been commenced on anti-convulsant medication prior to their pregnancy. However, many factors contribute to altered drug metabolism in pregnancy and result in a decrease in anti-convulsant drug levels. These include reduced compliance because of fears of teratogenicity, an increase in plasma volume, an increase in extra-cellular fluid volume and a reduced albumin concentration leading to increased clearance of the free drug.

A number of pregnancy complications have been associated with epilepsy including both antepartum and postpartum haemorrhage, pre-eclampsia, preterm delivery and low birth weight. The principal concern related to epilepsy in pregnancy is the increased risk of congenital abnormality. All anti-convulsant medication has been associated with fetal abnormality and there may also be an intrinsic link between epilepsy and fetal defects. Table 16.1 summarizes the major fetal abnormalities associated with anti-epileptic drug therapy. Many of these abnormalities are detectable by ultrasound and therefore all women should be offered the option of an expert scan.

Despite the risks of using anti-epileptic medication

(said to be about 2 per cent), failure to do so may lead to an increased frequency of epileptic fits resulting in both maternal and fetal hypoxia. Such patients therefore require careful pre-pregnancy counselling. Patients on multiple drug therapy should, wherever possible, be converted to the use of a single anti-convulsant drug and a 5 mg daily folic acid supplement. The patient should be reminded that uncontrolled seizures are more harmful to the fetus then the potential risks of drug therapy.

Monitoring of drug levels in pregnancy is difficult. The drug level is expected to fall, but in a majority of cases this is not associated with an increased frequency of fits. An increase in dosage to combat the anticipated fall may lead to an increased fetal risk. In the majority of cases, provided there is no increase in frequency of fits, most obstetricians would advocate not to alter the prenatal drug dosage. In the event of a prolonged seizure it is important to exclude other possible causes, particularly eclampsia. Causes include:
- eclampsia;
- epilepsy;
- encephalitis/meningitis;
- cerebral tumour;
- drug withdrawal;
- toxic overdose;
- metabolic disturbance.

In the postnatal period many of the anti-epileptic drugs have been shown to be competitive inhibitors of the prothrombin precursors resulting in deficiency of vitamin K-dependent clotting factors. It is essential that the neonate receive prophylactic vitamin K at delivery. Mothers may suffer from a marked loss of sleep in the postnatal period, which can predispose to fits. It is important to ensure good compliance at this time.

Migraine

Up to one-fifth of pregnant women will experience migraine, although 70 per cent of migraine sufferers feel that their migraine improves during pregnancy. Obstetric complications are not increased in migraine sufferers. For those women who develop migraine attacks during pregnancy they should be treated with analgesics, anti-emetics and where possible avoid factors thought to trigger the attack. Beta-blockade should not be routinely used because of its association with fetal growth restriction.

Bell's palsy

This is a unilateral neuropathy of the VIIth cranial nerve leading to paralysis of the forehead and lower face, and loss of taste on the ipsilateral anterior tongue may also occur. The incidence of this palsy is increased over three times during the third trimester of pregnancy. The outcome is generally good and complete recovery may be anticipated if the time of onset is within two weeks of the beginning of pregnancy. The only role for steroids is if they are given within the first 24 hours of the onset of symptoms. A reducing dose regime is used over a 10-day period. The palsy does not affect the pregnancy.

AUTOIMMUNE DISEASE

Systemic lupus erythematosus

Systemic lupus erythematosus (SLE) is a multisystem chronic autoimmune inflammatory disease. It is 5–10 times more common in women, particularly in black and Asian populations. It may cause disease in any system, but principally it affects the joints, skin, lungs, nervous system, liver and kidneys. The condition may be diagnosed prenatally or may be suspected for the first time during pregnancy, usually as a result of complications. The diagnosis is confirmed by the finding of a positive assay for antinuclear antibodies. The presence of antibodies to double-stranded DNA are the most specific for SLE.

SLE is a relapsing condition and it is not clear if pregnancy is a risk factor for increasing the risk of relapse. Approximately one-third of mothers with SLE will experience an exacerbation during pregnancy. The maternal and fetal risks of SLE are as follows:

Maternal
- Exacerbation of disease
- Worsening nephropathy/proteinuria
- Pregnancy-induced hypertension
- Thrombosis

Fetal
- Miscarriage
- Fetal death
- Growth restriction
- Preterm delivery

There is a strong association between SLE and both first and second trimester. Because of these significant risks pregnant women with SLE require intensive monitoring for both maternal and fetal indications. The mother should be seen frequently and baseline renal studies including a 24-hour urine collection for protein should be performed. Blood pressure should be monitored closely because of the association with pregnancy-induced hypertension. Serial ultrasonography is performed to assess fetal growth. In women with antiphospholipid or anticardiolipin antibodies who have suffered repeated pregnancy failures the use of aspirin and heparin has been shown to reduce the pregnancy loss rate. If antenatal treatment is required steroids may be given safely, for example in women with a renal nephropathy.

GASTROINTESTINAL DISORDERS

Acute fatty liver of pregnancy

This is a very serious disorder of liver function occurring in approximately 1 in 10,000 pregnancies. The condition typically is noted in primiparous women and develops in the third trimester or within a few days of a stillbirth. The presenting complaints are of abdominal pain, headache, nausea and vomiting which are shortly followed by progressive jaundice, encephalopathy and renal failure. The aetiology of the condition is unknown, but histologically a perilobular fatty infiltration of the liver cells is noted. There is a significant risk of maternal or fetal death. Following the onset of the condition there may a rapidly worsening cascade of problems and the situation is frequently complicated by hypertension and disseminated intravascular coagulation. Maternal death results from encephalopathy or overwhelming haemorrhage associated with the clotting defect. Fetal death is not uncommon and thought to be related to maternal liver failure and the metabolic disturbance.

The management relies on early diagnosis. Liver function tests are deranged and there may be evidence of renal failure. There is no place for a liver biopsy in view of the bleeding complications. Jaundice, vomiting, pruritus and malaise are worrying symptoms and hypertension may be present. Treatment is to deliver the baby as soon as possible. This will frequently be by Caesarean Section under general anaesthesia if clotting disorders prevent the use of an epidural. Supportive therapy with blood transfusion, fresh frozen plasma, platelets and dialysis may all be required around the time of delivery and in the immediate postnatal period. The management will require the input of several senior colleagues including a consultant physician and anaesthetist. Postnatally the liver function usually returns to normal over a few weeks and there is no evidence of long-term liver dysfunction.

Cholestasis of pregnancy

Cholestasis is an uncommon condition of pregnancy occurring in approximately 1:2000 pregnancies. Its incidence varies widely geographically, and it is especially common in certain South American countries, particularly Chile.

It presents most commonly in the late third trimester (after 36 weeks), with generalized itching, sometimes associated with reduced fetal movements. Upper abdominal pain, dark urine and steatorrhoea occur occasionally. It is crucial to recognize that a rash is not associated with cholestasis of pregnancy, although there may be marks associated with skin scratching. Occasionally, there may be jaundice, though this is usually in the later stages of the disease.

The importance of the condition is that it is associated with intrauterine growth restriction and

intrauterine death. The mechanism for this is not clear. Cholestasis is not as a rule associated with major maternal complications.

Complications of cholestasis

Maternal
- Haemorrhage
- Premature labour
- Steatorrhoea

Fetal
- Stillbirth
- Growth restriction
- Meconium staining of amniotic fluid

Maternal liver function is often mildly deranged, with raised transaminases. Bilirubin and bile acids may also be elevated, though not invariably so. Cholestasis must be differentiated from other causes of liver dysfunction in pregnancy. The major differential diagnoses are viral hepatitis, and cholestasis may be confused with early HELLP syndrome or acute fatty liver of pregnancy. Mothers with cholestasis are, however, usually reasonably well systemically.

Management of cholestasis

Symptomatic relief of itching can be provided by prescribing antihistamines, for instance oral chlorpheniramine. Bile acid binding resins such as cholestyramine and ursodeoxycholic acid given orally reduce maternal itching and can normalize liver function. Generally speaking, if there is any concern over fetal wellbeing (for instance, reduced fetal movements or growth) delivery is indicated. Similarly, it is unwise to allow a pregnancy to progress beyond 38 weeks because of the risk of intrauterine death. It is considered wise to give maternal oral vitamin K for a week prior to planned delivery; this is thought to reduce the risk of postpartum haemorrhage associated with a lack of clotting factors.

After delivery, maternal liver function returns to normal within days to weeks, as does pruritus. Cholestasis is reported to have a high recurrence risk in a subsequent pregnancy.

SKIN DISEASES IN PREGNANCY

There are extensive physiological changes to the skin during pregnancy. Increased pigmentation is usual, especially on the face (melasma), areolea, axillae and abdominal midline (linea nigra). Spider naevi are common, and broad pink linear striae (striae gravidarum) frequently appear over the lower abdomen and thighs. Striae gravidarum fade and become white and atretic after pregnancy but never disappear. Their appearance may be related to the increased levels of free cortisol during pregnancy. Pruritus without rash, can be a feature of normal pregnancy but liver function tests should always be performed with this symptom as it may be associated with cholestasis of pregnancy (which is a cause of increased perinatal mortality).

Pre-existing skin conditions such as eczema or psoriasis sometimes improve during pregnancy, perhaps because of increased levels of corticosteroids.

There are three principal dermatoses specific to pregnancy.

Polymorphic eruption of pregnancy

Polymorphic eruption of pregnancy (PEP), otherwise called pruritic urticarial papules and plaques of pregnancy (PUPP), is a pruritic eruption that appears late in the third trimester and affects about 1:200 pregnancies. The lesions occur mainly over the abdomen and upper thighs. Usually, the lesions run linearly along vertical striae. No side effects to the fetus are described, and the rash rapidly clears up after delivery. An aqueous cream of 2 per cent phenol in oily calamine and a sedative antihistamine afford symptomatic relief. Rarely, local or systemic steroids are required.

Pemphigoid gestationis

Pemphigoid gestationis (PG) was previously called herpes gestationis and is a rarer but more serious condition that is associated with an increased perinatal mortality. The eruption causes intense pruritus and begins in the peri-umbilical region,

Investigation of cholestasis

Maternal
- Liver function tests
- Clotting profile
- Renal function
- Hepatitis serology
- Autoimmune antibodies
- Bile acids (may allow disease progression to be tracked)

Fetal
- Ultrasound for growth, amniotic fluid and biophysical
- assessment
- CTG

spreading to the limbs, palms and soles. The eruption begins with papules and plaques, but these develop into vesicles and tense bullae after two or more weeks. The condition usually begins in the mid-trimester, and although there is frequently some improvement towards the end of pregnancy, there is typically flare postpartum with persistence for several months. The diagnosis is by direct immunofluorescence, which shows complement (C3) deposition in the basement membrane and confirms the nature of the lesion as an autoimmune condition possibly related to fetal antigens. The presence of complement distinguishes pemphigoid gestationis from PEP. This distinction is important because PG is associated with low birthweight, preterm labour and intrauterine death so intensive fetal monitoring is required. Treatment is with topical (e.g. 1 per cent hydrocortisone cream) or systemic (e.g. prednisolone 40 mg daily) steroids and sedative antihistamines.

Prurigo of pregnancy

This pruritic condition consists of groups of red or brown papules that cover the abdomen and extensor surfaces of limbs. It develops in late pregnancy and improves after delivery. No effects on the fetus are known and the condition usually responds to topical steroids. It should be distinguished from pruritic folliculitis, which is an acneiform eruption occasionally complicating pregnancy.

References for further reading

Barksy HE. Asthma and pregnancy. *Postgraduate Medicine* 1991; **89:** 125–32.

Jelsema RD, Cotton DB. Cardiac disease. In: James D.K., Steer PJ, Weiner C, Gonik B. (eds). *High risk pregnancy.* W.B. Saunders. 1994: 299–314.

Perry KG Jr, Morrison JC. The diagnosis and management of hemoglobinopathies during pregnancy. *Seminars in Perinatology* 1990; **14:** 90–102.

Sibai BM. Chronic hypertension in pregnancy. *Clinics in Perinatology* 1991; **18:** 451–61.

Vander Spuy ZM, Jacobs HS. Management of endocrine disorders in pregnancy. Part I: Thyroid and parathyroid disease. *Postgraduate Medical Journal* 1984; **60:** 245–52.

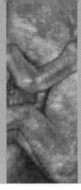

Chapter 17

Second trimester miscarriage

OVERVIEW

Second trimester miscarriage is a relatively common problem. It is particularly distressing to the woman and her family because her abdomen has been obviously growing, she has often felt fetal movements and her bonding with the baby has begun. It is considered to be an obstetric rather than a gynaecological disorder: this is important to note to achieve the correct philosophy of care. There are several causes of second trimester miscarriage, some of which are amenable to treatment.

Definition

Second trimester miscarriage is miscarriage that occurs between 12 and 24 weeks' gestation. After 24 weeks' gestation the baby is potentially viable and delivery then is preterm delivery. Miscarriage may be threatened, presenting with bleeding or few contractions and a cervix less than 3 cm dilated. When there is strong pain and a cervix dilated more than 3 cm then it is described as inevitable miscarriage. The presentation is particularly challenging when the membranes have ruptured and amniotic fluid is draining.

Incidence and epidemiology

In the UK, as in most other countries, there is no formal record of miscarriages. The incidence is unknown. There is a greater number of early miscarriages than late miscarriages and there are more preterm births than late miscarriages.

Miscarriage can be associated with major haemorrhage and sepsis. Maternal death is a rare but recognized consequence. Infective sequelae may lead to impaired fertility.

Aetiology

Risk factors

- Poor socio-economic status
- Smoking
- Infections, especially of the genital tract
- Previous miscarriage
- Previous premature birth

Local infection of the genital tract is thought to lead to damage to the chorio-amniotic membranes and consequent rupture. Systemic infection may also play a role particularly when the woman suffers a fever. Malaria may be one of the commonest associates with miscarriage. Persistent leakage of blood retro- or periplacentally over a period of time irritates the uterus resulting in contractions and possible damage to the membranes. An abnormal uterine shape of congenital origin may compromise the enlargement of the fetus. Fibroids may distort the cavity, however they are common and most pregnancies are successful in the presence of fibroids. If they degenerate or are submucous, are large or near the cervix they may cause miscarriage. Fetal abnormality does not cause miscarriage, however if polyhydramnios is a feature this may play a role. Severe polyhydramnios is rare in mid-pregnancy with the notable exception of twin-to-twin transfusion syndrome. Multiple gestation is clearly associated with mid-trimester miscarriage and preterm birth due to overdistension of the uterus.

The uterine cervix may be responsible, having been damaged previously through a conization or other surgical procedure. Previous late termination of pregnancy may also have damaged the cervix. There is speculation about the role of auto-antibodies such as antiphospholipid and anticardiolipin antibodies but their role it is not clear.

Clinical features

As with a threat of premature labour the membranes may be intact or ruptured at presentation. Miscarriage is often rapid without much labour pain. Presentation may be simply with backache and abdominal discomfort. There may be clear evidence of membrane rupture with few premonitory signs; this is a poor prognostic indicator especially if confirmed before 18 weeks' gestation.

History

The presenting history may be of general lower abdominal discomfort with backache, discomfort or pain from uterine contractions or vaginal loss. The vaginal loss may be mucus, blood or amniotic fluid. A history of being generally unwell, fever, or urinary

P | Understanding the pathophysiology

The uterus should be thought of as a distended sac filled with fluid, baby(ies) and placenta. There is one potential opening from it at the cervix. The cervix is usually at least 35 mm long and closed in mid-pregnancy. Various stimuli present over a period of weeks, resulting in contractions and shortening of the cervix (Fig. 17.1).

Multiple gestation (Fig. 17.2). The presence of more than one baby in the uterus may lead to overstretching, increased Braxton Hicks contractions and premature shortening and opening of the cervix.

Bleeding (Fig. 17.3). Disturbance at the utero-placental interface may lead to bleeding. This blood tracks down behind the membranes to the cervix. This stimulates uterine contractions and damages the membranes leading to membrane rupture.

Infection (Fig. 17.4). The uterine cavity is sterile but the vagina contains commensal bacteria. The distance between the vaginal organisms and the membranes decreases and the bacteria may ascend. The membranes gradually prolapse through the cervical canal and may eventually bulge before they rupture. It is thought that as this mechanism takes place fibronectin appears in the vaginal secretions.

Distorted uterus (Fig. 17.5). A uterus that is distorted by congenital malformation or fibroids in a low position may be less able to accommodate the enlarging fetus.

The cervix (Fig. 17.6). On account of previous damage or, rarely, a congenital defect the cervix may shorten and open prematurely. When this occurs as the primary phenomenon it is described as cervical weakness (a better term than cervical incompetence).

symptoms is also important. If a woman has had a previous miscarriage she is likely to present earlier in the process. A prior history of miscarriage, cervical cerclage, invasive prenatal diagnosis procedure, vaginal bleeding, fibroids or congenital uterine anomaly is relevant.

Always check the dating of the pregnancy clinically or by prior ultrasound examination and consider the possibility of pre-existing fetal death *in utero*. Ask if the baby has been and is moving.

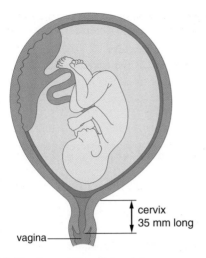

Figure 17.1 The uterus at 23 weeks' gestation.

cervix
35 mm long

vagina

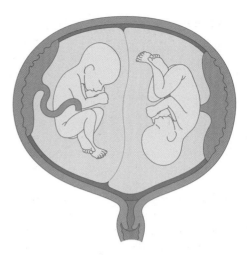

Figure 17.2 The uterus overdistended with twins or more.

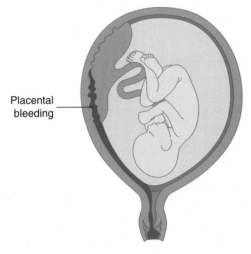

Placental
bleeding

Figure 17.3 Placental bleeding.

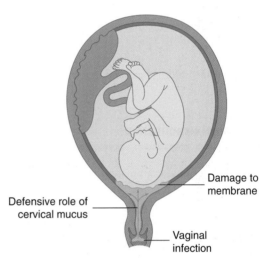

Damage to
membrane

Defensive role of
cervical mucus

Vaginal
infection

Figure 17.4 Ascending genital tract bleeding.

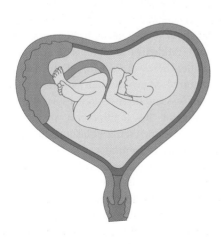

Figure 17.5 Septate uterus.

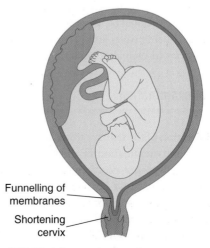

Funnelling of
membranes

Shortening
cervix

Figure 17.6 Weak (incompetent) cervix.

S Symptoms

- Abdominal discomfort and pain
- Backache
- Generally unwell
- Change in vaginal discharge
- Vaginal bleeding
- Vaginal blood loss

Signs

- Palpable contractions
- Vaginal loss of fluid, blood or mucus
- Cervical dilatation

Investigations

- Urine dipstick and mid-stream urine test (MSU) for culture and sensitivity
- Low vaginal swab for microbiology
- Full blood count
- Ultrasound scan (especially if the patient is unbooked) for fetal size, amniotic fluid assessment, level of presenting part and check placental site

Examination

General examination

A brief general examination of the woman is important. Is she unwell? Check her state of hydration, skin, conjunctiva and pulse rate. All this can be assessed while holding her hand in introduction. She will be anxious.

Abdominal examination

General abdominal examination is usually negative, however it must be done. There may be signs of a renal tract infection or of a gastro-intestinal problem. Gentle palpation of the lower abdomen for uterine contraction, irritability or tenderness may be revealing. Prior to 24 weeks the fetal parts cannot be felt and no attempt should be made to identify them. A hand-held Doppler device (often referred to as a Sonicaid) should be used to auscultate the fetal heart. Discreet enquiry should be made as to whether a sanitary towel is being worn and permission sought to inspect it prior to vaginal examination.

Vaginal examination

After inspection of the sanitary towel and any vaginal loss a speculum examination should be performed. A good light and proper positioning is important. A low vaginal swab should be taken, especially if the presentation is one of membrane rupture. The cervix is visualized. Any source of bleeding should be noted and any loss of fluid from the uterus sought by asking the woman to cough during the examination.

The cervix might already be opening and the membrane may be seen bulging through the cervical canal. If the cervix is opening or the membranes have ruptured then a digital examination should not be performed because this would exacerbate any infection present.

Treatment

A holistic approach to the situation is essential. Sympathy, pain relief and reassurance are essential. The ideal place for such women is a purpose-designed area not in the middle of the labour ward and not in a busy gynaecological ward. Beyond 18 weeks' gestation the labour ward philosophy becomes even more important. Midwives are prepared and skilled in looking after these women without much adaptation being required. Many hospitals now have a focus on pregnancy loss and there is often a specialist midwife coordinator for this. If the cervix was not initially dilated many women settle with supportive measures and the pregnancy continues.

Should the situation be one of membrane rupture then the situation is more difficult. Established chorio-amnionitis usually declares itself with contractions and delivery. With a history of fluid draining then membrane rupture should be confirmed by abdominal scan. If there are no contractions and no sign of infection then there is no urgency to interfere. The parents should be counselled in coming to terms with the inevitable situation of pregnancy loss. It is important that medical action only takes place when they are ready. Seeing the ultrasound scan screen may help by them realizing how little fluid remains inside the uterus. Some may want to wait for nature to take its course: others may want more immediate action. In both cases continuing support is important. No harm will come from conservatism as long as careful observation is made for signs of infection. Self-taken temperature and observation of changing vaginal discharge or lower uterine tenderness are recommended. This can be done at home.

If the option is taken to hasten the emptying of the uterus this is done with prostaglandin administration. Cervagem 1 mg vaginally every three hours for five times is usually effective. An oxytocin infusion (Syntocinon) may be necessary later in the process. Pain relief and indicated antibiotics should be given. In some hospitals with the requisite skills surgical evacuation of the uterus (dilatation and evacuation) in the operating theatre may be performed. This usually requires a general anaesthetic.

Should there be previous caesarean or other previous uterine surgery then special care should be taken when emptying the uterus in consultation with experienced doctors.

Antibiotics

Antibiotics are given for identified or strongly presumed infection, such as that of the urinary tract. Vaginal infection may be difficult to identify and there is some evidence that empirical antibiotics should be given. It seems that the best choice is erythromycin or metronidazole. This should be continued for a course of five days. Great care must be exercised if there is already clinical evidence of chorio-amnionitis or membrane rupture. In these cases nature may be saying that delivery is inevitable and to delay it may lead to further infection and consequent morbidity. Miscarriage is a sign of untreated infection. Treating has some delaying effect. However if the infection is low-grade and controllable then antibiotics, particularly in a situation of membrane rupture, may be helpful. The decision to use antibiotics or not requires appreciation of this delicate balance.

Tocolytics

There is currently no place for tocolysis in this treatment. Tocolytics are more effective in later pregnancy and are used to secure short-term prolongation of the pregnancy.

Cervical cerclage

There is a particular challenge when the cervix has opened and the membranes are bulging. Passing a supporting tape 'stitch' round the cervix to close it when it is opening seems logical. However the results of emergency cervical cerclage are poor. Every effort should be made to detect and treat other causes of the uterine instability. If persistent placental bleeding is leading to secondary opening of the cervix then closing the cervix with a stitch does not address the primary issue and is unlikely to be successful. It seems wise to delay insertion of a suture for 24 hours after admission. The only obvious issue during this time should be that the cervix has opened. Bleeding, contractions or infection are contraindications to cerclage. The woman should rest although not be on complete bedrest. When in bed it may be useful to elevate the foot of the bed. The chance of cerclage being successful is related to the cervical dilatation at insertion. A dilatation of more than 3 cm with an effaced cervix poses extreme difficulties even to the most experienced operator.

Cervical cerclage can be done under general or regional anaesthesia. There is greater safety in mid-pregnancy but the woman can make an informed choice about the method of anaesthesia. The woman is placed in lithotomy position and the labial area is shaved: this need not extend very far anteriorly. She is then washed and draped. The vagina and cervix are washed under direct vision after passage of an Auvard or Sims speculum. If the option selected is to insert a simple purse string suture (McDonald technique, Fig. 17.7) then infiltration of the tissues with dilute adrenaline is unnecessary. The membranes are reduced by the head down position and traction in the opposite direction with ring retractors on the anterior and posterior cervical lips. If the membranes appear particularly tense then a decompression amniocentesis is favoured by some at this point. Should the membranes still be bulging then a Foley

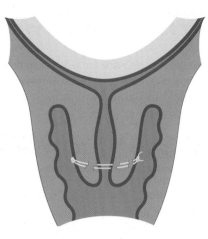

Figure 17.7 Cervical suture: McDonald technique.

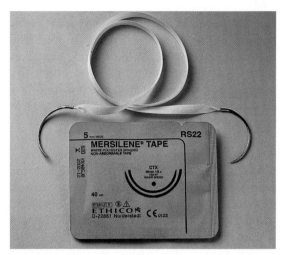

Figure 17.8 Photograph of Mersilene tape with needles at each end.

catheter with the balloon inflated to the appropriate distension and the tip cut off is passed through the cervical canal exerting counter traction against the balloon of membranes. At one point this is felt to 'pop' through the internal os. The Mersilene tape suture (Mersilene RS22, Ethicon, Edinburgh, Fig. 17.8) is then passed around the cervix taking bites at all four quadrants. As it is tied the Foley catheter balloon is deflated and the catheter is extracted as the knot is tied. The problem with this type of suture is that it is rather low on the cervical canal. An experienced operator may choose to use a Shirodkar technique with infiltration of the uterovesical vaginal fold and the posterior fornix with dilute adrenaline and a transverse incision anteriorly and posteriorly to achieve a high stitch placement (Fig. 17.9). The vaginal incisions are closed with 2/0 Vicryl. Depending on the dilatation of the cervix at the beginning the prospect of the pregnancy proceeding beyond 26 weeks may be as low as 50 per cent. Irrespective of the outcome of this pregnancy an interesting question will be what to do in the next pregnancy. Postoperatively the woman is observed for 24 hours, the fetal heart demonstrated to her the next day and she goes home on a course of antibiotics. If she is fortunate and the pregnancy goes to 37 weeks then in the absence of any obstetric indication for Caesarean Section the stitch is removed, again under anaesthesia, and a vaginal delivery pursued. The woman is warned to attend hospital at any time with abdominal pain, vaginal bleeding or ruptured membranes. Under such circumstances the stitch may be removed as an emergency.

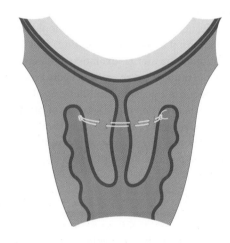

Figure 17.9 Cervical suture: Shirodkar technique.

Management of the miscarriage itself

If miscarriage and delivery is inevitable then certain points should be considered:
- Full attention is paid to maximize psychological support from caring staff.
- Adequate pain relief should be offered. These deliveries are usually quick but there is no contraindication to epidural anaesthesia. Patient controlled subcutaneous anaesthesia (PCA) is also ideal.
- Vaginal delivery will almost always occur even if there is a transverse lie or fetal malformation.

This is because of the relatively small size of the fetus.

- Unfortunately retention of the placenta or part of it is more common under these circumstances.
- If the pregnancy is close to 24 weeks then a paediatrician should be briefed and called to attend the delivery to assess viability at birth.
- The mother sees the fetus as a baby. She may want to touch the baby and hold the baby. Appropriate sensitivities should be exercised according to the choice of the woman and her partner.
- Follow-up by a senior member of staff and specialist midwife should be organized. This will lead on to discussion about a future pregnancy.

Later implications

During the follow-up discussion some clues to the aetiology of the loss will need to be considered. This is particularly so when the miscarriage is recurrent. Many women are given the idea that much mid-trimester loss is due to cervical weakness and the problem should be solved by a cervical suture, however the issue is more complicated than this. Each possible cause must be considered. If there was bleeding or a multiple gestation then it is unlikely that the same conditions will recur in another pregnancy. A cervical suture is therefore likely to be inappropriate. If infection seems to have played a prominent role then antibiotics may be important in a future pregnancy: often as one or two short courses.

If the pattern of the loss is one of cervical weakness then a prophylactic cervical suture may be appropriate in the next pregnancy. This is performed at 12–14 weeks' gestation. Two techniques are available as shown in Figures 17.7 and 17.9. It is thought that the Shirodkar technique may be superior. It is placed at an anatomical position close to the internal os which seems very logical and by virtue of its high position and being buried it is also more distant from potentially infective vaginal secretions. Some specialists use adjunctive antibiotics as short courses.

If a woman is of particularly high risk, having an extensive history of pregnancy loss and/or major cervical surgery, such as a large conization or a cervical amputation, then the unusual technique of transabdominal cervical suture may be used. This technique is invasive and should only be used by highly skilled operators. This technique is the one most likely to

achieve a high placement of the suture. A caesarean is necessary, however, if complications occur before viability then posterior colpotomy can be performed with removal of the suture and vaginal miscarriage. At Caesarean Section with a successful outcome the suture can be left in place for future pregnancies.

New developments

Bacterial infection: study continues on the role of infection and bacterial vaginosis. Treatment regimens of oral and vaginal applications continue.

Ultrasound scanning for cervical length: studies of the length of the cervix as determined on transvaginal ultrasound scan at 18–23 weeks' gestation are being conducted on high- and low-risk groups. Appearances of 'funnelling', shortening and opening are considered.

Fibronectin appears in the vaginal secretions in women threatening preterm birth. It may be predictive of progression of the process and is considered in conjunction with other tests.

Key Points

- Women with mid-trimester pregnancy loss require special consideration and treatment
- The differential diagnosis must be considered to plan logical treatment
- There is a role for antibiotics and cervical cerclage
- Sympathy and understanding are critical

Termination of pregnancy

Sadly, termination of pregnancy (abortion) becomes necessary in some pregnancies. In the second trimester this may be due to fetal malformation, fetal death or another compelling reason why the pregnancy cannot continue. In the UK it is done within the legislation of the Abortion Act (1967).

There are two options for this: medical termination or surgical termination. Surgical termination may not be available in some centres because it is a hazardous procedure requiring a large degree of skill. Medical termination takes at least one day of potential pain and suffering. The woman and her partner participate as in a labour and are able to see and hold the fetus if they wish. If it is a late medical termination beyond 22 weeks, then the process should be commenced with a fetocide. Surgical termination is a short procedure requiring a few hours in hospital but the family cannot see the fetal parts. Ideally both procedures should be available and the woman given a choice.

Medical treatment

This involves the use of a potent prostaglandin Cervagem (prostaglandin F2a). It is given vaginally as a 1 mg vaginal pessary three-hourly for five doses. In most cases this leads to active contractions and provokes miscarriage. More recently it has been supplemented with Mifepristone 200 mg orally 24–36 hours before the prostaglandin administration. This significantly shortens the induction delivery interval. Pain relief is a method of choice but patient-controlled opiate pump seems ideal. An ideal area for performing this procedure is often not available. It should be some form of transitional ward between obstetrics and gynaecology. A side room in the labour ward is often used and there is then the availability of sympathetic midwives. In most cases done before 22 weeks' gestation, a post-delivery uterine evacuation is appropriate as the placenta is often delivered in pieces. Secondary haemorrhage or return to hospital for evacuation is always a pity in these circumstances.

CASE HISTORY

Mrs M

22 years old

Second pregnancy: the first was a miscarriage at 18 weeks after rupture of the membranes

Now 20 weeks by early (12 week) ultrasound scan

Admitted to the labour ward with low back pain, feeling warm and slight vaginal blood loss followed by watery discharge

What is the likely diagnosis?

The combination of a previous mid-trimester loss and a history of a temperature, backache and vaginal loss make intrauterine infection (chorio-amnionitis) and cervical dilatation a strong possibility. This would be considered an 'inevitable miscarriage'.

What are the key points in examination and investigation of Mrs M?

Blood pressure, pulse rate and temperature	May be very pyrexial or even shocked
Abdominal examination	abdomen may be tender, suggesting chorio-amnionitis
Speculum examination	cervical dilatation, high vaginal swab (HVS)
MSU	exclude urinary tract infection
Ultrasound scan	fetal heart, amniotic fluid (may be absent or reduced)
Full blood count	white cell count important if raised

Further management:

On speculum examination, there were bulging membranes with some offensive amniotic fluid leaking. An HVS was sent. Mrs M became unwell with a temperature of 39.5°C and a tachycardia of 130/min. After counselling involving a neonatologist and obstetrician, a decision was taken to terminate the pregnancy in her interest, and a Syntocinon infusion was commenced. In addition, because of the risk of disseminated intravascular coagulation (DIC), a clotting profile and fibrinogen level were sent. Furthermore, she received opiate analgesics by subcutaneous infusion, IV rehydration and broad-spectrum antibiotics. She required close observation, with an indwelling catheter to monitor hourly urine output and the anaesthetist was closely involved in her management.

Mrs M delivered a baby with no signs of life eight hours after commencement of Syntocinon. She required an ERPC under ultrasound guidance by the consultant, but bled heavily following this (approximately 2,500 mL), requiring 8 units of blood and fresh frozen plasma. She developed severe DIC, and, because of the combination of haemorrhage, DIC and sepsis, became anuric. Acute renal failure was diagnosed and she required dialysis for three months, eventually making a full recovery.

Surgical treatment

Surgical termination of pregnancy presents increasing hazards proportionate to the gestational age. This is because the fetal parts are bigger and the risk of tearing the cervix or damaging the uterus is greater. The cervix should be prepared with a prostaglandin preparation or with Dilapan (Fig. 17.10). This absorbs moisture and swells up over 8–12 hours. The cervix is then already 12–14 mm dilated before the surgical procedure commences. The procedure should be performed with ultrasound available. This should be used to confirm the gestational age and guide insertion of the first instruments. It is also used

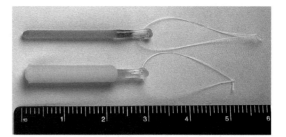

Figure 17.10 Dilapan before and after leaving in water for 12 hours.

at the end of the procedure to verify that the uterus is empty. Syntocinon is used to ensure the uterus is contracted after delivery.

Further reading

Flint S, Gibb D. Recurrent Second Trimester Miscarriage. *Current Opinion in Obstetrics and Gynaecology* 1996; **8:** 449–53.

Gibb D, Salaria D. Transabdominal cervicoisthmic cerclage in the management of recurrent second trimester miscarriage and perterm delivery. *Br J Obstet Gynaecol.* 1995; **102:** 802–06.

Kohner, N. *Miscarriage, stillbirth and neonatal...* Still birth and neonatal death society, UK, 1991.

Miscarriage Association booklets. Available from The Miscarriage Association, c/o Clayton Hospital, Northgate, Wakefield, West Yorkshire, UK

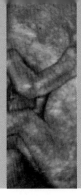

Preterm labour

OVERVIEW

Preterm labour is one of the commonest perinatal problems facing obstetricians. About 45 per cent of women presenting with 'threatened' preterm labour are in real labour, and go on to deliver within 48 hours; the remaining 55 per cent will stop contracting and not deliver imminently. Its cause is largely unknown and there is controversy over what investigations and treatments are necessary.

Definition

Preterm labour is labour occurring before 37 weeks' gestation. In practice, this means a labour occurring between 24 and 37 weeks; before 24 weeks the correct term is miscarriage rather than preterm labour. Preterm labour with intact membranes at presentation will be discussed in this chapter; this makes up at least half of the cases of preterm labour.

Preterm prelabour rupture of membranes with subsequent preterm labour is thought to have a different pathophysiological basis, much more related to infection, and is discussed separately (page 202).

Incidence and epidemiology

In the UK, approximately 7 per cent of labours are preterm. This figure is higher in inner city areas and lower in more affluent areas. With modern neonatal care, 30 per cent of babies born at 24 weeks' gestation will survive whereas almost 80 per cent survive at 27 weeks. Handicap risk is high in deliveries at 24 weeks (around 40 per cent), but this drops to less than 10 per cent at 27 weeks. So the period between 24 and 27 weeks is critical with respect to delivery, survival and handicap risk (Fig. 18.1).

Preterm delivery is associated with massive expenditure of neonatal resources. A neonatal intensive care cot in the UK costs at least £1000 per day in terms of staffing, drugs, equipment, etc. Remember that many neonates born at 24–28 weeks spend at least 10 weeks (70 days) in the unit. This has led to the extraordinary calculation in the USA that the neonatal and lifetime medical and support costs incurred for infants born weighing less than 900 g will exceed that individual's average lifetime earnings!

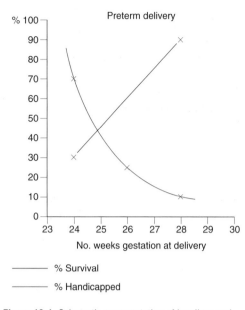

Figure 18.1 Schematic representation of handicap and survival rates following preterm delivery.

Risk factors

- Malnutrition
- Smoking
- Poor socio-economic status
- Genital infections, especially bacterial vaginosis (BV)
- Multiple gestation
- Uterine abnormality
- Recreational drug abuse
- Previous preterm labour
- Previous prelabour premature rupture of membranes (PPROM)

Aetiology

Often no cause is found for preterm labour; this is known as idiopathic preterm labour and makes up at least 75 per cent of cases. Local infection (chorio-amnionitis) is a cause of preterm labour in 10–20 per cent of cases with intact membranes (this figure is higher if labour follows PPROM, page 202), and is notoriously difficult to identify often until late in its natural history. Systemic infection, most commonly pyelonephritis, is also implicated. Antepartum haemorrhage (especially placental abruption) is a cause of preterm labour as blood leaking into the

P Understanding the pathophysiology

Many new theories have been put forward as to why preterm labour develops. None are proven, but all may explain how and why preterm labour develops. These include...

Infection: subclinical chorio-amnionitis may predispose to preterm delivery. However, infection will be associated with no more than 20 per cent, and most estimates suggest around 10 per cent, of uncomplicated preterm labours. The best link between preterm labour and infection is BV.

Disturbance of myometrial nitric oxide/prostaglandin balance: these agents act on smooth muscle cells and control myometrial contractility, and disturbance of this may lead to preterm contractions, hence labour. Nitric oxide is a vasodilator and smooth muscle relaxant; different prostaglandins can have relaxant or constrictor action.

The cervix as the initiator: far from being purely a mass of fibrous tissue, the cervix is a complex fibromuscular organ that can soften, hydrate and alter in form with dramatic rapidity. Changes in the cervix may alter the ordinary quiescence of uterine muscle, and predispose to preterm labour.

myometrium is a powerful stimulant of uterine irritability. Degenerating fibroids will also cause uterine irritability, which may in turn set off contractions. Multiple gestation is often associated with preterm labour; women with twins commonly go into labour between 34–37 weeks and triplets/quadruplets even earlier (although in those cases, Caesarean Section is almost always performed). Cervical incompetence (better termed 'weakness') may cause both late miscarriage and preterm labour. Less common causes include drug abuse (especially crack and cocaine), trauma to the abdomen or abdominal operations.

Clinical features

Labour may occur as it would at term; painful regular contractions followed by spontaneous rupture of the membranes (SROM). A diagnosis of preterm labour is made with regular uterine contractions accompanied by effacement and dilatation of the cervix, occurring between 24 and 37 weeks' gestation. There may or may not be rupture of the membranes (ROM); this does not however make the diagnosis. Sometimes preterm labour, especially in the 24–28 weeks' gestation band, may present as just abdominal pain or backache; these symptoms therefore warrant careful investigation.

History

There may be regular contractions or just vague backache. It is important to exclude gastro-enteritis or urinary tract infection as both may predispose to preterm labour. A history of nausea, vomiting or diarrhoea; urinary frequency, dysuria or haematuria is therefore relevant. Other factors pertinent to the history are amniocentesis, bleeding in early pregnancy and uterine anomalies.

Other important points are:

- Always check dates. Do menstrual dates agree with ultrasound dates? Is this preterm labour really preterm?
- Is the baby moving (concern about intrauterine death)?
- Has there been any bleeding (placental abruption)?
- Have the membranes ruptured (preterm prelabour rupture of the membranes, PPROM)?

General examination

This must include an assessment of the woman rather than just the uterus, as systemic disorders may predispose to preterm labour. Facial flushing or sweating may be a clue to systemic infection. Record vital signs: temperature, pulse rate and blood pressure.

S Symptoms

- Abdominal pain (not necessarily regular contractions)
- Backache
- Reduced fetal movements
- Nausea and vomiting
- Diarrhoea/increase in motion frequency
- Increase in vaginal discharge
- Vaginal bleeding

Signs

- Tachycardia
- Mild pyrexia (these two especially if associated with infection)
- Palpable contractions
- Cervical effacement and dilatation
- Membranes may be intact or ruptured

Assessment of skin turgor, dry mouth and tongue and sunken eyes will give an idea about hydration status.

Abdominal examination

Search for signs suggesting intra-abdominal pathology, rebound, guarding, localized tenderness. These may point towards pyelonephritis or appendicitis as a possible cause for preterm labour. Palpation of the uterus for tenderness, irritability and masses will help exclude placental abruption (tender, tense uterus with or without vaginal bleeding) or degenerating fibroid (tender 'lump' palpable within the wall of the uterus). A tender but soft uterus may be due to chorio-amnionitis.

In addition, no obstetric examination is complete without measuring the symphysis–fundal height, determining lie, presentation and engagement of the presenting part. Never forget to listen to the fetal heart and note its baseline rate.

Vaginal examination

If the membranes are intact, perform a gentle digital vaginal examination. You should note cervical dilatation and effacement, presence or absence of membranes and bleeding. If the membranes are ruptured, speculum examination under aseptic conditions is advisable.

Treatment

Treatment is directed at making the woman comfortable and reducing ambient stress levels, giving antibiotics, correcting dehydration and dealing with

(see later)

Investigations

- Urine 'dipstick'; if positive then send mid-stream urine test (MSU) for culture and sensitivities (MC&S). If dehydrated, ketones may be present
- High vaginal swab (HVS)
- Full blood count (WCC relevant in case of infection)
- Blood cultures if pyrexial >38.5°C
- C-reactive protein/erythrocyte sedimentation rate (ESR) if membranes ruptured or suspicion of infection
- If infection of the chorion or amnion is suspected, then amniocentesis and/or cordocentesis may be carried out to determine the presence of bacteria or white cells
- A transvaginal ultrasound scan of the cervix (see later) may be a good predictor of preterm delivery

any suspected infection. Analgesia may be oral, for example paracetamol/codeine combinations, however if these are likely to be poorly tolerated or abdominal pain is a major feature then intramuscular opiates such as pethidine and diamorphine are often used. There is some evidence that acute dehydration can predispose a woman to preterm labour, and even if she is not vomiting and/or pyrexial, rehydration with normal saline or Hartmann's solution (1 litre over 60 minutes initially) is considered a useful adjunct to treatment.

Many women's contractions appear to settle after these relatively simple management techniques; these 'general' points of therapy should be effected before determining whether tocolytics are appropriate.

Antibiotics

More specific treatments include antibiotics (preferably IV for prompt action) if urinary tract infection (UTI) is suspected. UTI is often associated with preterm labour; whether the mechanism is via a systemic immune-mediated reaction involving cytokines hence precipitating contractions or causing uterine irritability because of the close anatomical proximity of the kidneys and uterus is unknown. The best antibiotics for UTI are those with Gram-negative spectrum, hence a second or third generation cephalosporin rather than amoxycillin, to which resistance is now common among *E. coli*.

Chorio-amnionitis (much more common after PPROM), may lead to preterm labour and delivery; in this situation antibiotics are given generally to avoid dangerous maternal sepsis rather than any hope of countering the intrauterine infection. The choice of antibiotic in this situation might include the combination of amoxycillin, or a cephalosporin together with metronidazole.

Steroids

Steroids must be given to any woman at high risk of preterm delivery. Two commonly used examples are dexamethasone or betamethasone. These are given intramuscularly and orally respectively, in two doses twelve hours apart. They aid fetal lung maturation and their administration has been shown to reduce the incidence of respiratory distress syndrome (RDS) in the neonate (see New developments, page 278).

Tocolytics

This is a disparate class of drugs that are used to reduce uterine contractility, i.e. stop uterine contractions. Most act as smooth muscle relaxants, and have a place in particular for transfer of women in preterm labour to another hospital, or for 'acute' use of less than 48 hours, whilst the beneficial effect of maternally-administered steroids is awaited. Contraindications to their use include rupture of membranes, any evidence of chorio-amnionitis, fetal anomaly and antepartum haemorrhage. These drugs should be used sparingly, under close supervision and include:

- Beta-agonists such as ritodrine, salbutamol and terbutaline (given IV or orally): these act on beta-2 adrenergic receptors on muscle causing relaxation. In therapeutic doses they cause tachycardia, sweating, headache and, rarely, life-threatening cardiovascular compromise with pulmonary oedema.
- Calcium channel blockers such as nifedipine (given orally): this class of drug acts as a smooth muscle relaxant. Side effects are maternal and generally mild, including headache and flushing.
- NSAIDs such as indomethacin (given orally or rectally): block prostaglandin production and hence reduce myometrial contractility. Maternal side

effects are not pronounced, but fetal side effects include oligohydramnios, intraventricular haemorrhage and a risk of a patent ductus arteriosus in the neonate requiring surgical ligation. These side effects are uncommon if only 24-hour therapy is used, and increase in severity and frequency depending on how long indomethacin is used for.

- Glyceryl trinitrate (GTN) (transdermal or IV administration): GTN is a nitric oxide donor, causing smooth muscle relaxation. It appears relatively safe and well tolerated and at least as effective as other tocolytics. However, it is relatively new and is yet to be formally assessed in trials.

Choice of tocolytic is difficult, as there is no real certainty that any of these substances prolong gestation much more than placebo. We know that ritodrine has been shown in a large randomized controlled trial to reduce the number of deliveries within 48 hours of commencement of treatment in women with preterm labour, compared to placebo. This did not lead to a statistically significant prolongation of gestation. The side effect profile of many tocolytics, particularly ritodrine, precludes their more widespread use. Nifedipine and GTN seem to be the least harmful and best-tolerated tocolytics. Tocolytic combinations do not work better than single agents and simply lead to multiplication of side effects.

Management of the labour itself

If labour becomes established, then certain points differ from the management of term labour:

- The mother must be fully aware of what is likely to happen in her labour and ideally she should have had the chance to speak to the neonatologist. Good analgesia and hydration must be maintained. An epidural anaesthetic may be wise, especially if a Caesarean Section is likely, however this is to be avoided if there are signs of systemic infection.
- Cardiotocograph monitoring should be continuous. A preterm baby is more likely than a fully grown one to become distressed in labour.
- The membranes should not be ruptured until as late as possible in the labour. The cushioning effect of the amniotic fluid may protect the fragile fetal body from birth trauma. Occasionally, very premature babies may be delivered in their sac.

- If the baby is breech, or there are twins or higher order multiple gestation then Caesarean Section may be indicated. The hazards of preterm breech delivery include cord prolapse, and head entrapment by an incompletely dilated cervix. This occurs because before 34 weeks, the baby's head is proportionately larger than the abdomen (especially in intrauterine growth restricted babies) and therefore the baby's abdomen may slip through the cervix whereas the head gets caught and can lead to fetal demise or intracranial trauma.
- Caesarean Section may be performed through a classical (longitudinal) rather than lower segment (transverse) uterine incision. This is more likely in extreme prematurity, when the lower uterine segment is not properly formed
- The second stage of labour must not be extended. Sometimes, forceps are used at delivery of the head; it is believed that this avoids intracranial trauma. Ventouse should not be used below 34 weeks.

Additional points in management

You should remember to liaise closely with your neonatology colleagues. If there is no neonatal cot available, then consider an '*in utero*' transfer (i.e. transfer before delivery occurs) to the nearest neonatal facility. '*In utero*' transfer carries a better prognosis for the baby than '*ex utero*' transfer. The best incubator for the baby is the mother's womb.

Arrange for an ultrasound scan. This will give useful information on presentation, estimated fetal weight, amniotic fluid volume, and will exclude major anomaly. An ultrasound is essential in the case of 'late bookers' or those who have not had a previous ultrasound in this pregnancy.

New developments

Predicting preterm labour
Screening for BV: BV is an abnormal colonization of the vagina by anaerobic bacteria and *Trichomonas vaginalis*. This means that the pH of the vagina becomes more alkaline (>4.5) and may lead to preterm prelabour rupture of membranes (PPROM) or preterm labour. The condition

may be treated with oral metronidazole or clindamycin.

Scanning for cervical length: a short cervix (less than 2.5 cm) at 22–24 weeks assessed on transvaginal ultrasound is predictive for preterm labour. Other factors such as 'funnelling' of the membranes through the internal cervical os may also be predictive (Fig. 18.2).

Assay of fetal fibronectin (fFN) in cervicovaginal fluid: fFN is a marker of membrane disruption and the test

may be positive in women at high risk of delivery beyond 24 weeks or so. If fFN is positive, especially if there are other clinical and screening investigation (see above) grounds to be concerned, then admission may be arranged, steroids given to reduce the risk of respiratory distress syndrome (RDS) and liaison with neonatal services to determine the best place for delivery, should this occur (Fig. 18.3).

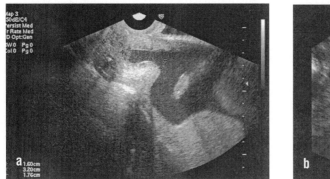 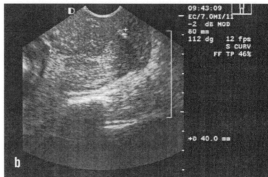

Figure 18.2 (a) Cervical length and funnelling on ultrasound, (b) normal cervix.

CASE HISTORY

Mrs R A

28 years old, married, Nigerian

Non-smoker, works as a catering manager in a school

Gravida 3 para 1: 1 termination of pregnancy at 10 weeks, age 18

1 SVD at 30+5 weeks following preterm labour, age 27. Baby born weighing 1.6 kg in good condition and required five weeks in the neonatal unit.

Knife cone biopsy 3 years ago

Normal cervical smear 2 years ago

No history of pelvic inflammatory disease

Otherwise fit and well, taking iron supplements

Appendicectomy aged 26

Lives in her own home (bought) with husband (building society manager)

Now eight weeks pregnant, seen in the antenatal booking clinic and concerned about her risks of having a further episode of preterm labour.

Discussion

What risk factors does Mrs A have for preterm labour?

Termination of pregnancy in the first trimester is unlikely to predispose towards preterm labour.

However, having had a previous preterm labour and

delivery at 30+5 weeks is a definite risk factor and puts her in the 'high risk' category.

A knife cone biopsy is probably more traumatic to cervical competence than the more commonly performed LLETZ (long loop excision of the transformation zone) procedure and may have affected cervical function leading to an increased risk of preterm labour. Mrs A is therefore at high risk of having a preterm delivery.

What care should Mrs A receive?

In view of her high risk of preterm delivery, she should receive consultant-led care in a hospital. It may be a good idea for her to meet a neonatologist, and be shown around the neonatal unit. Some units, especially in the USA, utilize home monitoring of contractions (tocography) to assess the possible onset of preterm labour.

How can her risk be more accurately assessed?

Clinical risk factors for preterm labour, as described above, are only good enough to be a vague guide as to likelihood of preterm delivery. Further measures that may allow not only greater predictive accuracy, but the chance of intervening to improve outcome, include screening for BV, scanning for cervical length and fetal fibronectin assay (see section above: New developments).

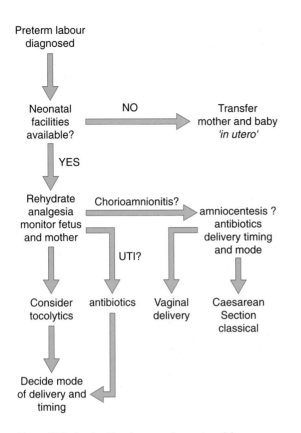

Preterm labour
diagnosed

Neonatal facilities available? — NO → Transfer mother and baby *'in utero'*

YES

Rehydrate analgesia monitor fetus and mother — Chorioamnionitis? → amniocentesis ? antibiotics delivery timing and mode

UTI?

Consider tocolytics | antibiotics | Vaginal delivery | Caesarean Section classical

Decide mode of delivery and timing

Figure 18.3 An algorithm for managing preterm labour.

The role of antenatal steroids

There is now no doubt that administration of steroids to the mother at least 24–48 hours before a preterm delivery reduces the risk of severe RDS once the baby is born. RDS is the major killer of preterm babies. Steroids work by increasing surfactant production from type II pneumocytes in the fetal lung.

This evidence, dating back to the 1970s, much of it from placebo-controlled randomized trials (grade A evidence), now makes it very difficult for any obstetrician

not to give steroids to a mother at high risk of preterm delivery. If a woman is at really high risk of preterm delivery, it is becoming standard practice to administer steroids every 10–14 days (this dosage regime has not, however, been proven) until approximately 34 weeks, when the risk of RDS is much less. Additionally, artificial surfactant is often given, by neonatologists, immediately following delivery to babies at risk of RDS.

In certain cases, steroids should be given up to 36 weeks' gestation:

- twins or triplets
- diabetic mothers
- doubt about dates

Steroids are generally well tolerated. They may cause psychological changes immediately after administration, but these are usually mild mood changes or euphoria. Diabetic women, or those with impaired glucose tolerance, need close observation of blood sugar levels for up to 48 hours after steroid administration and may need an insulin 'sliding scale' infusion until stabilized. This is because steroids antagonize the effect of insulin.

🔑 Key Points

- Preterm labour occurs in roughly 7 per cent of pregnancies
- Only about 50 per cent of women in threatened preterm labour ultimately deliver before 37 weeks
- Preterm prelabour rupture of membranes is associated with a high infection rate
- The aetiology of preterm labour is unknown in more than 50 per cent of cases
- Tocolytics may be used to gain time for steroids to work, though they are only moderately effective
- Preterm labour is a risk factor for preterm labour in a future pregnancy
- Measurement of the cervical length at 22–24 weeks may predict women at high risk of preterm labour

References for further reading

Iams J D, Paraskos J, Landon M B, Teteris J N, Johnson F F. Cervical Sonography in Preterm Labor. *Obstet Gynecol* 1994; **84:** 40–6.

Canadian Preterm Labour Investigators Group. Treatment of preterm labor with the beta-adrenergic agonist ritodrine. *N Engl J Med* 1992; **327:** 308–12.

Hagan R, Benninger H, Chiffings D, Evans S, French N. Very

preterm birth - a regional study. Part 1: Maternal and obstetric factors. *Br J Obstet Gynaecol* 1996; **103:** 230–38. Part 2: The very preterm infant. *Br J Obstet Gynaecol* 1996; **103:** 239–45.

Morales W, Schoor S, Albritton J. Effect of metronidazole in patients with preterm birth in preceding pregnancy and bacterial vaginosis: a placebo-controlled, double blind study. *Am J Obstet Gynecol* 1994; **171:** 345–49.

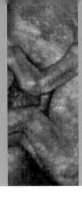

Operative intervention in obstetrics

OVERVIEW

The best outcome of pregnancy is a healthy mother and baby, ideally following a normal vaginal delivery with an intact perineum. Sadly, for many women and babies, the hazards of childbirth are a serious risk. Indeed, operative obstetric intervention to manage these hazards has come to be regarded as a mainstay of safe motherhood.

Millions of women have died and more women continue to die in childbirth. Although now not a problem seen frequently in Western labour wards, in the nineteenth century maternal mortality in England was called a 'dark continuous stream'. The risk of dying then was nearly a hundred times greater than it is today. In the absence of skilled attendants and facilities for intervention this figure remains accurate today for 'death in childbirth' in many parts of the world.

Sepsis, haemorrhage and eclampsia were, and remain, the leading causes of death. There can be no doubt that operative vaginal and abdominal delivery, and surgical management of placental and uterine complications have all contributed to the dramatic improvements seen in maternal risk and outcome in the West.

Ironically, at the close of the twentieth century, the issues of 'over-intervention' are more topical in the West. Indeed, as operative interventions carry their own risks of mortality and morbidity, this chapter maintains the principle of 'avoiding unnecessary operative intervention wherever possible' (*primum non nocere*).

The material included in this chapter is based on a systematic review of the literature. It is intended to give the reader an introduction to operative procedures in as relevant and practical a way as possible.

For that reason a large component of each section is 'how to do it'.

General principles that should be adhered to in all situations where interventions are contemplated are as follows.

- A diagnosis should be recorded and examination or operative findings clearly documented.
- The most appropriate intervention should be chosen.
- At all stages details of planned procedures should be discussed with the mother, who should remain free to make informed choices.
- Documentation should be legible, timed, dated and signed.
- Full details of operative procedures and complications should be recorded.
- Always count and record swabs.

PERINEAL CARE

Episiotomy

Definition

Episiotomy is a surgical incision of the perineum made to increase the diameter of the vulval outlet during childbirth.

History and epidemiology

Although introduced as an obstetric procedure over 200 years earlier, in general, obstetricians only came to favour episiotomy at the beginning of the twentieth century. It was then thought that all primigravidae should receive an episiotomy to protect the fetal head and the pelvic floor. By the 1970s episiotomy rates were as high as 90 per cent. Further research carried out over the last 20 years has shown the problems associated with the procedure, which include unsatisfactory anatomical results, increased blood loss, perineal pain and dyspareunia. These studies have concluded that the routine use of episiotomy should be abandoned. The WHO recommends an episiotomy rate of 10 per cent for normal deliveries.

How to avoid an episiotomy/perineal trauma

Alternate positions of the woman during labour may prevent perineal damage, e.g. kneeling, a supported

---

Indications for an episiotomy

Absolute indications
- Previous perineal reconstructive surgery
- Previous pelvic floor surgery

Relative indications
- Shoulder dystocia
- Short or rigid perineum
- Fetal distress
- An instrumental or breech delivery

---

squat or all fours. Physiological pushing and an upright position may allow the presenting part to descend and stretch the perineum gently. Fetal distress can sometimes be rectified by change of maternal position and may prevent a ventouse or forceps delivery. A constant caring companion reduces the incidence of episiotomy and perineal trauma. Alternatives to epidurals for pain relief should be considered. When instrumental delivery is required the use of the vacuum extractor rather than forceps is associated with a decrease in perineal trauma.

Technique

There are two different techniques widely used (Fig. 19.1):
1. Midline (common in USA): this is cut vertically from the fourchette down towards the anus.
2. Mediolateral (standard in the UK): this starts in the midline position at the fourchette but is then directed diagonally outwards to avoid the anal sphincter.

The advantages of the midline episiotomy are:
- less blood loss;
- it is easier to repair;
- the wound heals quicker;
- there is less pain in the postpartum period;
- the incidence of dyspareunia is reduced.

However, the major disadvantage that it carries is a high risk of it extending to involve the anal sphincter (third/fourth degree tear).

Anaesthesia

Prior to an episiotomy being performed adequate anaesthesia must be administered. If the woman has an epidural it must be topped-up accordingly or the perineum must be infiltrated with local anaesthetic.

Performing the episiotomy

Large, sharp straight scissors are the instrument of choice. If the episiotomy is performed too far laterally it will not increase the diameter of the vulval outlet but may cause damage to the right Bartholin's

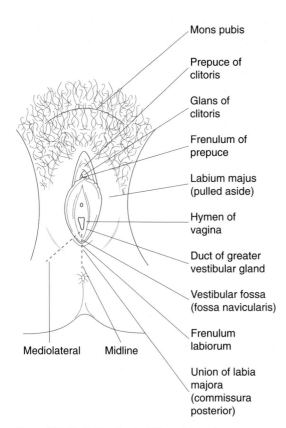

Mons pubis

Prepuce of clitoris

Glans of clitoris

Frenulum of prepuce

Labium majus (pulled aside)

Hymen of vagina

Duct of greater vestibular gland

Vestibular fossa (fossa navicularis)

Frenulum labiorum

Union of labia majora (commissura posterior)

Mediolateral   Midline

Figure 19.1 Mediolateral and midline episiotomies.

gland. This could predispose to a decrease in vaginal lubrication or cyst formation. If it is made too small, it will not increase the diameter of the vulval outlet sufficiently to facilitate delivery and it may form a weak point in the perineal tissues from which a tear could extend.

The episiotomy must be made in one single cut. If it is enlarged by several small cuts, a zigzag incision line will be produced which will be difficult to repair. The episiotomy should begin in the midline at the fourchette.

Complications

Cuts that begin more laterally are likely to be more painful and more complicated to suture. Any episiotomy may extend and cause a third degree tear to the anal sphincter. An episiotomy can bleed heavily. Haemostasis should be achieved, with pressure or arterial clamps if necessary. Infection is more likely when the episiotomy is contaminated. Prophylactic antibiotics may be indicated.

🔑 Key Points

- The episiotomy rate should be kept under 20 per cent
- Use mediolateral cut — but must begin in midline
- Refer for experienced opinion if episiotomy extends

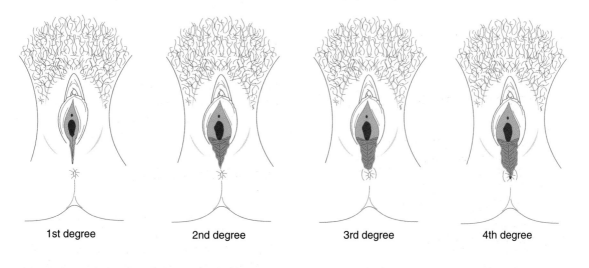

1st degree   2nd degree   3rd degree   4th degree

Figure 19.2 Perineal anatomy with schematic graded injuries.

Perineal repair

Definition of perineal injury (Fig. 19.2)

- First degree: involves skin only.
- Second degree (includes most episiotomies): involves perineal muscle.
- Third degree: secondary tear with partial or complete disruption of the anal sphincter.
- Fourth degree: third degree tear with anal epithelium.

History and epidemiology

Perineal injuries have occurred since childbirth began and surgical attempts at repair have been documented across a wide range of cultures, starting with crude juxtaposition described in ancient Egypt.

In the UK today approximately 750,000 women give birth each year and of these 525,000 (70 per cent) will sustain perineal trauma and will require stitches. The majority of these women will experience perineal pain in the immediate period following delivery and over 100,000 will have long-term problems such as superficial dyspareunia. If the repair is performed perfunctorily or inadequately it may leave women suffering from perineal pain which they describe as being far worse than the pain of childbirth.

Long-term perineal morbidity, associated with failure to recognize or to repair adequately trauma to the external anal sphincter, can lead to major physical, psychological and social problems.

Technique

Review of the literature reveals that the skill of the operator, the technique of repair and the type of suturing material used are all identified as contributing factors to perineal pain during the healing process.

Some first degree tears, will not require suturing and others will simply require one or two interrupted sutures. For second degree tears, women who have their perineum repaired by continuous subcutaneous sutures experience fewer problems in the immediate

postpartum period than when interrupted transcutaneous sutures are used.

Absorbable synthetic suture material is better than traditional materials such as catgut or silk.

Complications

Missing the apex of the tear or episiotomy may allow continued bleeding or the development of a paragenital haematoma. Deep sutures including rectal mucosa could lead to fistula formation. Over enthusiastic tight suturing can lead to significant later discomfort. Closure of the skin over the fourchette sometimes leads to formation of a bridge of tissue that can make intercourse very uncomfortable. Malaligned repairs lead to distortions in healing and increased scarring.

🔧 Key Points

- Absorbable synthetic suture preferable
- If possible, do a subcutaneous stitch
- If extensive tear, may need regional/general anaesthetic

Overzealous repairs can, paradoxically, lead to more complications

Third/fourth degree tear repair

History and epidemiology

Traditionally this has been thought to be a complication affecting relatively small numbers of women (0.5–2 per cent). More recent work has shown that unrecognized complete disruption of the anal sphincter is much more common than this. Long-term incontinence affects 5 per cent of women.

Technique

As the anal sphincter (like the levator ani muscle), is normally in a state of tonic contraction even at rest, disruption will result in retraction of the muscle ends. In order to bring the muscle ends together, adequate muscle relaxation with regional or general anaesthesia is essential. Some surgeons juxtapose the ends of the sphincter; others overlap them. A non-absorbable material (such as nylon) should be used. Antibiotics and laxative agents are prescribed to prevent secondary infection and constipation.

Complications

Up to half the women who sustain a third/fourth degree tear develop bowel symptoms (including incontinence) despite a postpartum primary anal sphincter repair. The most probable explanation for the poor outcome is either inexpertise of the operator or inappropriate repair technique. It is for this reason that the most experienced person available should be involved.

ASSISTED DELIVERY

Instrumental vaginal delivery

Definition

Delivery of a baby vaginally using an instrument for assistance.

History and epidemiology

Instrumental vaginal delivery is the hallmark of the specialty of obstetrics and the 'man-midwife'. Prior to the sixteenth century childbirth was predominantly the domain of traditional (female) birth attendants. Barber-surgeons and others with appropriate skills were involved in the management of obstructed labour (usually by destructing the fetus). A variety of single-bladed instruments were also used as levers to deliver the fetal head. With the discovery of forceps (first used, and kept secret, by the Chamberlen family in London) a means to end the suffering of obstructed labour and a tool for delivering babies alive became available. Used exclusively by

men, this allowed them to achieve, and maintain, a position of authority until this century.

Hundreds of different sorts of forceps have been invented and continue to be used around the world. Some forceps in current use were designed in Victorian times and others in the previous century (e.g. 'Simpson' [Fig. 19.3] and 'Neville-Barnes'). Although they have undoubtedly been used to save many lives, they are also associated with many maternal deaths. Particularly dangerous were 'high-forceps' deliveries; sometimes these were attempted by GP obstetricians at home. Where the delivery failed the woman would be referred to the hospital as an 'FFO' ('failed forceps outside'). To ensure that GPs did not try high deliveries, Wrigley, before the Second World War, introduced a new design with short shanks/arms. Kjelland's (see Fig. 19.3) forceps are another important development from the turn of the century. These forceps did not have a 'pelvic curve' and could be turned around in the vagina to rotate an 'occipito-posterior' position.

In the 1950s the vacuum extractor (or ventouse) was invented in Sweden and is now more widely used worldwide than forceps. Current evidence suggests that when assisted vaginal delivery is required, the ventouse should be chosen first, principally because it is significantly less likely to injure the mother.

Worldwide, assisted vaginal delivery remains an integral part of the obstetrician's duties. Although it may occur as infrequently as 1.5 per cent of deliveries (Czech Republic), in other countries it occurs as often as 15 per cent (Australia and Canada). Discrepant rates may be related to differing management of labour.

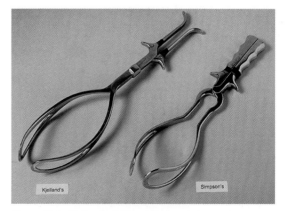

Figure 19.3 Kjelland's (left) and Simpson's (right) forceps.

How to lower instrumental vaginal delivery rates?

Various techniques may help in achieving low instrumental delivery rates, e.g. companionship in labour, active management of the second stage with Syntocinon, upright posture in the second stage and undertaking fetal scalp sampling (rather than a delivery) when fetal heart rate decelerations occur. Letting the epidural wear off or having a more liberal attitude to the length of the second stage when an epidural is being used will also reduce the risks of needing an assisted delivery.

Ventouse delivery

Types of ventouse cup

The metal cups most widely used are the 'Bird-modification' ones. These have a central traction chain and a separate vacuum pipe. The anterior cups come in 4, 5 and 6 cm sizes. The posterior cup is designed to be inserted higher up in the vagina than the anterior cups. This is to allow correct placement over the occiput when the head is deflexed. More recently a number of soft cups have been developed, one example of which is the silicone-rubber cup (Fig. 19.4). The soft cups are smoothly applied to the contour of the baby's head and do not develop a 'chignon'.

It has been shown that successful delivery is most likely with the ventouse when the cup is applied in the midline over the occiput. A well-placed cup will result in a well-flexed head, whilst failure to put the cup far enough back will result in deflexion.

Technique

To minimize the chances of any fetal damage the prerequisites and basic rules for delivery with the ventouse should be followed.

Prerequisites for delivery with the ventouse
- Dilatation of the cervix and full engagement of the head.

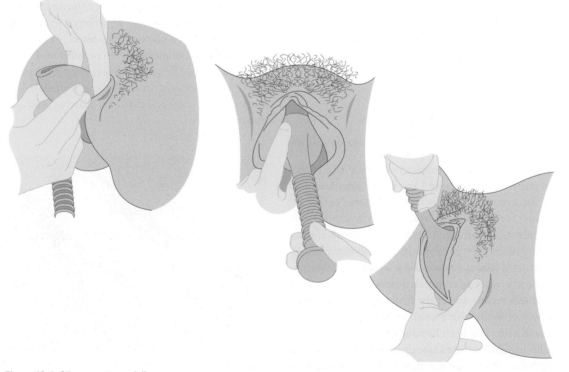

Figure 19.4 Sil-cup ventouse delivery.

Indications and contraindications for delivery with the ventouse

Indications for delivery with the ventouse
- Delay in the second stage
- Fetal distress in the second stage
- Maternal conditions requiring a short second stage

Contraindications for delivery with the ventouse
- Face presentation
- Gestation less than 34 weeks
- Marked active bleeding from a fetal blood sampling site

- Cooperation of the patient.
- Good contractions should be present.

Basic rules for delivery with the ventouse
- The delivery should be completed within 15 minutes of application.
- The head, not just the scalp, should descend with each pull.
- The cup should be reapplied no more than twice.
- If failure with the ventouse occurs despite good traction the forceps should not be tried as well.

Examination
Firstly, the patient should be carefully examined. The size of the baby should be estimated per abdomen and the head should be fully engaged (none of the head should be palpable above the pubic symphysis). The position of the vertex and the amount of caput should be determined by vaginal examination, which should include a description of the attitude of the presenting part. In a 'flexed' attitude only the posterior fontanelle can be felt, whilst any situation where the anterior fontanelle can be felt or where the posterior fontanelle cannot be found is 'deflexed'.

Preparation
There is no need to catheterize the patient (unless there is another indication e.g. epidural). No additional anaesthetic is required (perineal infiltration will suffice if an episiotomy is planned). Lithotomy is the commonest position used but delivery may be possible in dorsal, lateral or squatting positions. The appropriate cup should be chosen. It should be connected to the pump and a check should be made for leakages prior to commencing the delivery.

Delivery with the ventouse
The vacuum extractor cup is gently inserted into the vagina with one hand whilst the other hand parts the labia. The pressure is taken to 0.8 kg/cm^2, beginning traction with the next contraction after this pressure has been achieved.

Traction should be along the pelvic axis (downwards at 45°) for the duration of the contraction (Fig. 19.5). One hand should rest on the bell of the cup whilst the other applies traction. Malmstrom, who invented the ventouse, said, 'Vacuum extraction is a matter of co-operation between the traction hand and the backward-pressing hand'. The hand on the cup detects any early detachment and also indicates whether the head moves downwards with each pull. The fingers on the head can promote flexion and can help to guide the head under the arch of the pubis by using the space in front of the sacrum. As the head crowns the angle of traction changes upward through an arc of over 90°. At this point either an episiotomy is cut or, if the perineum is stretching as normal, it is simply supported with the hand that was on the bell.

The difficult ventouse
Each of the following factors contributes to failures:
- Failure to use the correct cup type. Failures with the silicone-rubber cup group will be common if it is used inappropriately when there is deflexion of the head, excess caput, a big baby or a prolonged second stage of labour.
- Inadequate initial assessment of the case:

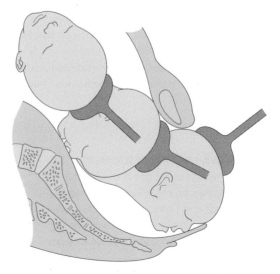

Figure 19.5 Traction down the pelvic axis.

the head being too high. A classic mistake is to assume that because caput can be felt below the ischial spines the head must be engaged. Mis-diagnosis of the position and attitude of the head. Attention to simple detail will minimize the occurrence of this problem.

- Either too anterior or lateral placements will increase the failure rate. If the cup placement is found to be incorrect, it may be appropriate to begin again with correct placement midline over the occiput.
- Failures due to traction in the wrong direction. These may be amenable simply to a change in angle of traction.
- Excessive caput. Rarely, even with the metal cups, adequate traction is not possible because of excessive caput. Careful consideration in these cases must be given to delivery by Caesarean Section unless the head is well down, in which case forceps can be used.
- Poor maternal effort. There is no doubt that maternal effort can contribute substantially to the success of the delivery. Adequate encouragement and instruction should be given to the mother.
- The incidence of (true) failure is low and usually secondary to outlet contraction.

Complications

With good technique and adherence to guidelines the risk of complications to mother or baby are small. Trauma to the genital tract is the commonest maternal complication. Unrecognized injury of the cervix leading to serious haemorrhage has been reported. Most babies will have a chignon (oedematous skin bump) at the site of the cup application. Some will also have a cephalhaematoma (subpe-

riosteal bleed). Rare serious intracranial injuries will be more likely to occur if multiple attempts at delivery are made (especially if a variety of instruments are used).

Forceps delivery

Technique

1. It is essential the head is fully engaged on abdominal palpation. This is particularly true with face presentation (which will appear to be engaged on vaginal examination sometime before the head is actually engaged).
2. It is generally advised that catheterization and an episiotomy are required for forceps delivery.
3. It is essential that the position of the head is carefully noted. If occipito-transverse or occipito-posterior, complications are more likely.
4. It is essential that the operator check the forceps pair that they have been given. It may be useful to check the maximum diameter between the two blades as well (a pair that is not true will have a maximum diameter of as little as 7 cm; the maximum diameter should be at least 9 cm).
5. The left-handed blade is applied first.
6. It is held in the operator's left hand (like a pen).
7. Insertion (downwards, then inwards) is guided by the right hand (Fig. 19.6).
8. Exactly the same procedure is followed for the other blade.
9. The blades must lock easily. They should not be forced to close.

Key Points

- Ensure head is fully engaged abdominally
- Use the correct size and type of ventouse cup
- If forceps indicated ensure use of a matching pair
- Unless head is on perineum, DO NOT use an alternative instrument after failure with ventouse or forceps
- DOCUMENT carefully. Count and document swabs

Indications and contraindications for forceps rather than ventouse

Indications
- Face presentation
- Bleeding from fetal blood sampling site
- After-coming head of the breech
- Delivery before 34 weeks' gestation

Contraindications to a vaginal assisted delivery
- Head not fully engaged
- Cervix not fully dilated

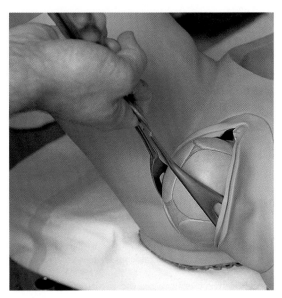

Figure 19.6 Application of forceps (using model).

10. The first pull is downward and then upward. If the head does not descend, the station may be higher than first thought or the position may be occipito-posterior.

Complications

Traumatic vaginal and uterine injuries can occur with forceps delivery. This would often be the result of undue traction or rotatory forces. As in ventouse delivery serious injuries to the baby can occur when excessive force is used or when multiple attempts are made.

Breech delivery

Definition

The three different types of breech presentation (extended, flexed and footling) are illustrated in Figure 19.7.

History and epidemiology

Three per cent of all term pregnancies present as breech. This may be due to fetal (congenital abnormality), placental (cornual or praevia), amniotic fluid (increased) or uterine (bicornuate or septate) factors.

Breech delivery has an important part in the history of childbirth. Before the discovery of forceps it was sometimes possible to deliver a baby in obstructed labour by internal podalic version and breech extraction. This technique was also used, prior to the use of Caesarean Section, to try to stem the bleeding from a placenta praevia. Internal version and breech extraction are no longer practised except in very specialized situations. Indeed clinicians skilled in the art of breech delivery are becoming rarer as more women with a term breech pregnancy have an elective Caesarean Section.

Figure 19.7 Different breech types (extended, flexed and footling).

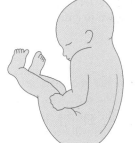
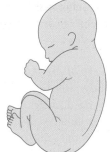
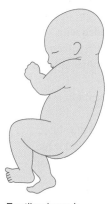

Extended breech   Flexed breech   Footling breech

Caesarean Section or vaginal breech?

No controlled trials of adequate breadth comparing elective Caesarean Section and planned vaginal delivery have been carried out. The two small studies that do exist show an increase in short-term morbidity in those babies delivered vaginally. On the other hand there was increased maternal morbidity due to the Caesarean Section in the elective procedure arm of the studies. Much of the remaining evidence supporting elective Caesarean Section comprises hospital audit, revealing outcomes for vaginal breeches and for those delivered by Caesarean Section. These studies may be biased by the inclusion of undiagnosed breeches delivering vaginally and very rapid deliveries where Caesarean Section could not be performed. A large prospective multicentre trial comparing Caesarean Section and vaginal delivery for the term breech is currently underway.

Prerequisites for vaginal breech delivery

Fetomaternal
- The presentation should be either extended (hips flexed, knees extended) or flexed (hips flexed, knees flexed but feet not below the fetal buttocks).
- There should be no evidence of fetopelvic disproportion with a pelvis clinically thought to be adequate and an estimated fetal weight of ≤3500 g (ultrasound or clinical measurement).
- There should be no evidence of hyperextension of the fetal head and fetal abnormalities should have been searched for.

Management of labour
- A trial labour should only be precluded with medical/obstetric complications that are likely to be associated with mechanical difficulties at birth (e.g. unable to push).
- Careful monitoring of fetal wellbeing and progress of labour.
- Epidural analgesia is not essential and may be associated with prolongation of the second stage.
- In selected cases induction or augmentation may be justified.
- Fetal blood sampling from the buttocks provides an accurate assessment of the acid-base status, (when the fetal heart rate trace is suspect).

Skilled operator
- There should be an operator experienced in delivering breech babies available in the hospital.
- All operators should be given training to be able to undertake a symphysiotomy should the head be entrapped.

Although much emphasis is placed on adequate case selection prior to labour, a recent survey of outcome of the undiagnosed breech in labour managed by experienced medical staff showed that safe vaginal delivery can be achieved.

Technique

Breech delivery epitomises the position of 'masterly inactivity' (hands-off). Problems are more likely to arise when the obstetrician tries to speed up the process (by pulling on the baby).

Delivery of the buttocks
In most circumstances full dilation and descent of the breech will have occurred naturally. When the buttocks become visible and begin to distend the perineum preparations for the delivery are made. The buttocks will lie in the anterio-posterior diameter. Once the anterior buttock is delivered and the anus is seen over the fourchette (and no sooner than this), an episiotomy can be cut.

Delivery of the legs and lower body
If the legs are flexed they will deliver spontaneously. If extended they may need to be delivered using 'Pinnard's manoeuvre'. This entails using a finger to flex the leg at the knee and then extend at the hip, first anteriorly then posteriorly. With contractions and maternal effort the lower body will be delivered. Usually a loop of cord is drawn down to ensure that it is not too short.

Delivery of the shoulders
The baby will be lying with the shoulders in the transverse diameter of the pelvic midcavity. As the anterior shoulder rotates into the anterior–posterior diameter, the spine or the scapula will become visible. At this point a finger gently placed above the shoulder will help to deliver the arm. As the posterior arm/shoulder reaches the pelvic floor it too will rotate anteriorly (in the oppositie direction). Once

the spine becomes visible, delivery of the second arm will follow. This can be imagined as a 'rocking boat' with one side moving upwards and then the other. Loveset's manoeuvre (see Chapter 9) essentially copies these natural movements. However, it is unnecessary and meddlesome to do routinely (one risks pulling the shoulders down but leaving the arms higher up, alongside the head).

Delivery of the head

The head is delivered using the Mauriceau-Smellie-Veit manoeuvre (the baby lies on the obstetrician's arm with downward traction being levelled on the head via a finger in the mouth and one on each maxilla) (Fig. 19.8). Delivery occurs with first downward and then upward movement (as with instrumental deliveries). If this manoeuvre proves difficult, then forceps need to be applied. An assistant holds the baby's body aloft whilst the forceps are applied in the usual manner.

Complications

The greatest fear with a vaginal breech is that the baby will get 'stuck'. Interference in the natural process by inconsiderate use of oxytocic agents or by trying to pull the baby out (breech extraction) will (paradoxically) increase the risk of obstruction occurring. When delay occurs particularly with delivery of the shoulders or head, then the presence of an experienced obstetrician will reduce the risk of death or serious injury.

CAESAREAN SECTION

History and epidemiology

Caesarean Section to deliver the baby of a mother who has died has been documented in ancient Egypt, Asia and Europe. The first caesarean carried out on a live woman is thought to be that of the wife of Jacob Nufer, a sixteenth century Swiss pig-farmer. She was in obstructed labour and her life was saved by the procedure. The history of the operation thereafter is fascinating with a wide range of isolated cases being documented with various techniques being investigated to try to lower the enormous risks of death due to haemorrhage and sepsis. By the early twentieth century the 'classical' (midline vertical uterine incision) operation had become quite widespread for

Figure 19.8 Mauriceau–Smellie–Veit manoeuvre for delivery of the head.

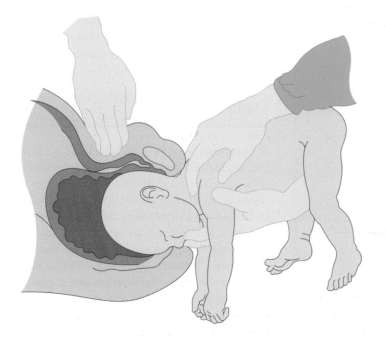

obstructed labour and placenta praevia. When Munro–Kerr introduced the concept of a 'lower segment operation' in the 1920s the profession was derisive. Nevertheless he persisted with the new procedure which has now become the standard intervention for complicated labour worldwide.

Preparation for Caesarean Section

All patients being transferred to theatre must be in left lateral position with a wedge under the right buttock (to prevent 'supine hypotension' and fetal distress). Premedication with antacid is standard. In theatre, the operating table must also be kept in left lateral tilt position until after the delivery. Thromboprophylaxis should be considered for all patients and prophylactic antibiotics should be given.

Operative procedure

Double gloving reduces the likelihood of needle puncture and use of a clear plastic shield reduces exposure

Indications for Caesarean Section

- Obstructed labour, malpresentation, malposition, multiple gestation
- Fetal distress/prolapse cord
- Maternal medical conditions requiring urgent/controlled delivery
- Obstetric complications e.g. placenta praevia
- Previous caesarean section

The 'classical' operation is still undertaken occasionally (less than 1 per cent of cases), for specific indications (shown below).

Classical caesarean section: possible indications

- Preterm delivery with poorly formed lower segment
- Placenta praevia/abruptio with large vessels in lower segment
- Premature rupture of membranes, poor lower segment and transverse lie
- Transverse lie with back inferior
- Large cervical fibroid
- Severe adhesions in lower segment reducing accessibility
- Postmortem caesarean section

of the face. A transverse suprapubic skin incision should be used. The bladder should be reflected inferiorly before incising the uterus. It is possible to injure the baby as the uterine wall is opened, accordingly considerable care needs to be taken. Delivery of the placenta should be by continuous cord traction. The uterus should be left inside the abdomen for repair. Securing both angles of the uterine incision first will reduce the risk of 'missing an angle' and having post-surgical bleeding. Reperitonealizing may cause more harm than good and is not required.

Postmortem Caesarean Section

If a pregnant woman has a cardiac arrest and the fetus is viable, postmortem Caesarean Section should be carried out without delay. For speed this would be best done via midline skin and uterine ('classical') incisions. Not only can a baby's life be saved but, resuscitation of the mother is facilitated (less pressure on the diaphragm and improved venous return).

Complications

Overall the risks of both early and long-term complications are increased in women delivered by Caesarean Section, when compared with the outcomes after normal vaginal delivery. The risks are surgical and anaesthetic. The main problems are thromboembolism, infection and haemorrhage, which can be minimized by appropriate prophylaxis and surgical skill.

TWIN DELIVERY

Twin pregnancy has an overall incidence of 1 in 80 in the population but with increasing numbers of babies resulting from artificial conception, the incidence of twins and greater multiple gestation is increasing. Overall perinatal mortality is increased and the risks are greater for monozygotic than dizygotic twins. Complications in labour are more common with multiple gestations. These include premature birth, abnormal presentations, prolapsed cord, premature separation of placenta and postpartum haemorrhage. Judiciously managed, labour is generally considered to be safe. It may require considerable expertise and is the only situation where internal podalic version is still practised in obstetrics.

Analgesia during labour

Epidural analgesia is recommended. Indeed, if the presentation of twins is anything other than vertex–vertex, the use of an epidural can be justified in terms of analgesia for possible intrauterine manipulations required in the second stage for delivery of the second twin. Alternatively, having an anaesthetist present and ready to administer anaesthesia if complications arise is a satisfactory alternative.

Vaginal delivery of vertex–vertex

Although this combination is considered low-risk and will most frequently be delivered by a midwife, an obstetrician should be present as complications with delivery of the second twin can occur. Delivery of the first twin is undertaken in the usual manner and thereafter the majority of second twins would have been delivered within 15 minutes.

After the delivery of the first twin, abdominal palpation should be performed to assess the lie of the second twin. It is helpful to use ultrasound for confirmation, which is also useful for checking the fetal heart rate. If the lie is longitudinal with a cephalic presentation, one should wait until the head is descending then perform amniotomy with a contraction. If contractions do not ensue within 5–10 minutes after delivery of the first twin, then an oxytocin

infusion should be started. If an assisted delivery becomes necessary, then the vacuum extractor has a number of advantages.

If the second twin is non-vertex, which occurs in about 40 per cent of twins, numerous studies have shown that vaginal delivery can be safely considered.

If the second twin is a breech, the membranes can be ruptured once the breech is fixed in the birth canal. A total breech extraction may be performed if fetal distress occurs or if a footling breech is encountered but this requires considerable expertise. Complications are less likely if the membranes are not ruptured until the feet are held by the operator. Where the fetus is transverse, external cephalic version can be successful in over 70 per cent of cases. The fetal heart rate should be closely monitored and ultrasound can be helpful to demonstrate the final position of the baby. If external cephalic version is unsuccessful, given that the operator is experienced, an internal podalic version can be undertaken.

Internal podalic version (Fig. 19.9)

A fetal foot is identified by recognizing a heel through intact membranes. The foot is grasped and pulled gently and continuously into the birth canal. The membranes are ruptured as late as possible. This procedure is easiest when the transverse lie is with the back superior or posterior. If the back is inferior or if the limbs are not immediately palpable, ultrasound may help to show the operator where they would be found. This will minimize the unwanted experience of bringing down a fetal hand in the mistaken belief that it is a foot.

Non-vertex first twin

Many clinicians choose Caesarean Section when the first twin presents as a breech, because of concern about 'interlocking'. However, this complication is extremely rare (approximately 1 in 1000 twin pregnancies).

Preterm twins

Even in low birth weight twin gestations, the method of delivery in relation to fetal presentation will have little or no effect on neonatal mortality and

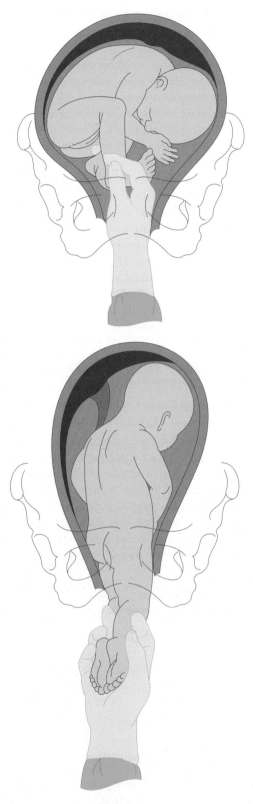

Figure 19.9 Internal podalic version.

subsequent neonatal developmental outcome. No significant differences in perinatal outcome exist when comparing breech-extracted second twins to those delivered by Caesarean Section.

PLACENTAL COMPLICATIONS

Retained placenta

Incidence

Retained placenta is found in 2 per cent of deliveries. The frequency of retained placenta is markedly increased (twenty-fold) at gestations <26 weeks and even up to 37 weeks it remains three times more common than at term. At term 90 per cent of placentas will be delivered within 15 minutes. Once the third stage exceeds 30 minutes there is 10-fold increase in the risk of haemorrhage.

Management

When the placenta is delivered, it should be inspected for completeness because, if there is a suggestion of retained segments, manual exploration of the uterine cavity is required. This will need to be undertaken under anaesthesia.

If the placenta is retained as a whole, it is often worth checking prior to induction of anaesthesia that it has not detached spontaneously. Not infrequently, a placenta is found in the cervical canal or vagina at this time. If it is still within the uterus, the operator (wearing a 'gauntlet' glove) should use the fingers of one hand, held as a 'spatula', to lift the placenta, whilst the hand on the abdomen balances these movements with downward pressure on the uterus. If there are retained fragments, then further manual exploration (with a gauze swab around the exploring fingers) of the uterine cavity will need to be undertaken. If retained fragments cannot be removed in this manner, curettage with a blunt instrument may be required. Small remaining fragments of placenta can be left if there is no haemorrhage, provided there is adequate antibiotic cover and follow-up. Antibiotics should be routinely administered as there is a significant association between manual removal of the placenta and postpartum endometritis.

Placenta accreta

Definition

Placenta accreta is a retained placenta that is morbidly adherent to the uterine wall.

Epidemiology

Placenta accreta is a serious cause of haemorrhage. It is becoming more common, and over the last 40 years, the incidence has increased ten-fold. This phenomenon is due to the fact that lower segment Caesarean Section appears to increase the risk of subsequent placenta praevia, and there is a well-documented association between placenta praevia and previous Caesarean Section and placenta accreta. In recent reviews, up to a quarter of women undergoing Caesarean Section for placenta praevia, in the presence of one or more scars, subsequently underwent Caesarean hysterectomy for placenta accreta.

Management

If placenta accreta with haemorrhage is encountered, and if the woman has no intention to bear further children, hysterectomy is the procedure of choice. However, if hysterectomy is considered a last resort, then other measures may be successful in up to 50 per cent of women. These procedures range from simple excision of the site of trophoblast invasion

🔧 Key Points

- Anticipate haemorrhage, site IVI, take blood for full blood count, group, save and catheterize
- Check that placenta is not in the cervical canal or vagina prior to giving anaesthetic
- Give prophylactic antibiotics
- Carry out manual removal — call senior help if accreta and/or heavy bleeding

with oversewing of the area to uterine or internal line vessel ligation.

Uterine inversion

Incidence

Uterine inversion (Fig. 19.10) occurs approximately once every 2000 deliveries. It is more likely to occur with vigorous cord traction and with Crede's manoeuvre (manual compression of the uterus to encourage delivery of the placenta) but can occur in the absence of 'mismanagement'. It is more likely in primiparous patients and where there is a fundal placenta.

Diagnosis

Uterine inversion is associated with haemorrhage in over 90 per cent of cases and shock is its most common complication (40 per cent). The appearance of shock out of proportion to the amount of blood loss may be explained by increased vagal tone in response to the inversion.

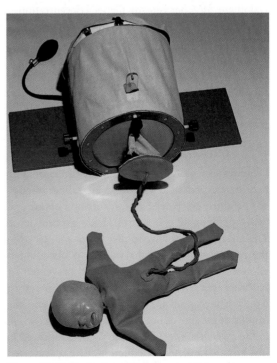

Figure 19.10 Uterine inversion (using model).

The uterus most commonly presents as a pelvic mass, sometimes protruding from the vagina, but in cases where it does not protrude from the vagina, it may go undetected resulting in a subacute or chronic inversion.

Management

Manage shock

The treatment of hypovolaemia and shock should be addressed immediately and appropriate senior obstetric and anaesthetic assistance should be summoned.

Reposition the uterus

An attempt should be made to reposition the uterus, manually via the vagina, without attempting to remove the adherent placenta first. The earlier the restoration, the more likely the success. In one-third of patients, manual reposition is successful without the use of uterine relaxants.

Uterine relaxation

If repositioning of the uterus is not readily accomplished, uterine relaxation may be attempted with a tocolytic. When available, general anaesthesia using Halothane at 2 per cent or higher concentration is effective.

Removal of the placenta

Once the uterus is in position, the attendant's hands should remain in the endometrial cavity until a firm contraction occurs. The placenta can carefully be removed at this point.

If simple repositioning fails

O'Sullivan suggested treating uterine inversion with hydrostatic pressure. Two litres of saline at body temperature are placed on an infusion stand and kept approximately 2 metres above ground level. The nozzles of two long rubber tubes are placed in the posterior fornix of the vagina. Whilst fluid is allowed to flow quickly, its escape is prevented by blocking the introitus by using the operator's hands. The vaginal walls begin to distend and the fundus of the uterus begins to rise. After correction of the inversion, the fluid in the vagina is allowed to flow out completely. Reduction of the inverted

Key Points

- Can happen even with 'proper' third stage care
- The sooner the inversion is replaced the better
- Do not remove the placenta, if adherent (until uterus replaced)

uterus is usually achieved in 5–10 minutes after commencement of this technique. These methods are successful in the vast majority of cases. Very rarely a laparotomy is required to reposition the inversion surgically. Once replaced, IV oxytocics should be administered.

Complications

Regardless of the method of uterine replacement employed, careful manual exploration afterwards is essential to rule out the possibility of genital tract trauma.

SURGICAL MANAGEMENT OF OBSTETRIC HAEMORRHAGE AND RUPTURED UTERUS

Vulval and paravaginal haematomas

Definition

Haematomas are divided into those that lie above and those that lie below the levator muscle (Fig. 19.11). Infralevator haematomas include those of the vulva and perineum, as well as paravaginal haematomas and those occurring in the ischiorectal fossa. Supralevator haematomas spread upwards and outwards beneath the broad ligament or partly downwards to bulge into the walls of the upper vagina. These haematomas can also track backwards into the retroperitoneal space.

Incidence and associations

Criteria used to define a haematoma vary widely and

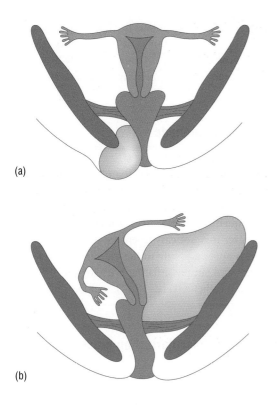

(a)

(b)

Figure 19.11 (a) Vulval (b) paravaginal haematoma.

because of this a range of frequencies have been reported. An acceptable definition would be any haematoma greater than 4 cm in diameter. The incidence of these would be approximately 1:1000 deliveries.

The injury is frequently related to episiotomy but in some series nearly 20 per cent of patients developed a significant haematoma despite delivery with an intact perineum. Overall, half of the women who develop a genital haematoma do so following a spontaneous delivery.

Diagnosis

Although a vulval haematoma is usually obvious, a paravaginal haematoma may be missed, with no symptoms until shock develops. In general, the symptoms depend upon the size and rate of haematoma formation. Some genital haematomas may be up to 15 cm in diameter.

Management

The management of an infralevator haematoma usually necessitates, in addition to resuscitative measures, surgical evacuation of the haematoma. However, this depends on the size. If the haematoma is less than 5 cm in diameter and not expanding, most obstetricians would simply recommend observation using ice-packs and pressure dressings to limit haematoma expansion. Appropriate analgesia should be given and markings should be made on the skin to establish whether the peripheral margins of the mass are expanding. For haematomas larger than 5 cm in diameter or those that are rapidly expanding, surgical intervention is recommended.

Technique

Where possible, the incision should be made via the vagina to minimize scar formation. If distinct bleeding sites are seen, these can be clamped but more commonly there is no distinct bleeding. If a figure of eight suture does not achieve haemostasis, then either a drain or a pack can be used.

Key Points

- A trap for the unwary — beware occult haemorrhage in 'collapsed' postpartum patient
- Large vulval haematomas benefit from drainage
    Leave the wound open
    Leave a drain
- Broad ligament haematomas are usually managed conservatively

Subperitoneal haematomas

Incidence and associations

A subperitoneal haematoma (broad ligament) is much less common than a genital haematoma: 1 in 20,000 deliveries. They follow either spontaneous vaginal delivery, Caesarean Section or forceps operations. Approximately 50 per cent of subperitoneal haematomas are discovered virtually immediately, whereas the other half only present after 24 hours. Patients presenting immediately tend to show signs of lower abdominal pain and haemorrhage.

Management

A conservative approach is recommended with 'expectant' management. If it is not possible to maintain a stable haemodynamic state, prompt surgical exploration is recommended and a hysterectomy may be indicated.

MASSIVE OBSTETRIC HAEMORRHAGE

Definition

Massive obstetric haemorrhage is variously defined both quantitatively (>1000 mL) and qualitatively (shock) (see also Chapter 20).

Causes of massive obstetric haemorrhage

The majority of cases are due to an atonic uterus but a variety of important causes need to be ruled out.
- Retained placenta/placenta accreta.
- Perineal, vaginal or cervical laceration.
- Ruptured uterus.
- Vulval, paravaginal and broad ligament haematomata.

Initial management

1. Resuscitation (two large-bore IV cannulae)
2. Adequate fluid/blood replacement
3. Adequate monitoring (O_2 saturation monitor, continuous pulse and blood pressure measurement)
4. Urinary catheterization
5. Senior involvement: anaesthetist and obstetrician

In most cases of massive haemorrhage, it will be appropriate to stimulate further uterine contractions by given additional oxytocic agents (ergometrine/prostaglandins). Arrangements will be made for an examination (probably under anaesthesia), in theatre.

Uterine tamponade

Bimanual compression of the uterus has long been practised as initial management of an atonic uterus. Uterine packing continues to be recommended as the subsequent surgical management of preference. However it is not easy to ensure that firm compression is applied evenly to the bleeding surface of the uterus and simply inflating a urological hydrostatic balloon catheter (Fig. 19.12) will be quicker and more effective.

Uterine devascularization procedures (Fig. 19.13)

Bilateral uterine artery ligation is the simplest procedure and in some series has been reported to be very helpful. If bleeding continues bilateral ovarian vessel ligation should be tried.

Bilateral internal iliac artery ligation is successful in avoiding hysterectomy in approximately half of the cases associated with uterine atony and placenta accreta. Because of collateral circulation the uterus will not become ischaemic. However, delay (e.g. due to inexpertise) in carrying out the procedure and

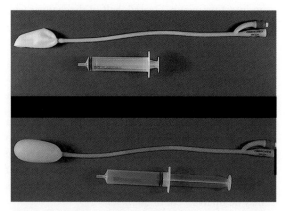

Figure 19.12 Balloon catheter (for haemostatic tamponade).

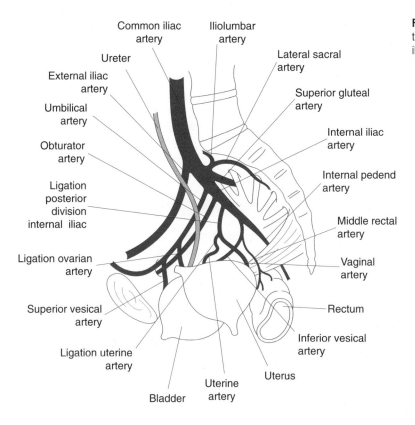

Figure 19.13 Uterine devascularisation procedures (with other anatomy illustrated).

Common iliac artery

Iliolumbar artery

Ureter

Lateral sacral artery

External iliac artery

Superior gluteal artery

Umbilical artery

Internal iliac artery

Obturator artery

Internal pedend artery

Ligation posterior division internal iliac

Middle rectal artery

Ligation ovarian artery

Vaginal artery

Superior vesical artery

Rectum

Ligation uterine artery

Inferior vesical artery

Bladder

Uterine artery

Uterus

therefore delay in hysterectomy carries a poorer prognosis.

RUPTURED UTERUS

Incidence

Complete ruptured uterus can be a life-threatening emergency. Fortunately, however, the condition is rare in modern obstetrics, despite the increase in Caesarean Section rates. The incidence is about 0.3 per cent.

The risk of uterine rupture is significantly increased with a combination of risk factors, e.g. when an oxytocic agent is administered to multigravid patients with a previous Caesarean scar.

Principle risk factors for ruptured uterus

- Previous Caesarean Section (particularly 'classical')
- Multiparity
- Oxytocic agents
- Previous gynaecological surgery (e.g. myomectomy)
- Congenital abnormality of the uterus (e.g. septate)

Diagnosis and outcome

The commonest finding (70 per cent) is fetal distress. Bleeding and pain are surprisingly uncommon (<10 per cent). Once fetal distress occurs it is likely that significant neonatal morbidity will be found if more than 18 minutes elapse before delivery.

Findings

Lower uterine segment dehiscence is the commonest current finding. The rupture of the lower segment may extend anteriorly into the back of the bladder or laterally towards the region of the uterine artery, or even into the broad ligament plexus of veins, causing extensive haemorrhage and damage. Posterior rupture of the uterus is uncommon but can occur with previous uterine surgery or intrauterine manipulation.

Management

- Total hysterectomy (see below).
- Sub-total hysterectomy.
- The choice of sub-total hysterectomy may be dictated by the individual's situation. For example, where the risks to the bladder and ureter are grave, the choice of sub-total hysterectomy would be preferable.
- Simple repair. The choice of simple uterine repair would depend on the size of the injury and on the wishes of the mother.

🔧 Key Points

- Most common associated feature is fetal distress
- Most often previous Caesarean Section and/or oxytocic agents in multiparous patient
- Often an acute emergency if baby is to be saved

INJURIES TO THE CERVIX

After a vaginal delivery, the majority of women will have lacerations and/or bruising of the cervix. Minor cervical lacerations are therefore extremely common. Usually these remain undetected. However, bleeding which does not appear to be arising from the vagina or perineum and which continues despite a well-contracted uterus, is an indication for examining the cervix. Deep lacerations and particularly those that involve the vaginal vault need to be managed in theatre under anaesthesia. A laceration into the vault could extend forward to the bladder or laterally towards the uterine artery at the base of the broad ligament.

Management

Prompt recognition of the injury and action to control the bleeding is essential.

Repair

For repairing a cervical tear, good visibility using right angle retractors is essential. Using two pairs of ring forceps applied to the cervix at any one time, it is possible to inspect the whole circumference accurately. Identification of the apex of the tear is essential before commencing repair.

🔧 Key Points

- Often looks damaged
- Very rarely associated with bleeding
- Ventouse prior to full dilatation has been implicated

CAESAREAN HYSTERECTOMY

Incidence

Emergency indications for Caesarean hysterectomy are less common than in the past as there are now alternative treatments available (0.01–0.05 per cent).

Indications

The relative risk of emergency hysterectomy is increased with caesarean delivery, previous Caesarean birth, placenta praevia, placenta accreta and uterine atony.

The majority of hysterectomies are done for haemorrhage where conservative medical and surgical measures have been unsuccessful. Increasingly, placental problems account for a larger proportion of cases.

🔧 Key Points

- Anticipate problems, e.g. accreta in placenta praevia and previous Caesarean Section
- Try medical (and possibly surgical) alternatives
- Consent patient for this, if in doubt prior to inducing anaesthesia

RARELY PERFORMED BUT IMPORTANT OPERATIVE INTERVENTIONS

Symphysiotomy

Symphysiotomy is considered of some value for the management of cephalo-pelvic disproportion in selected situations in developing countries and it has also been recommended as the treatment of choice for a trapped after-coming head of a breech.

It has a very low maternal mortality with no procedure-related deaths in a series of nearly 2000 women. In contrast, Caesarean Section in rural developing world hospitals may be associated with a mortality of up to 5 per cent and a reported incidence of uterine scar rupture in subsequent pregnancies of up to 6.8 per cent. However, in symphysiotomy subsequent symptoms such as pain in the symphysis pubis and groin are common. A major advantage is that the majority of women (73 per cent) will have an uncomplicated vaginal delivery in a subsequent pregnancy.

Indication

Symphysiotomy can be considered in cases of cephalo-pelvic disproportion with a vertex presentation and a living fetus. At least one-third of the fetal head should have entered the pelvic brim. It may also

---

CASE HISTORY

Miss M S

1.80m tall, 76 kg at booking

First pregnancy: spontaneous labour at 39 weeks' gestation

Abdominal examination: average size baby, estimated around 3.6 kg

Vaginal examination: Vertex presentation

After a slow labour, finally reached full dilatation of the cervix after 10 hours

Normal, reactive cardiotocograph baseline 135/min; clear liquor draining

After one and a half hour's active pushing, the station of the head is +1 cm below the ischial spines (0/5 palpable on abdominal examination), there is caput and moulding. The position of the head is occipito-anterior.

Should Miss S have an assisted delivery?

After a long labour and prolonged maternal efforts at pushing in the second stage of labour, an assisted delivery is quite appropriate. Hopefully, the baby can be delivered vaginally as there is no evidence of fetal compromise and the vertex is at station +1 below the ischial spines.

What features suggest that an assisted delivery might be difficult?

Caput and moulding suggest that the baby's head is being squeezed tightly through the pelvis; this might mean an assisted delivery would be trickier than first thought and the operator must be sure of the exact position of the head prior to attempting delivery.

Which instrument should be chosen?

Either ventouse or forceps would be reasonable. Many obstetricians would use ventouse in the first instance to reduce maternal soft tissue trauma. Equally, it could be argued that the presence of caput would make ventouse more likely to fail, and a non-rotational forceps (such as Neville Barnes') could be used.

Should the delivery be performed in the Obstetric Theatre?

If there is any concern that the delivery might not succeed easily, or there is fetal distress, then Miss S should be moved to the operating theatre for a 'trial of ventouse/forceps'. Should the delivery not be completed simply and rapidly, a Caesarean Section might be required. In this situation, a Caesarean Section would be most unlikely unless the fetus were to become compromised and attempted vaginal delivery was more difficult than at first thought. One important question depends on the skill of the obstetrician. Is the true position of the vertex (taking into account the boggy caput) at +1 cm and is the fetal head really occipito-anterior? If this was in fact occipito-posterior, and the baby's head was at the spines (0 cm) then in many cases a Caesarean might be performed.

What risks are there for Miss S after delivery?

Postpartum haemorrhage is always more common after an assisted delivery due to the risk of uterine atony and vaginal or cervical lacerations. In this situation, these risks are compounded by a long labour. The appropriate steps should be taken to anticipate and deal with this: IV access, blood sent for haemoglobin estimation and grouping and saving, oxytocin/ergometrine at delivery and an intravenous oxytocin infusion for four hours after delivery.

be indicated for the trapped after-coming head of a breech and has been described as an intervention in a 'desperate case' scenario of shoulder dystocia.

Destructive operations

Destructive operations may be required where the fetus is dead and where a vaginal delivery is either the only delivery that can be managed in that particular situation or it is the only route by which the mother wishes to be delivered. The three commonest destructive procedures are craniotomy, perforation of the after-coming head and decapitation.

Craniotomy

Craniotomy is indicated for the delivery of a dead fetus when labour is neglected and obstructed in a cephalic presentation.

After-coming head of the breech

This can be managed similarly, by craniotomy with perforation of the head through the occiput. Where there is hydrocephalus and accompanying spina bifida, cerebrospinal fluid can either be withdrawn by exposing the spinal canal and passing a catheter into the canal and up into the cranium or the hydrocephalic head can be decompressed transabdominally using a spinal needle.

Decapitation

In cases of neglected obstructed labour with shoulder presentation and a dead fetus, decapitation might be the treatment of choice.

References for further reading

de Swiet M, Chamberlain G. (eds). *Basic Science in Obstetrics and Gynaecology. 2nd edition.* London: Churchill Livingstone, 1996.

O'Dowd MJ, Philipp EE. *The history of obstetrics and gynaecology.* New York, London: Parthenon Publishing Group, 1994.

Myerscough PR. *Munro-Kerr's Operative Obstetrics.* 10th edition. London: Ballière-Tindall, 1982.

Pregnancy and Childbirth Reviews. In: The Cochrane Database of Systematic Reviews. The Cochrane Library. Update Software. Oxford. (4 issues each year)

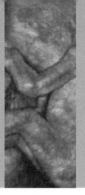

Chapter 20

Obstetric emergencies

OVERVIEW

Obstetric emergencies require quick and decisive action to save the life of the mother and the child. Severe hypertensive disorder, haemorrhage and embolism all threaten the life of the mother. The fetus is directly threatened by umbilical cord accidents, other forms of hypoxia and mechanical delivery problems. Death of the mother was frequent in the early part of the twentieth century in the UK and occurs daily throughout the world today.

The Taj Mahal was built by Shah Jahan in memory of his wife Mumtaz Mahal who died of a postpartum haemorrhage after the birth of their fourteenth child (Fig. 20.1).

Definition

An emergency is defined as a situation or occurrence of a serious and often dangerous nature, developing suddenly and unexpectedly, and demanding immediate attention. Hypertensive disorder (pre-eclampsia and eclampsia) remains one of the leading causes of maternal death along with haemorrhage and embolism (thrombotic or amniotic fluid). In an emergency the fetus is threatened by interruption to its lifeline of the placenta and the umbilical cord. Any emergency is initially treated according to the ABC principle: Airway, Breathing, Circulation.

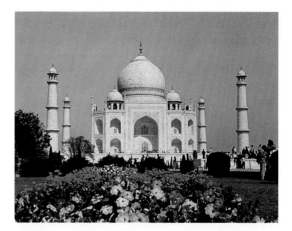

Figure 20.1 The Taj Mahal was built by Shah Jahan in memory of his wife Mumtaz Mahal who died of a postpartum haemorrhage after the birth of their fourteenth child.

Hypertensive disorder

Severe high blood pressure, whether part of pre-eclampsia or not, is a serious threat to the health of the pregnant woman and her baby.

Severe pre-eclampsia and eclampsia

Definition

Pre-eclampsia (or proteinuric hypertension in pregnancy) is a disease of pregnancy characterized by a blood pressure of 140/90 or above on two separate occasions with a preceding normal blood pressure in early pregnancy. This is associated with significant proteinuria (>300 mg in a 24-hour urine collection) and often clinically evident tissue oedema. The condition is progressive. Eclampsia is the same condition that has proceeded to the presence of convulsions. Imminent eclampsia/fulminating pre-eclampsia is the transitional condition characterized by increasing symptoms and signs. See also Chapter 11.

Incidence and epidemiology

Eclampsia is relatively rare in the UK. During 1992 eclampsia occurred in nearly one in 2000 pregnancies in the UK and was associated with the death of nearly 1 in 50 of the women and a perinatal mortality of 56/1000 births. Thirty-eight per cent of the cases occurred antepartum, 18 per cent intrapartum and 44 per cent post-delivery. The Confidential Enquiry into Maternal Deaths in the United Kingdom, published in 1996, recorded 20 deaths due to hypertensive disorders of pregnancy in the triennium 1991–1993: of these 11 were due to eclampsia. Eclampsia is a leading cause of maternal death in all countries. Severe pre-eclampsia is more common than eclampsia. Any form of hypertensive disorder, often mild, occurs in at least 10 per cent of the pregnant population.

Aetiology

An empty plinth at the Chicago Lying-In Hospital awaits the name of the person who discovers the secret of pre-eclampsia. It is uniquely a disease of pregnancy and is only definitively treated by emptying the uterus. It is a multisytem disorder because the vascular changes occur in all organs (Fig. 20.2). The renal effects cause proteinuria, the cerebral effects cause eclampsia, the haematological effects cause coagulation changes, the hepatic effects cause liver dysfunction and the placental effects cause utero-placental insufficiency, intrauterine growth restriction (IUGR) and placental abruption. The placental effects correlate with defects in the utero-placental circulation.

Risk factors in pre-eclampsia/eclampsia

- Nulliparity
- Multiple gestation
- Extremes of reproductive age
- Diabetes mellitus
- Chronic hypertensive disease
- Afro-Caribbean ethnicity
- Family history of hypertension

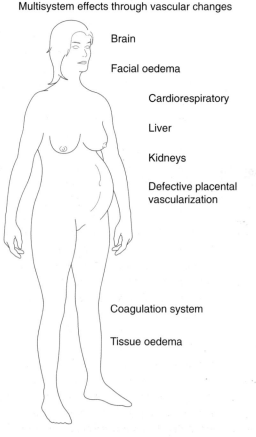

Multisystem effects through vascular changes

Brain

Facial oedema

Cardiorespiratory

Liver

Kidneys

Defective placental vascularization

Coagulation system

Tissue oedema

Figure 20.2 Pathophysiology of pre-eclampsia/eclampsia.

P Understanding the pathophysiology

This multisystem disorder cannot occur outside of pregnancy although it seems to be the trophoblastic tissue that prevents the stimulus. The disorder also occurs in hydatidiform mole without a fetus.

Defective invasion of the spiral arterioles is at the origin of the macroscopic process.

All arterioles are affected therefore there is the potential for all organs to be affected.

Clinical manifestations arise particularly from effects on brain, kidneys, liver, cardiorespiratory and haematological systems.

The immunological system has an ill-defined role.

S Symptoms in fulminating pre-eclampsia/ imminent eclampsia

- Headache
- Visual disturbance
- Epigastric pain
- Generally unwell and nauseated
- Restlessness, tremulousness and twitching
- Swelling
- Poor urine output

Signs in fulminating pre-eclampsia/ imminent eclampsia

- Agitation
- Hyperreflexia
- Facial and peripheral oedema
- Right upper quadrant tenderness

Clinical features

Eclampsia is obvious as a grand mal convulsion. However epileptic convulsions do occur in pregnancy and must be considered in the differential diagnosis.

A preceding scenario of pre-eclampsia is highly suggestive. Should this not be present then a normal blood pressure after the convulsion is not reassuring as the effect of the convulsion is to temporarily lower the blood pressure. In these circumstances heavy proteinuria and tissue oedema suggest an eclamptic aetiology. Any convulsion in pregnancy should be considered to be eclampsia until proved otherwise. Women developing this condition may report vague symptoms generally of headache and sometimes tissue oedema also manifesting as weight gain. If placental effects are significant then she may complain of being small and having reduced fetal movements. Usually the blood pressure will have been normal early on pregnancy but she is quite likely to give a family history of hypertension in female relatives. In an emergency situation there is little time for eliciting a detailed history.

Examination

The woman may have a general sense of unease and appear unwell. Facial oedema may be evident more often to family who see her daily. Peripheral oedema may be marked although 'dry' pre-eclampsia certainly exists: it may be a more severe form of the disease. The blood pressure will be raised and if the diastolic pressure is above 110 m of mercury it merits the description of 'severe'. Soon after a convulsion the blood pressure may be normal. Upper abdominal tenderness and hyperreflexia are classical features. The abdomen may be smaller than expected and there may be a suspicion of oligohydramnios with reduced fetal movements.

Investigations

In an emergency situation there is little time for investigation but the following should be requested.
- Urine for protein testing.
- Haematological and clotting indices.
- Renal function tests.
- Liver function tests.

Treatment

First aid is important during a convulsion:
- Turn the woman on her side with head down.
- Ensure airway is protected.
- Give oxygen by face mask.
- Magnesium sulphate 5 gm IV over a few minutes.

The definitive treatment is delivery, however the woman's condition must be stabilized first. The anaesthetist should be involved at an early stage. A maintenance infusion of magnesium sulphate should be commenced to prevent a further convulsion. This should be adjusted depending on urine output and reflexes. Diazepam is a poor second choice. The blood pressure is likely to rise and the drug of choice to control this is hydralazine IV; diazoxide may be kept in reserve. A urinary catheter should be passed to facilitate the careful management of fluid balance. The retained fluid goes to the extravascular space and the intravascular volume is depleted. Diuretics are of limited value. Should oliguria become a problem the central venous pressure measurement and infusion should be undertaken. A decision is then required to move towards delivery. The fetal condition should be verified by ultrasound examination and cardiotocography. Unless labour is well-established in progess then caesarean delivery under carefully controlled circumstances is appropriate. If the baby is dead, which is unusual, then an attempt at vaginal delivery may be appropriate. In the most severe cases at an early gestation (22–26 weeks) then even with fetal demise Caesarean Section may be necessary in the maternal interest.

Post-delivery

Eclampsia and pre-eclampsia are recognized to occur after delivery. When this occurs, or after delivery in such a situation, surveillance should not be relaxed. The infusions should be continued until 12 hours after the symptoms, proteinuria and raised blood pressure have subsided. The resolution often mirrors the development. In spite of the seriousness of this disease resolution is often complete and the chance of recurrence in subsequent pregnancy is rather low.

New developments

The association of abnormal utero-placental blood flow with this condition has been fully explained in Chapter 11. This may have increasing significance in prediction and diagnosis.

The serious nature of this condition requires highly skilled care by experts. Care in a darkened room to remove extraneous stimuli has no place. Intensive care and surveillance is what is required. The Maternal Mortality report has suggested that regionalization of specialized opinion should be organized. Transfer to a referral centre or the provision of telephone support is appropriate in this situation.

Magnesium sulphate has become the anticonvulsant drug of choice in this situation. Although popular for many years in North America it had only been used by a few hospitals in the UK. A paper published in 1995 of a randomized trial has led to its widespread acceptance specifically for eclampsia. It seems likely that what is appropriate for eclampsia is also appropriate for severe pre-eclampsia although this remains to be confirmed by further study.

Haemorrhage

Definition

Any blood loss from the vagina during pregnancy, greater than a show, is abnormal: blood loss after delivery that is excessive is also abnormal.

P Understanding the pathophysiology

The haemochorial nature of human pregnancy places the pregnant woman at particular risk of haemorrhage (Fig. 20.3). The placental cotyledons are directly bathed in maternal blood. Any disruption at this interface may lead to blood loss. This is initially retro- or periplacental. It will often be concealed and may extend. There are important differences in clinical presentation depending on whether the placenta is normally sited or low-lying (placenta praevia). The conditions underlying antepartum haemorrhage have been covered in Chapter 14. Resolution of haemorrhage depends essentially on haemostasis at the placental bed. This is achieved by constriction of the bed by myometrial contraction. Coagulation factors and platelets are secondary to this process. Final resolution of placental bleeding antepartum can only be achieved by delivery. Post-delivery there is also the question of the anatomical integrity of the tissues that have been exposed to surgical treatment. Effective management of major haemorrhage demands aggressive supportive measures at the same time as measures to resolve the bleeding.

Obstetric blood loss is almost always maternal in origin. The only exception is in the cases of vasa praevia antenatally. A pregnant woman can tolerate more than 500 mL of blood loss without decompensation, however the same amount would exsanguinate a term fetus.

origin. PPH, depending on the definition, occurs in 3–5 per cent of women. In the Confidential Enquiry into Maternal Deaths published in 1998 there were 12 deaths due to haemorrhage; three were due to placenta praevia, four to abruption of the placenta and five to PPH.

Antepartum haemorrhage

The focus of this chapter is on the management of obstetric haemorrhagic shock. In developed health care systems the placental site will be known from previously documented ultrasound examination. A full understanding of the implications of this is important. The essential comparison of haemorrhage from placenta praevia with that from placental abruption is important (Table 20.1).

If the cardiotocograph (CTG) is very abnormal with a relatively small amount of bleeding then fetal bleeding from vasa praevia is likely. This is a particularly urgent emergency to resolve by delivery in the fetal interest.

The elements of treatment concerning resuscitation in antepartum haemorrhage (APH) are similar in APH and PPH, however in APH final resolution is only achieved through emptying the uterus. The method of delivery depends on the circumstances. If there is no placenta praevia and the maternofetal condition is reasonable then vaginal delivery is desirable. Should there be major placenta praevia, heavy blood loss or maternofetal compromise then Caesarean Section by a senior obstetrician is appropriate.

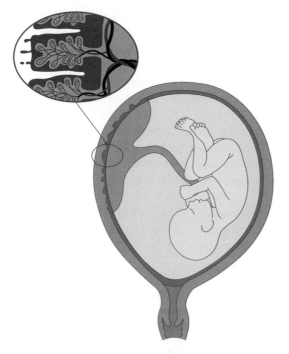

Figure 20.3 Haemochorial placentation.

Incidence and epidemiology

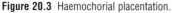

Vaginal bleeding after delivery is relatively common. Any vaginal bleeding occurs in about 10 per cent of women but major haemorrhage is less common, occurring in about 0.5 per cent due to placenta praevia, possibly 1 per cent due to placental abruption. There are other bleeds of unspecified

Table 20.1 – Comparison of haemorrhage from placenta praevia with that from placenta abruption

Placenta praevia	Placental abruption
Painless	Painful
No precipitating factor	Sometimes precipitating factor
Less distressed	Agitated and distressed
Soft abdomen	Tender, tense abdomen
Abnormal lie and presentation	Normal lie and presentation
Less likely abnormal CTG (hypoxia)	More likely abnormal CTG (hypoxia)
Random association/pre-eclampsia	More marked association/pre-eclampsia
Coagulation defect later	Coagulation defect sooner

Postpartum haemorrhage

Excessive blood loss after delivery is defined as primary or secondary postpartum haemorrhage (PPH). Primary PPH is the estimated loss of greater than 600 mL in the first 24 hours after delivery. Estimation is very difficult. Signs of haemorrhagic shock irrespective of amount of blood loss are important.

Secondary PPH is excessive vaginal bleeding from day one until six weeks after delivery.

There are two main categories of PPH: atonic and traumatic. Atonic (90 per cent of cases) is due to failure of the uterus to contract; traumatic (10 per cent of cases) is due to damage to the genital tract. The comparison of clinical background is important.

The uterus that is slow to contract before delivery will also be so after. Atonic haemorrhage is commoner in a uterus that is overstretched by multiple fetuses, polyhydramnios or a big baby. Induced labour or augmented labour, particularly when it has become very prolonged, is a clear association. Traumatic haemorrhage is associated with traumatic delivery, assisted or not, and previous uterine surgery. There may well be a combination of atonic and traumatic haemorrhage. Both must be carefully considered in the acute situation.

Management

Immediate management is life-saving. A call for help to mobilize senior staff from obstetrics, midwifery, anaesthetics and haematology is important.

Because poor uterine contraction is likely to be contributing, a hand should placed on the lower abdomen and the fundus of the uterus rubbed to stimulate a contraction. Irrespective of whether nothing, oxytocin or ergometrine has already been given as part of routine management, ergometrine 0.5 mg should be given intramuscularly.

IV access must be secured. A large bore cannula of at least 16 gauge should be inserted into a forearm vein. Blood is withdrawn for haemoglobin estimation and crossmatch of blood. Immediate infusion of one litre of Hartmann's solution is given. An infusion of normal saline with 100 units of Syntocinon added to one litre should be commenced at 20 drops per minute. In the proportion of cases that are due to poor contraction this first series of manoeuvres will stop the bleeding. If significant further bleeding occurs more detailed examination of the genital tract is necessary. Traumatic damage is likely and the source must be found. Problems arise because of delays in treatment moving to the next step.

- A further 0.5 mg of ergometrine should be given IV.
- Fundal massage is continued.
- Good lithotomy and analgesia is obtained for detailed vaginal and cervical inspection.
- Trauma is repaired as indicated.

Prostaglandin F2 alpha (haemabate) is used as a second line oxytocic. It can be injected systemically or into the myometrium through the anterior abdominal wall.

Intravenous (IV) therapy

If haemorrhage is severe or persistent then a central venous pressure line should be placed.

Fluid replacement

Initial infusion may be of Hartmann's solution or normal saline, but a colloid becomes necessary in order to maintain volume within the intravascular space. Haemaccel (Hoechst) or Gelofusine (Consolidated Chemicals), which are both chemically modified solutions of degraded gelatin, is the best choice initially, but should be followed by whole blood and fresh frozen plasma. The only difference between them is that Haemaccel contains over 10 times more calcium than Gelofusine. The calcium can lead to clotting in warming coils when Haemaccel is mixed with citrated blood or fresh frozen plasma. In cases of massive, rapid haemorrhage, uncrossmatched group 0 negative blood should be given. In the face of massive haemorrhage with a developing coagulation defect, fresh, whole blood is ideal but is no longer available because of the difficulties of screening for infection (such as AIDS) in donated blood while it remains fresh. A substitute of its component parts should be given as:

- packed red cells;
- fresh frozen plasma;
- platelets (after 5 or 6 units of blood).

The collaboration of the duty haematologist is important. Accurate fluid management with central venous pressure measurement, urinary catheterization and careful fluid balance recording is critical.

CASE HISTORY

Mrs O

29 years old, married Nigerian.

Non-smoker, social worker assistant

4th pregnancy: 1 termination of pregnancy at 8 weeks

1 SVD at 39 weeks, 3.2 kg baby, no problem.

1 LSCS for 'fetal distress', 3.4 kg baby, well.

Sickle cell trait

Husband, normal haemoglobin (Hb) electrophoresis

Normal cervical smear 1 year ago

Fit and well, weight 97 kg.

Lives in three-bedroomed rented house with husband and children.

Current pregnancy

Booked at 22 weeks: Hb 10.1 g/dL, 23 weeks scan showed normal fetus but low placenta covering the os. Currently taking iron and folate supplements. Repeat scan at 32 weeks showed placenta remained mainly anterior. Type 3 placenta praevia covering the cervical os. Further scan arranged for 37 weeks and then elective caesarean section at 38 weeks.

At 37 weeks at 04:30 admitted to labour ward complaining of vaginal bleeding of about 300 mL. Pulse rate 100 beats per minute, blood pressure 110/70 mmHg. There were irregular uterine contractions that settled. Baby moving and CTG normal. Blood was taken for haemoglobin and crossmatch 6 units of blood.

Discussion

What risks does Mrs O face?

Mrs O faces the life-threatening risk of further haemorrhage before, during and after delivery. High-risk delivery should not be undertaken at 06:00 unless it is life-saving. The condition was stable and review by the consultant was due at 09:00. This was undertaken and the Caesarean planned for that morning with a consultant anaesthetist and consultant obstetrician present. Consent was taken for Caesarean Section and any other procedure including, specifically hysterectomy, if required.

The senior registrar, assisted by the consultant, performed an ultrasound scan to assess the obstruction presented by the placenta before commencing the operation. At operation the placenta was found as predicted under the knife as the uterus was incised. The amniotic cavity was opened 'above' the upper placental edge and the baby delivered in excellent condition. The placenta was delivered in several pieces. There was bleeding from venous sinuses of the uterus that was controlled by ligation and diathermy coagulation. A transfusion of three units of blood was considered prudent and commenced. The operation was completed and Mrs O returned to the recovery area with her baby, accompanied by her husband.

Two hours later the midwife called the registrar because there had been a PPH. The pulse rate was 120 beats per minute, the blood pressure was 80/40 and there was a substantial amount of blood on the bed.

What should be done?

This is a serious emergency. The blood infusion was increased to a maximum rate. An additional litre of Hartmann's solution was infused. The registrar called for help and massaged the fundus of the uterus. Ergometrine 0.5 mg was given IV. An infusion of 100 units of Syntocinon in normal saline was commenced at 30 drops per minute. With a good light a speculum examination was performed. Blood clot was removed from the vagina and there was persisting bright red bleeding.

What is the next step?

Speedy resolution of the problem is important. Maternal mortality is associated with tardiness in the decision-making process. A probable source of the bleeding is the uterine incision. An examination in the operating theatre is important.

This was performed and initially a blood clot was removed from a poorly contracted uterus. The bleeding continued and so a laparotomy was performed. Prior to laparotomy the woman and her partner were advised of the possibility of a hysterectomy. Six further units of blood were prepared as well as fresh frozen plasma. At laparotomy the uterine incision was inspected and found to be intact. The uterus was noted to be poorly contracted. Prostaglandin (haemabate) was injected directly into the uterine muscle. Direct pressure was applied to the uterus bimanually for 20 minutes. Her condition was stable and the operation was completed. At the end of the operation the vaginal loss was observed for 20 minutes and was not excessive. She was observed on the intensive care unit for 12 hours and then returned to the maternity ward where she made a good recovery.

She was grateful to have conserved her uterus and hopes to have another child.

Serious sequelae develop because of too slow a response to the danger signals.

Further treatment

Continuing haemorrhage necessitates an examination under anaesthesia, initially vaginally followed by laparotomy if indicated. At laparotomy a senior doctor will have to decide whether arterial ligation is possible. The ultimate solution is hysterectomy; in an emergency situation this may have to be subtotal. The family is kept fully informed of the decision-making.

New developments

The avoidance of hysterectomy is important in a woman whose family is not yet complete. Packing of the uterine cavity can be effective but balloon tamponade is a more attractive proposition. A Sengstaken-Blakemore tube placed per vaginam or at laparotomy is effective. It should be left in place for at least 24 hours.

Embolization of the pelvic vasculature with absorbable gelatin sponge or polyvinyl particles by an interventional radiologist has also been reported. The organization of this would be difficult in an emergency situation: it requires to be set up prospectively.

Synthetic oxygen-carrying products such as fluorocarbon and haemoglobin solutions are in the process of development. Platelet substitutes are also being developed. Ease of availability and their acceptance by religious groups that do not accept blood transfusion make this an important development.

Embolism

A pregnant, or labouring woman, is in a particularly precarious condition if her respiratory function is compromised. This occurs with venous thromboembolism and amniotic fluid embolism.

Venous thromboembolism (see also Chapter 14)

Incidence and epidemiology

There is little data concerning the incidence of thromboembolic complications in pregnancy but it

S Symptoms of pulmonary embolism

- Acute breathlessness
- Chest pain
- Haemoptysis

Signs of pulmonary embolism

- Tachycardia
- Cyanosis
- Hypotension

might be about 0.3 per cent. However it attains great significance as the leading cause of maternal death in the United Kingdom with 48 deaths between 1994 and 1996.

Aetiology

Pregnancy causes a hypercoagulable state. Additional factors such as age (greater than 35 years), obesity (body weight greater than 80 kg), parity of four or more, gross varicose veins, current infection, pre-eclampsia and immobility predispose to thrombosis. Bedrest in pregnancy can be dangerous. Special risks are present when there is a family history of thrombosis, pulmonary embolism, thrombophilia and antiphospholipid syndrome.

Investigations and treatment

A major pulmonary embolism requires urgent treatment at the same time as investigation.

Investigations for embolism

- Arterial blood gases.
- Chest X-ray.
- ECG.
- Ventilation/perfusion scan.
- +/-Pulmonary angiogram.

Treatment

In collaboration with a physician and a haematologist, heparin and rarely streptokinase should be given IV. As in any maternofetal emergency the first priority is to resuscitate the mother.

- Oxygen
- Ventilatory support
- Cardiopulmonary resuscitation

If her condition is fully stabilized then a decision may be taken to proceed to delivery in the maternal interest. This should be by Caesarean Section under conditions of intensive care.

New developments in thromboembolism

Greater awareness of the risks of immobilization in pregnancy has led to less bedrest, less admission to hospital and more mobilization.

The Royal College of Obstetricians and Gynaecologists has issued a recommendation with respect to thromboembolism and Caesarean Section. This is reproduced below:

Risk Assessment Profile for Thromboembolism in Caesarean Section

LOW RISK - Early mobilization and hydration
• Elective Caesarean Section - uncomplicated pregnancy and no other risks factors.

MODERATE RISK - Consider one of a variety of prophylactic measures
• Age >35 years
• Obesity (>80 kg)
• Para 4 or more
• Gross varicose veins
• Current infection
• Pre-eclampsia
• Immobility prior to surgery (>4 days)
• Major current illness, e.g. heart or lung disease, cancer, inflammatory bowel disease, nephrotic syndrome
• Emergency Caesarean Section in labour

HIGH RISK - Heparin prophylaxis +/- leg stockings
• A patient with three or more moderate risk factors from above
• Extended major pelvic or abdominal surgery, e.g. Caesarean hysterectomy
• Patients with a personal or family history of deep vein thrombosis, pulmonary embolism or thrombophilia or paralysis of lower limbs
• Patients with antiphospholipid antibody (cardiolipin antibody and/or lupus anticoagulant)
Management of different risk groups
• Low-risk patients – Patients undergoing elective Caesarean Section with uncomplicated pregnancy and no other risk factors required only early mobilization and attention to hydration.

• Moderate-risk patients – Patients assessed as at moderate risk should receive subcutaneous heparin (doses are higher during pregnancy but not following Caesarean Section) or mechanical methods.
• High-risk patients – Patients assessed as at high risk should receive heparin prophylaxis and, in addition, leg stockings are beneficial.
• Prophylaxis until the 5th postoperative day is advised (or until fully mobilized if longer).
• Many units suggest the continued use of anti-embolism/pneumatic boots during Caesarean Section.

Amniotic fluid embolism

Definition

This condition occurs when amniotic fluid enters the maternal circulation. It causes acute cardiorespiratory compromise as well as a coagulation defect, which is often severe.

Incidence and aetiology

This is a rare, serious condition (1:30,000) which occurs when amniotic fluid enters the maternal circulation. This has been associated with rupture of the membranes, rapid labour, vaginal delivery and Caesarean Section. The mechanism appears to be the access of amniotic fluid presumably at a higher pressure than usual, directly into the maternal circulation through a defect somewhere near the placental site. This embolism of amniotic fluid is unpredictable and has catastrophic consequences due to:
• acute cardiorespiratory embarrassment;
• coagulation failure.

There were 10 histologically confirmed deaths from amniotic fluid embolism between 1991-1993 in the Report of Confidential Enquiries (HMSO, 1996).

S Symptoms of amniotic fluid embolism

The patient experiences the sudden onset of severe chest discomfort and difficulty in breathing. She may become pale and cyanosed with signs of cardiovascular collapse.

👁 Signs of amniotic fluid embolism

- Venous congestion may be obvious with a raised jugular venous pressure.
- Output failure becomes evident with tachycardia, hypotension and peripheral vasoconstriction.
- Haemorrhage with coagulation failure may be suggested by petechial skin haemorrhage, bleeding at puncture sites and vaginal bleeding. Coagulopathic signs may be the presenting features without other symptoms

Investigations

There is no time for investigation as these patients are critically ill and 30 per cent will die in the first hour. A high index of suspicion is necessary when a previously normal patient suffers cardiorespiratory collapse during labour or soon after delivery. The diagnosis can only be confirmed at postmortem by finding the pulmonary vasculature packed with amniotic debris and trophoblast or by aspirating blood from the pulmonary artery from a Swan-Ganz catheter and examining it for trophoblastic tissue. The differential diagnosis includes venous thromboembolism.

A coagulation profile should be requested urgently as dramatic haemorrhage with coagulopathy is common if the patient survives the initial embolism. Indeed together with coagulopathy the condition is unresponsive to oxytocics and surgical haemostasis.

Management

Artificial ventilation, cardiopulmonary resuscitation and circulatory support are the first measures and IV dopamine and steroids may be useful. Acidosis should be corrected and aggressive treatment of the coagulopathy pursued. If the patient survives, comprehensive intensive care should be instituted with a central venous line, arterial lines peripherally and to the pulmonary artery. A life-support system is necessary. Detailed analysis of the coagulation status by a haematologist may permit the use of anticoagulants or antifibrinolytics to improve the circulation.

The baby is unlikely to survive such a major insult. Delivery should be undertaken after stabilization of the maternal condition. In such a dangerous maternal state vaginal delivery is preferable if there is any reasonable prospect of it.

Prognosis

The maternal mortality of amniotic fluid embolism is more than 90 per cent. Death should only be attributed to amniotic fluid embolism when histological proof has been obtained by the pathologist.

In such a serious condition, prevention has to be considered when a cure is unusual. Excessive uterine contractions with oxytocin administration must be avoided. In the Report on Confidential Enquires (HMSO, 1989), death from amniotic fluid embolism in four multiparous women was associated with the use of oxytocic drugs. There were fewer such deaths more recently. Attention must always be focused on the nature of uterine contractions. More research is needed into this condition.

New developments in amniotic fluid embolism

Unfortunately there are none to report in this difficult and lethal condition. Study of this condition is complicated because of its rarity. There is a fair correlation between amniotic fluid embolism and medical intervention in labour especially with oxytocic drugs. Such intervention should always be circumspect and careful.

There is a national register of amniotic fluid embolism that has been started, based in Bradford.

Postpartum collapse

Definition and aetiology

Physiological adaptation during normal delivery is very considerable. Nutritional intake will have been restricted during labour with the consequent development of dehydration, ketosis and mild pyrexia. Changes in circulating volume, shivering and the emotional climax of delivery all contribute to the picture. Reassurance, a warm drink and analgesia will counter these changes. If a pathological event supervenes the situation becomes dramatic with shock and its attendant symptoms.

Postpartum collapse is most commonly associated with PPH. However, other possibilities of an obstetric nature are amniotic fluid embolism, thromboembolism, uterine inversion and sepsis. Other intra-abdominal catastrophies such as a ruptured aneurysm of the hepatic artery, splenic artery or the

S Symptoms of postpartum collapse

The patient's condition suddenly deteriorates with faintness, dizziness, vomiting and a general feeling of unease. In embolism of either type, chest pain and difficulty in breathing will be seen often with dramatic onset

👁 Signs of postpartum collapse

Collapse manifests by pallor, cyanosis, tachycardia, hypotension, poor peripheral perfusion and alteration in consciousness is obvious

aorta itself, ruptured liver or spleen or complication of associated pelvic disease are rare but recognized. Associated causes such as cerebrovascular accident and myocardial infarction are unusual: they can occur at any time.

Investigation

Cardiorespiratory symptoms and signs direct attention to that area with a request for urgent chest X-ray, electrocardiogram, blood gases, haemoglobin and serum electrolytes. Persistent alteration of consciousness, or loss of consciousness without cardiorespiratory signs, suggests a neurological or metabolic problem. Serum electrolytes and investigation of intracranial structures are necessary. Detailed neurological examination should be undertaken; serum electrolytes and imaging of the brain are important. The computerized axial tomography (CAT) scan has been a great advance in this area.

Although external bleeding will be an obvious cause of postpartum collapse two occult aetiologies must be considered: internal bleeding and uterine inversion.

Internal bleeding

Internal bleeding may be localized in the broad ligament, peritoneal cavity, paravaginal tissues and perineum. A surprisingly large volume of blood can accumulate even in apparently enclosed spaces and is associated with acute pain and discomfort. Shock with consequent need for resuscitation, transfusion of several units of blood and surgical evacuation of the haematoma is common. Generalized peritoneal bleeding may require specialized surgical help if from a non-pelvic site.

Internal bleeding may be due to uterine damage related to a previous uterine scar (Caesarean Section or myomectomy) or spontaneous rupture during delivery. Rupture during delivery is a significant risk in the multiparous woman treated with oxytocics. Rapid labour and abnormal fetal heart rate pattern may also have been features. Great caution must be exercised in treating such patients as rapid, untreated labour may also result in uterine damage. A posterior position of the occiput, strong contraction and vigorous multiparous expulsive effort before and at full dilatation of the cervix set the scene for this. Abdominal (peritoneal) pain is usually a feature of intraperitoneal bleeding, circulatory changes inconsistent with the external signs are seen and serial girth measurements will reveal a gradual increase. A real-time ultrasound scan will show free fluid in the peritoneal cavity.

Uterine inversion

Uterine inversion (Fig. 20.4) must be excluded in postpartum collapse. This is a rare condition and specific management points are discussed in Chapter 19, on operative obstetrics.

It may be recognized by the appearance of the inverted uterus at the vulva or by finding it on vaginal examination performed because of postpartum haemorrhage or collapse. As soon as it is recognized

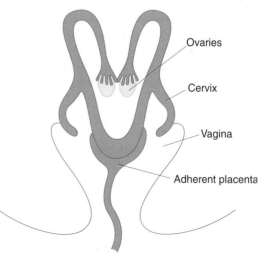

Figure 20.4 Inverted uterus.

an attempt should be made to replace it by manual compression with the placenta still attached. An oxytocic is then given and the placenta removed manually. Should this fail then it can be tried under general anaesthesia with a bolus of a betamimetic such as ritodrine being given to relax the constriction ring of the cervix.

Hydrostatic replacement or more extensive surgical manipulation may not be necessary.

Management

In the absence of embolism, the most likely causes of postpartum collapse are abdominopelvic. Resuscitation and concomitant elucidation of the cause must be quickly conducted. The Airways, Breathing, Circulation (ABC) drill is followed with a large-bore cannula inserted to immediately infuse 1000 mL of normal saline. Establish IV access with a large-bore IV cannula of normal saline. Even if there is uncertainty about the cause of collapse 1000 mL of normal saline is unlikely to be harmful to the young, otherwise healthy, parturient and may be life-saving if hypovolaemia is present.

Immediate vaginal examination may reveal accumulation of blood or uterine inversion. Uterine inversion is more easily replaced the shorter the time of inversion. Venous congestion, oedema and bruising develop later. Firm digital pressure to pass the fundus back through the constriction ring is often successful. Subsequently, an IV infusion of oxytocin should be given to maintain contraction for several hours. If there is difficulty which is due to the tight constriction ring then, rather than considering cumbersome methods of mechanical replacement or incising the cervix, a bolus of a tocolytic drug or halothane inhalation should be considered. This immediately relaxes the construction ring and the uterus can be replaced. This should be followed up by an infusion of oxytocin (at least 100 milliunits per minute).

If blood accumulation is found in the soft tissues of the pelvis then resuscitation, anaesthesia, evacuation and haemostasis are necessary. It is often impossible to locate a specific bleeding vessel and oversewing with obliteration of the space has to suffice. If no blood is found in the lower genital tract then peritoneal bleeding must be considered. Abdominal ultrasound scan is a useful investigation in these circumstances. Laparotomy and internal haemostasis is then necessary. Support from a general surgical colleague should be ensured.

Prognosis

This depends on the cause of the collapse.

Acute fetal compromise and uterine rupture

For consideration of acute 'fetal distress' reference is made to Chapter 9, Labour.

Emergency situations requiring immediate Caesarean Section are placental abruption, umbilical cord prolapse and prolonged fetal bradycardia. In these circumstances the baby should be delivered within 30 minutes from a 'cold' start (woman presents directly from home) and within 20 minutes from a 'hot' start (woman is already an inpatient on the labour ward).

Intact utero-placental circulation is important for placental function and fetal wellbeing. In rare circumstances the circulation may collapse with implication for the mother as well as the fetus. The uterus stops contracting after uterine rupture. The maternal circulation is interrupted and there is fetal distress. If this is significant it may not be possible to save the fetus and the uterus may be damaged. If the uterus is ruptured it may be repaired but left weakened to support a future pregnancy.

Umbilical cord accidents

Definition and aetiology

Umbilical cord presentation is the presence of a segment of umbilical cord at the cervical os as the presenting part. Prolapse is present when the membranes have ruptured and the segment of cord may be at any level from the upper vagina to outside the introitus. This occurs in about 1:500 deliveries. The stage preceding cord presentation is the presence of cord beside the presenting part and may manifest as variable decelerations of the fetal heart. The fetus is totally dependent on oxygenated blood delivered through the compressible umbilical vein in the cord. The probability of cord accidents is related to the length of the cord, which is unknown before delivery, the fit of the presenting part in the pelvic brim and abnormal cord insertion into a placenta which is partly sited in the lower segment as type 1 or type 2 placenta praevia. Clinically, therefore, cord accidents are more common in abnormal lie, breech

S Symptoms of umbilical cord accident

The only symptom is that in cord prolapse the woman may have felt a gush of fluid and subsequently seen or felt a loop of cord in or outside the vagina

👁 Signs of umbilical cord accident

The only characteristic sign is the finding of palpable or visible cord in the vagina. The other main sign is found on investigation of the nature of the fetal heart rate

presentation especially flexed or footling and placenta praevia with marginal cord insertion.

Investigations

Fetal heart rate monitoring may already have been in progress showing deep variable decelerations. Once cord accident has been diagnosed no further investigation is necessary other than to ascertain fetal condition and review the likelihood of rapid vaginal delivery. Under these circumstances, palpation of the cord for pulsation is more difficult than it may seem. Care should be taken to ensure it is not the pulsation in the examiner's own finger that is felt. If the patient has been admitted with a prolapse that may have been present for some time the baby may already be dead. A good quality fetal monitor or a portable ultrasound machine should be used to clarify this if necessary.

Management

Cord accident is an indication for immediate Caesarean Section if the baby is alive and vaginal delivery cannot be effected immediately. In all cases blood should be taken for haemoglobin and crossmatch; an IV infusion of Hartmann's solution is sited for access. If the fetal heart is absent and the lie longitudinal, normal delivery should be anticipated. This may at some stage include oxytocic treatment. The absence of life in the baby should be explained to the mother and appropriate management undertaken.

When the baby is alive and the cervix fully dilated in a nullipara or nearly fully dilated in a multipara, vigorous attempts to secure vaginal delivery should be made whilst preparations are made for Caesarean Section.

Maximal flexion of the hips in lithotomy is useful, great maternal explosive effort is exhorted and forceps applied if the head is showing signs of descending through the birth canal with each contraction. This is more likely to occur in a multipara. If the presentation is breech in a nullipara, Caesarean Section should be performed as breech extraction would be very hazardous. If the woman is a multipara having had average or good size babies previously, then breech extraction is an option in skilled hands.

When the cervix is not fully dilated and the baby is alive, immediate Caesarean Section is arranged. The person making the diagnosis should:

1. Call for immediate Caesarean Section and reassure the mother.
2. Pass a urinary catheter.
3. Position the patient in knee–chest or exaggerated Sims' position.
4. Maintain digital pressure to keep pressure off the cord especially during contractions.
5. Replace exposed cord in the vagina to keep it warm and prevent vasospasm.

Although this is an undignified posture for the patient, maintenance of these measures until delivery may save the baby's life. Assistants should at the same time:

- establish IV access with 16 gauge or large-bore cannula; and
- take blood for haemoglobin crossmatch;
- give an H2 receptor agonist and/or antacid;
- assist the anaesthetist.

Delivery by Caesarean Section should pose no difficulty. The operator's fingers may touch those of the person applying pressure through the vagina.

Postoperatively, antibiotics should be given on account of these manipulations.

Prognosis

The outlook for the baby, when there has been compression or cord presentation, should be good if the baby was not already growth restricted, has not been stressed for too long and if delivery is uncomplicated.

The condition of a well-grown baby that has suffered cord prolapse in hospital and when management has been appropriate should also be good.

The condition of a baby that has suffered cord prolapse at some distance from medical help is likely to be very bad if it is not already dead at diagnosis.

w developments in umbilical cord ccidents

Management requires the presenting part to be kept from compressing the umbilical cord. Some have suggested passing a urinary catheter and filling the bladder to achieve this. Others have suggested the use of a bolus dose of a betamimetic drug such as ritodrine to achieve the same result. For obvious reasons neither suggestion had been tested by a randomized controlled trial. Whatever technique is suggested it should not lead to further delay in delivery in this emergency situation. In a multiparous woman where the cervix is nearly fully dilated 'aggressive' vaginal examination and strong encouragement to push should resolve the problem. This may be particularly helpful if this situation arises during a home birth.

Shoulder dystocia

Definition and aetiology

Shoulder dystocia means difficult delivery of the shoulders. The shoulders should follow the head with the same, or the following, contraction. If they do not the difficulty can range from slight to complete obstruction of delivery. The incidence is 0.2–1.2 per cent depending on the definition. The baby is usually big (greater than 4 kg) and the mother smaller than average. Shoulder dystocia is the most frightening

S Symptoms in shoulder dystocia
The woman feels intense pressure and stretching of the birth canal

👁 Signs in shoulder dystocia
The head has emerged and then may have retracted on the perineum

and threatening obstetric emergency. Delay beyond five minutes leads to hypoxia and ultimately fetal death. Undue haste and traction leads to damage to the cervical plexus nerve roots of the baby. The need is to be prepared both in anticipation and practice.

Babies that are abnormal, such as those with anencephaly or hydrops fetalis are unusual causes of shoulder dystocia.

Management

The preparation in practice involves having a prepared plan of action (shoulder dystocia drill). This should be discussed frequently and practised in advance.

Post-delivery

The paediatrician should examine all such babies for soft tissue, bone or nerve damage. Erb's palsy may be a consequence. Full discussion should take place with the family.

Risk factors in shoulder dystocia

Anticipation (antenatally)
- Large baby
- Small mother
- Excessive maternal birthweight
- Maternal obesity
- Diabetes mellitus
- Postmaturity
- Previous shoulder dystocia or big baby

Anticipation during labour
- Big baby/small mother
- Prolonged first stage of labour
- Prolonged second stage of labour
- Forceps or vacuum extraction

Shoulder dystocia drill

- Don't panic and don't pull excessively
- Reposition: on all fours or full flexion and abduction of the hips (McRobert's position)
- Supra pubic pressure laterally toward the baby's face
- Liberal episiotomy
- Manipulation to rotate shoulders internally
- Attempt to deliver posterior shoulder

In theory fracturing the fetal clavicle, performing a symphysiotomy or replacing the fetal head followed by Caesarean Section (Zavanelli manoeuvre) may all be effective but few doctors have any experience of these techniques

Conclusion

An obstetric emergency rapidly converts a happy, normal event to a potential catastrophe. Labour wards must be organized to deal with this. Risk assessment must be an integral part of the management of each pregnancy and preventive measures should be in place. Women at high risk of operative delivery should have an H2 receptor agonist and an antiemetic in labour. The risk factors for thromboembolism should be constantly borne in mind. The appropriate level of staff in an interdisciplinary team should always be available. Given such precautions birth can be made as safe as possible.

Key Points

- Obstetric emergencies can lead to maternal and fetal compromise
- Some emergencies can be anticipated according to risk classification
- Guidelines are important
- Action should be rapid and decisive
- Senior staff involvement is critical
- Remember the ABC: Airway, Breathing, Circulation
- Reassure the family

References for further reading

Report on Confidential Enquiries into Maternal Deaths in the United Kingdom. London; HMSO, 1994–1996, 1998.

Eclampsia in the United Kingdom (British Eclampsia Survey Team BEST Report). *BMJ* 1994; **309:** 1395–9.

Eclampsia Collaborative Group. Which Anticonvulsant for women with eclampsia? Evidence from the Collaborative Eclampsia Trial. *Lancet* 1995; **345:** 1455–63.

Chapter 21

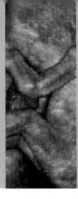

Psychiatric disorders in pregnancy and the puerperium

OVERVIEW

Pregnancy affects mental illness in a complex way. It is vital for obstetricians, midwives and other healthcare professionals to be alert to the sometimes subtle indications of impending mental illness and to be aware of the issues surrounding diagnosis and treatment in pregnancy and the puerperium. Remember that pregnancy is one of the greatest factors for mental illness in a woman's life.

THE IMPORTANCE OF PSYCHIATRY TO OBSTETRICS

Healthy women experience marked psychological and emotional changes during pregnancy and, in particular, after delivery.

There is a great variation in the range of emotional and behavioural changes during pregnancy. In general, the second and third trimesters of pregnancy are associated with a feeling of emotional wellbeing. However, it is relatively common for women to feel more nauseated and emotional during the first trimester of pregnancy particularly if the pregnancy is unwelcome or associated with social adversity or emotional conflict. States of emotional distress and of minor depression are relatively common, some studies suggesting that up to 15 per cent of pregnant women are affected in the first trimester. Emotional stability and a sense of wellbeing usually improve as the pregnancy progresses. First-time mothers and those with well-founded anxieties about the wellbeing of their pregnancy may experience relatively high levels of anxiety during the later stages of pregnancy but will usually respond to reassurance based on information and explanation. A heightened emotional state and anxiety about the impending delivery are common in the latter stages of pregnancy.

In contrast to the variability of emotional changes during pregnancy, the majority of women experience a sequence of marked emotional and behavioural changes following delivery. For the first 24 to 48 hours following delivery, it is very common for women to experience an elation of mood, a feeling of excitement, some overactivity and difficulty sleeping. This has been called 'the pinks'. It is important to ensure adequate rest and to guard against overactivity in this phase. There has been a suggestion that women who experience a marked elevation of mood following delivery are more likely to experience a severe state of 'the blues' and are perhaps more likely to experience a postpartum mood disorder.

Between the 3rd and the 10th postpartum day, the mother's mood state changes to being low, tearful and labile. Frequently they experience irritability, insomnia and a tendency to be oversensitive to criticism with transient bouts of despair and catastrophizing (blowing things out of proportion). This is known as the 'the blues', the commonest day of onset is day 5. The severity of the 'blues' varies from being relatively mild to quite distressing but it is essentially a normal, and probably inevitable, consequence of childbirth and should not be confused with mental illness. Unlike mental illness, it usually only lasts 48 hours. It responds to kindness and reassurance and does not deteriorate over the following days as postnatal depression does. Tearful and anxious episodes may recur on occasion for a number of weeks following childbirth particularly when the mother is tired or when the baby is difficult to settle. It is important that all professionals involved in the care of newly delivered mothers know of the timing, characteristics and essentially benign nature of the 'blues'. It is also important that women themselves and their partners are made aware of this phenomenon during antenatal classes.

Psychiatric morbidity in childbirth

Childbirth contributes a substantial risk to the mental health of women (Table 21.1). In the year following childbirth, women who were previously well have a greatly elevated risk of being admitted to a psychiatric hospital, being referred to a psychiatrist, suffering from a psychotic illness or suffering from a severe depressive illness. This risk is higher than their lifetime risk, and is much greater than for other women or men. At least 10 per cent of all women delivered will suffer from a depressive illness severe enough to meet the criteria for DSM'III'R major depressive illness. If less severe cases are included then the incidence of postnatal depression is even higher: between 15 and 20 per cent of all deliveries. Approximately 3–5 per cent of all women delivered will meet the criteria for moderate to severe depressive illness (of a type that requires antidepressant medication). Just below 2 per cent of all women delivered will be referred to a psychiatrist in the postpartum year. Four

Table 21.1 – Incidence of postpartum mental disorders

15–30%	'depression'
10%	major depressive illness
3–5%	moderate/severe depressive illness
1.7%	referred
4/1000	admitted
2/1000	admitted psychosis

per thousand deliveries will be admitted to a psychiatric hospital, of whom half (2 per 1000) will be suffering from a psychotic illness. Over 80 per cent of these women will be suffering from their first, ever psychiatric illness but 20 per cent will have had a previous postpartum illness or non-childbirth-related psychiatric disorder.

In contrast to the increased risk of serious psychiatric disorder following childbirth, a woman is less likely to be seriously mentally ill, to be referred to a psychiatrist, to take an overdose, commit suicide or be admitted to a psychiatric hospital during pregnancy. However, a significant minority of pregnant women has mental health problems and the obstetrician will be required to manage women who have become pregnant whilst suffering from a mental illness and receiving treatment. A significant minority of women becomes mentally ill during pregnancy (15 per cent in the first trimester, 8 per cent in the second and 5 per cent in the third). The majority of these conditions is not serious and will resolve as the pregnancy progresses. However some will not, with implications for the mental health of those women after delivery. Women may also present at booking clinic currently well but with past histories of psychiatric disorder, and will be concerned about the effect that childbirth might have upon their mental health. Thus a substantial minority of patients seen by obstetricians and the maternity services (between 15 and 20 per cent of all patients) will have mental health problems which have to be taken into account in their management.

Pregnancy in mentally ill women

For women with an existing psychiatric disorder, childbirth poses a predictable risk of relapse and, for those with chronic disability, concerns about their ability to care for their child.

With the exception of anorexia nervosa no psychiatric condition is associated with a reduction in biological fertility. Therefore all forms of psychiatric disorder may present associated with pregnancy. Women whose stability of mental health and social functioning depends upon taking regular medication pose a particular problem for the psychiatrist and obstetrician.

Effectiveness of treatment

For those mothers who become mentally ill for the first time following childbirth the diagnosis is likely to be that of a variant of an affective disorder. These range in severity from the most severe and rarest, puerperal psychosis (a form of manic-depressive or bipolar disorder) through severe depressive illness to less severe and milder forms of depression. Effective treatments are available for all of these conditions. There is evidence to suggest that postpartum affective disorder is particularly sensitive to treatment, has a shorter illness duration and better lifetime prognosis. Approximately half of these women will become ill following subsequent childbirths.

Consequences of lack of treatment

If postnatal depression is untreated, adverse sequelae may arise (see box below).

Although the majority of these illnesses are self-limiting and will recover by six months postpartum, 30 per cent of women are still ill at one year postpartum and over 10 per cent at two years postpartum. Long-standing postnatal depressive illness affects mother–infant attachment and relationships, and interferes with the social and cognitive development of their children. Such adverse effects can be detected in the child, beyond the resolution of the mother's illness, up to the age of 5 to 7 years old. These effects are particularly marked in boys and when combined with social and marital adversity. Prolonged postnatal mental illness may also lead to the breakdown of marriages. These adverse consequences of postnatal mental illness underline the importance of early detection and vigorous treatment. Psychiatric morbidity and hazard to mother and infant may be reduced to a minimum by speedy diagnosis and referral for treatment by obstetricians, midwives and general practitioners.

Prediction of risk

The risk factors for serious mental illness are listed in the box (below).

Women with a previous history of postnatal depression or puerperal psychosis are at 1:2 risk of developing such a condition following every subsequent childbirth. The illness is likely to present at about the same time as before, thus allowing the woman's medical attendants and family to be aware of the necessary period of vigilance. Women with a previous history of non-postpartum affective disorder are also at increased risk of becoming ill following childbirth. If the illness was manic-depressive (bipolar) the risk is also 1:2. If the illness was a

---

Adverse sequelae of postnatal depression

Immediate
- Physical morbidity
- Suicide/infanticide
- Prolonged psychiatric morbidity
- Social attachments to infant
- Emotional development of infant

Later
- Social/cognitive effects on child
- Psychiatric morbidity in child
- Marital breakdown
- Future mental health problems

Risk factors for serious mental illness

Primiparity
- Past psychiatric history
- Family psychiatric history
- Past obstetric/gynaecologic complication (loss)
- Caesarean Section (primipara, only for psychosis)

Trend
- Higher social class
- Higher age
- Longer marriage/birth intervals

non-psychotic depressive illness or other neurotic condition the risk is also elevated and is thought to lie between 1:5 and 1:3. Women with chronic schizophrenia may not be at a particularly elevated risk of relapse, either during pregnancy or during the early postpartum period but may face later problems with the stresses of child-rearing.

Women with a family history of serious affective disorder are at increased risk of developing such an illness following childbirth.

Some of the risk factors for a primiparous woman developing a mild postnatal depressive illness are also known. However, they are less specific or useful in predicting individuals at risk, more for identifying a vulnerable population. They include such factors as:

- Single
- Young
- Short relationship
- Early deprivation
- Chronic life difficulties
- Social adversity
- Lack of a confidant
- Past psychiatric history
- Question termination of pregnancy index
- Antenatal admission (non-serious conditions)
- Prior social services involvement
- Ambivalence about the pregnancy

Structured contact with maternity and primary healthcare services

Pregnant and postpartum women are in frequent and regular contact with medical services. With a little adjustment these contact points could be modified so that risk factors for developing illnesses could be identified at booking clinic and during the pregnancy. The postnatal check at six weeks could be modified to include screening of all women for postnatal depression, early identification and prompt treatment.

Mental illness in pregnancy

There is probably a slightly increased risk of minor (neurotic) mental illness during the first trimester of pregnancy, with about 15 per cent of pregnant women suffering from such conditions having been previously well prior to conception (a new episode).

These illnesses usually resolve spontaneously as the pregnancy progresses. Women who develop a minor illness (usually anxiety or reactive depression) in the first trimester of pregnancy are not thought to be at increased risk of developing postnatal depression after delivery. However those very few women who develop such an illness in the last trimester of pregnancy may be at increased risk of postnatal depression and should be followed up. Psychotropic medication is not usually required for women who develop minor mental illness in pregnancy. Counselling and improving social supports is the preferred and effective treatment.

The risk of developing a new episode of major mental illness (manic depressive illness or schizophrenia) is low during pregnancy and probably lower than at other times in a woman's life. This is in contrast to the dramatic increase in risk following childbirth. Similarly women with a past history of major psychiatric disorder are probably not at increased risk of relapsing during pregnancy. However on the rare occasion that they do or when such an illness develops for the first time in pregnancy these illnesses will require treatment. For severe depressive illnesses tricyclic antidepressants (for example, dothiepin 150 mg daily) can be used but they will need to be reduced by 25 mg per two weeks so that the mother is receiving less than 75 mg or preferably has stopped the antidepressant before delivery. This is because there have been some reports of babies born to mothers receiving a full therapeutic dose of tricyclic antidepressants suffering from neonatal jitteriness and anticholinergic side effects. Once delivered the antidepressant can be gradually increased back to a therapeutic level. This is to guard against the substantial risk of the mother developing a postpartum relapse. Very rarely a new episode of mania can occur during pregnancy. This can be treated as is usual with chlorpromazine or another neuroleptic in the smallest possible dose that effects resolution of the symptoms. Again this will need to be reduced to a minimum possible dose before delivery. There have been some reports of mothers suffering from hypotensive episodes following delivery on large doses of neuroleptics. There have also been reports of babies suffering from hypotonia and extrapyramidal side effects. Once delivered the neuroleptic should be increased again to mitigate against the substantial risk of a manic relapse following delivery.

Lithium should not be used in pregnancy as it is teratogenic in the first trimester (it causes cardiac defects) and in the last trimester has been associated with fetal hypothyroidism. However if the mother is not breastfeeding lithium may be re-introduced after delivery aiming at a therapeutic serum level by day 5. This has been shown in non-randomized clinical studies to be very effective at preventing a postpartum manic relapse.

The risk to the fetus from receiving psychotropic medication *in utero* has to be balanced against the risk posed by maternal disturbance.

Manic depressive illness

If a woman has a history of multiple episodes of manic depressive illness she may be receiving a combination of one or more of the following groups of drugs: antidepressants, neuroleptics and lithium. She may often be given the advice to stop these drugs before conceiving and may face therefore not only a dramatic increase in risk of relapsing following delivery (1:2) but also of relapsing during pregnancy in the weeks following cessation of medication. If at all possible such women should discuss with their psychiatrist before conception the likely effects of stopping their medication and of childbirth on their mental health. If the patient, family and psychiatrist have every reason to believe that given a stable mental state she can meet the needs of the developing child then she will need assistance to manage her condition. She should be advised to gradually reduce her lithium before conception. If necessary her mental state will need to be stabilized with antidepressants (if she becomes depressed) or with a small dose of neuroleptic (if she become hypomanic). Her mental health should then improve as the pregnancy progresses. Once delivered she should be restarted on her normal regime and if she wishes to breastfeed this should include a neuroleptic. If she does not wish to breastfeed then lithium can be started on the first postpartum day.

Chronic schizophrenia

Women suffering from chronic schizophrenia will usually be maintained either on an oral neuroleptic or commonly an intramuscular depot injection of the neuroleptic, such as fluphenazine decanoate (modicate) or flupenthixol (depixol). If this medication is stopped they run a substantial risk of having a relapse in their schizophrenic illness within three months. Again ideally these women should discuss with their psychiatrist their capacity to parent as well as the effects of pregnancy and the postpartum period on their mental health. If when well and stable even on medication they have the resources to effectively parent a child then they should be advised not to stop their medication in order to conceive or during pregnancy. However as they approach delivery their medication should be reduced to the minimum possible level compatible with mental health and then increased on the day of delivery to the normal regime. Women with chronic schizophrenia may benefit from a period of in-patient admission on a mother and baby unit to help them get off to the best possible start with their infant and provide an opportunity to assess their capacity to care for the child. Providing medication is continued the risk of relapse in the immediate postpartum period is not high. However such women may remain vulnerable to the stresses and strains of child-rearing for some months and years to come.

Aetiology of postpartum mood disorders

It is generally assumed that biological factors are the most important aetiological factors for the severe illnesses (postpartum psychosis and severe depressive illness) and psychosocial factors the most important for mild postnatal depressive illness.

Neuroendocrine factors

The constancy of incidence across cultures and, over time, the close temporal relationship of the onset of childbirth and the more recent findings of a high risk of subsequent postpartum illness and a lowered risk of non-postpartum episodes would tend to suggest a neuroendocrine basis for the severe condition. Changes in cortisol, oxytocin, endorphins, thyroxine, progesterone and oestrogen have all been implicated in the causation of this condition. Comparable dramatic changes in steroidal hormones outside of the postpartum period have a well-known association with affective psychoses and mood disorders. A plausible recent theory is that the sudden fall in oestrogen triggers a hypersensitivity of D2 receptors in a predisposed group of women and may be responsible for the severe mood disturbance that follows. The occurrence and severity of the postnatal blues are thought to be related to both the absolute level of progesterone and to the relative drop from a prepartum level. However there is no clear association between the postpartum blues and affective psychoses and no evidence as yet to implicate progesterone in the aetiology of these conditions.

Obstetric factors

Caesarean Section has been shown to be associated with postpartum psychosis in first-time mothers. Previous obstetric loss has been associated with severe postnatal depressive illness as has infertility and an adverse experience of childbirth. However, there is no direct evidence to suggest that other obstetric complications predispose to severe psychiatric illness.

Social factors

Severe postpartum illness can affect women with much wanted babies from happy and stable marriages, who live in comfortable, economic circumstances. It can also affect the deprived and vulnerable. Apart from a family history and personal history of psychiatric disorder, there is little to distinguish women suffering from severe mental illness from other postpartum women.

However, women suffering from minor postnatal depression do show significant differences when compared to well women and to women suffering from severe postnatal depression or puerperal psychoses. The risk factors for mild postnatal depression appear to be predominately psychosocial. They include being young, either single or with a short marriage or relationship, lack of a female confidante, chronic social adversity, marital discord, previous psychiatric history, prior social services involvement and antenatal admission in the last trimester of pregnancy. They are significantly more likely than other women to have been admitted on multiple occasions but for non-serious conditions, usually abdominal pain with no explanation or unfounded concerns about restricted fetal growth.

CLINICAL SYNDROMES

The majority of women who have become mentally ill following childbirth will have been well previously (a new episode). Most of these women will be suffering from their first mental illness (lifetime first episode). However some women have had a previous postpartum illness or an illness at another time in their life from which they have recovered. The overwhelming majority of these 'new' illnesses are affective (mood disorders) which vary in severity from the mildest (minor postnatal depression) through to moderate to severe postnatal depression to the most severe form, puerperal psychosis (a variant of manic-depressive or bipolar disorder).

It should be remembered that other conditions such as panic disorder, anxiety states and obsessive compulsive disorder can occur following childbirth.

The problems faced by women with enduring mental health problems who become pregnant can usually be identified before conception or during the pregnancy and these women require a special approach. The risk of developing a new episode of mental illness (usually affective disorder) following childbirth is substantial and is elevated over lifetime risk. Women run a sixteen-fold increased risk of being admitted to a psychiatric hospital suffering from puerperal psychosis, a ten-fold increase in risk of suffering from a severe depressive illness, a five-fold increase in risk of suffering from non-psychotic postnatal depression and of being referred to a psychiatrist.

Postpartum (puerperal) psychosis

This is the most severe form of affective disorder (manic-depressive or bipolar illness) (see signs box). Up to one-third of these patients will be manic and two-thirds will suffer from a depressive psychosis. The onset is very abrupt, rarely before the 3rd postpartum day, the commonest day of onset is day 5. They therefore need to be carefully distinguished from 'the blues', which will be experienced by over half of all women. The blues will settle, usually within 48 hours.

Postpartum psychoses will rapidly deteriorate. The majority of postpartum psychoses will have presented before the 16th postpartum day. In the first few days these abrupt onset psychoses take the form of an acute undifferentiated illness, hallmarked by restless agitation, perplexity, confusion, fear and suspicion, insomnia, not eating and drinking and rapidly forming delusional ideas about themselves and their babies. After three to five days the illness becomes more clearly that of an affective psychosis. However, many of these women will also experience first-rank symptoms of schizophrenia with frightening hallucinations and delusions so that the diagnosis is often that of a schizo-affective psychosis. Despite this and the fact that they are very seriously disturbed it is important to remember that the treatment and prognosis is that of an affective psychosis and that the majority of these patients will recover quickly and fully, although the risk of recurrence after subsequent childbirth is approximately 1:2.

Management

The patient should be referred urgently to a psychiatrist and will usually require admission to a psychiatric unit. If possible this should take place in a specialized setting where the mother and her infant can be managed together (a psychiatric mother and baby unit). The immediate priority will be to sedate the patient with neuroleptic medication to a level that allows her to be safely contained within her environment. Such medication will also reduce the perplexity, fear and distress and over a period of 48 hours should begin to make some impact on hallucinations and delusions. Patients with first onset postpartum psychoses or those with postpartum-only psychoses are often effectively treated with smaller doses of neuroleptics than would be usual for non-postpartum conditions. A suggested initial regime

---

👁 Signs

Puerperal psychosis
- Risk factors:
    Family/personal history
    Caesarean Section
- Abrupt onset 80 per cent 3–14 days
- Rapidly changing clinical picture
- 99 per cent manic-depressive/schizo-affective
- Good prognosis
- Admission with baby; vigorous treatment
- Risk for next baby is 1:2

---

would be 50 mg of chlorpromazine three times daily or its equivalent of haloperidol 5 mg bd or trifluoperazine 5 mg bd. The dose can be titrated up or down to an equivalent of 150 mg of chlorpromazine, three or four times a day. These medications are also available as intramuscular injections or syrups, which may aid compliance in a highly disturbed state. These drugs commonly induce extra pyramidal side effects, particularly in postpartum women, both parkinsonism and acute dystonias. These can be prevented or treated by using an antiparkinsonian agent such as procyclidine 10 mg bd. Lithium carbonate can also be used to treat acute episodes of mania, as well as its more familiar use as a prophylactic against recurrence of manic-depressive illness. For severe depressive psychoses electroconvulsive therapy (ECT) is the treatment of choice. Antidepressants, because they take between 10 and 14 days to begin their effect, are rarely appropriate as a first line treatment for a severely disturbed depressive psychosis.

Puerperal psychosis usually responds very quickly to treatment. There should be substantial improvement within days, with recovery taking place within two weeks for mania and four to six weeks for the depressive psychoses. In the latter case antidepressants will need to be started to maintain recovery after the cessation of ECT.

Risk of relapse

Although early onset puerperal psychoses respond very well to treatment, patients frequently relapse after recovery. Continuation of medication is therefore very important for six months following recovery. A patient who has presented with a manic psychosis may relapse with a depressive psychosis or a further episode of mania. If this happens on more than one occasion the clinician may well think of using lithium carbonate in order to stabilize the mood for as long as six months to one year postpartum. If the patient has suffered from a previous episode of non-postpartum manic depressive illness prophylaxis should be continued for two years following delivery.

Risk of recurrence

The risk of recurrence is now estimated at 1:2 following any subsequent childbirth. The risk is likely to be highest if the patient has a baby within two years of recovery from her illness. Such patients should therefore be advised to delay their next pregnancy until they have been well for at least two years.

Severe major postnatal depression

Severe major postnatal depression affects between 3 and 5 per cent of all women delivered. It too develops in the early weeks after delivery but does not show the abrupt onset of the puerperal psychosis, developing more slowly. A third of the patients present within the first three weeks after delivery and they are the most severely disturbed. However, two-thirds present later between 10 and 12 weeks postpartum. Most of these women would have been diagnosable at the six-week postnatal check and are often missed and go untreated.

Women with severe postnatal depression have the classical biological syndrome of early morning wakening, a mood which is worse in the morning, impaired appetite, concentration and interests. They are often indecisive and find it uncharacteristically difficult to cope with everyday life. Their mood is profoundly lowered. They feel flat, empty and weary, there is a loss of zest and interest in life and a loss of the ability to feel pleasure or enjoyment (anhedonia). They feel guilty and incompetent and about one-third have intrusive obsessional thoughts of harm coming to their children. They are often frightened that they are bad mothers. Women with severe postnatal depression are frequently very anxious and some may experience panic attacks.

Management

Antidepressants
The biological syndrome and the severity of the depressed mood predict a response to antidepressants. Tricyclic antidepressants are usually the treatment of choice, unless there is a contraindication or a previous response to another class of antidepressant. A suggested initial regime would be dothiepin, starting at 75 mg at night increasing over a few days to 150 mg nocte. Improvement can be expected within two weeks and resolution of the illness between four to six weeks. Antidepressants will need to be continued for six months following recovery before gradually reducing.

Hormones
See New developments on page 328.

Risk of relapse

Providing medication is continued for at least six months, the majority of women can expect to fully recover. However, some will need to continue their medication for longer. The risk following future pregnancies is 1:2–1:3 for those women who have postpartum-only illnesses. The risk of recurrence outside of childbirth is lower than previously thought. However, for those women who have had episodes outside of childbirth the risk following subsequent births is lower, but the risk of non-postpartum episodes is elevated compared to women with postpartum onset disorder.

Mild postnatal depression ('the blues')

This is the commonest condition following childbirth. At least 7 per cent of women will reach the

---

S **Symptoms**

Features of severe postnatal depression
- Onset in first two weeks, more gradual
- Two peaks presentation:
  - 2–4 weeks
  - 10–12 weeks
- Early presentation (often missed because atypical)
- Atypical covert classical symptoms:
  - Early morning wakening
  - Diurnal variation of mood
  - Slowing and impaired concentration
  - Overt guilt/worthlessness
  - Anomie (low socio-economic status)
  - Ruminative worry
  - Anxiety
- Treatment:
  - Antidepressants/counselling
  - Good prognosis
- Risk 1:2–1:3 next baby

CASE HISTORY

Mrs A

Aged 32, graduate teacher with a stable marriage and comfortable social circumstances.

Her father had a severe depressive illness, aged 50 years and was treated with ECT.

She developed an acute onset psychosis on 7th postpartum day following delivery at 37 weeks of twins. The pregnancy was otherwise uncomplicated. She was admitted to a mother and baby unit. For the next three days she had severe behavioural disturbance and had hallucinations, delusions and an elevated mood. This state responded to haloperidol 5 ng bd. On 11th postpartum day her mood and cognitions became clearly depressed and she wouldn't eat or drink. She was treated with ECT. Within a week (after two treatments) she had recovered and remained well and was a devoted and competent mother.

Four years later she was re-admitted to the mother and baby unit on 8th postpartum day following a full-term normal delivery of a singleton. Her mental state was identical to the previous episode. She and her husband asked for ECT. She was fully recovered by the second postpartum week.

Ten years later she has had no further babies and no further psychiatric episodes.

S Symptoms of mild postnatal depression

- Vulnerable 'at risk'
- Insidious onset in first week
- Presents three months to one year postpartum
- 'Understandable'
- Unhappy and tearful, i.e. depressed
- Most express problems with mothering
- In addition are symptoms of anxiety and phobias
- Treatment comprises counselling and social support

criteria for mild major depressive illness and many more would meet the criteria for minor depressive illness. This form of depression tends to affect a vulnerable population and usually presents later in the postpartum year. The symptoms are variable and the patient is often tearful, having difficulty in coping, particularly with the infant (see box), complains of irritability and lack of satisfaction with motherhood. Symptoms of anxiety, initial insomnia and a sense of loneliness and isolation are common. The patient is often distractible and better in company. She frequently has social and marital problems. The full biological syndrome of major depressive illness is absent.

Management

Psychological treatments are as effective as antidepressants, and more effective than standard care for this group of patients. Six weekly sessions of specific counselling by a trained health visitor are effective treatment, as is a similar course of cognitive psychotherapy. The latter form of treatment would appear to be particularly popular with patients and confers some benefit to those patients who are suffering from depression only within the context of childbirth and to their children. Social support and practical help from a female confidante improves the mental health and wellbeing of the mother and the child both as a preventative and treatment strategy. This form of common depression often associated with social adversity and marital conflict may become chronic and have adverse effects on the child. Social and psychological interventions are particularly important but are likely to take place in primary care. Preventative strategies, using modified antenatal classes, could possibly reduce morbidity in this group in their next pregnancy.

Breastfeeding and psychotropic medication

Many women who present with mental illness early in the puerperium are breastfeeding and its continuation is usually very important to them. Depressed women are often advised to stop breastfeeding, partly because it is commonly believed that psychotropic medication adversely affects the infant and partly because it is commonly believed that the mother's mood will improve. However, there is no evidence that stopping breastfeeding in itself improves the mother's mental state. In reality it often adds to the burden of guilt they feel. Continuing breastfeeding, particularly when depressed, often helps to maintain a relationship with the baby and a feeling of usefulness and may protect the infant (particularly boys) from the effects of maternal depression. Continuing to breastfeed requires a great deal of skill on the part of the psychiatric nurse when women are so very disturbed. Totally breastfeeding the infant may not be possible in the first few days of a severe puerperal psychosis. Nonetheless, it should be possible to maintain lactation with a combination of expressing the milk and frequent suckling of the infant.

When it is clearly important to continue breastfeeding, the choice of psychotropic medication becomes very important (Table 21.2). Lithium should probably not be given to breastfeeding women. The available evidence suggests that tricyclic antidepressants in full dosage are safe for breastfeeding. They are present in only very small amounts in breast milk and significant quantities are not detectable in the infant's serum.

The use of neuroleptics is more contentious. Phenothiazine, such as chlorpromazine (in single dosage of 50 mg and not more than 200 mg a day) and trifluoperazine (in a single dosage of 5 mg and not more than 15 mg a day) are also probably safe for breastfeeding mothers. However the long-term effects on the developing child and adult are unknown. The infant should be closely monitored and the breastfeeding suspended if the baby is drowsy, does not wake and cry for its feeds, or does not suckle strongly. If the severity of the mental state requires the use of parenteral medication, or a single dosage of more than the equivalent of 100 mg of chlorpromazine, it is probably safer to suspend breastfeeding for a period of 12–24 hours and express the milk.

Paediatric advice should be sought if the baby is premature, of low birth weight or jaundiced.

Prevention

For the small minority of women with predictable risk factors, particularly those who have had a previous postpartum illness or serious mental illness, an

Table 21.2 – Psychotropic medication and breastfeeding

Medication	Indicated in breastfeeding
Tricyclic antidepressants	Yes
SSRIs	
fluoxetine	No
fluvoxamine	Probably no
paroxetine	No
sertraline	No
MAOIs	Probably no
Lithium	
Neuroleptics	
moderate/oral	Probably yes
high/IM	No
Benzodiazepines, alcohol, cannabis	Best avoided

exciting opportunity exists for prevention, both psychological and pharmacological interventions (*vide infra*). Secondary prevention is a reality now (screening, early detection and prompt treatment).

Several strategies are involved in prevention.
- Counsel women with chronic severe mental illness about pregnancy.
- Manic depressive illness: consider restarting treatment after delivery.
- Chronic schizophrenia: maintain medication throughout pregnancy.
- Previous history puerperal psychosis/severe postnatal depression: close contact in the first few weeks following delivery.
- Consider prophylaxis after delivery.
- Assess all women at six-week postnatal check for postnatal depression.

New developments

The role of ovarian hormones in postnatal affective disorder

Both oestrogen and progesterone are popularly thought to be related to female mood disorders, postnatal depression, premenstrual syndrome and perimenopausal depression.

Scientifically ovarian steroids are widely hypothesized to influence mood, cognition and behaviour, although most of the neuroscientific evidence comes from animal studies.

Oestrogen influences the sexual differentiation of the fetal mammalian brain, the development and maintenance in the mature brain of monoamine neurones and pathways (both dopamine and serotonin). Oestrogen receptors are found in greatest numbers in the same part of the brain thought to be responsible for mood and cognition. Oestrogen increases the number of 5 HT (serotonin) receptor sites and both intra- and extracellular levels of serotonin. Oestrogen increases the number of dopaminergic receptor sites and changes in oestrogen levels result in an increased sensitivity of D2 receptors. Oestrogen also, by influencing neurotrophin production and by acting as an antioxidant exerts a protective effect on neurones.

Progesterone receptor sites are found in large numbers in the areas of the brain where the GABA (gamma-aminobutyric acid) receptors are sited and exerts a sedative effect. Progesterone increases dopaminergic activity in the oestrogen-primed brain. There is some evidence that progesterone reduces extracellular levels of serotonin in the brains of rats.

Theoretically oestrogen is an antidepressant and progesterone potentially a depressant. Both changes in oestrogen level (premenstrually, postnatally and perimenopausally) and relatively 'low' levels of oestrogen could be linked to depression particularly in situations where progesterone levels are relatively high. The neuroprotective effect of oestrogen is thought to contribute to the relatively low rates (compared to men) of neurodevelopmental disorders and schizophrenia. The withdrawal of this protection perimenopausally is thought to contribute to the female excess of late onset schizophrenia, Alzheimer's disease and the risk of developing tardive dyskinesia.

There is however no evidence to suggest that the absolute levels of progesterone or oestrogen are any different in women who suffer from postnatal depression than in those who are well. The 'blues' an essentially normal and benign condition postpartum is thought to be linked to both the absolute (low) level of progesterone and the relative drop from prepartum levels. There are some clinical studies suggesting that oestrogen is an effective antidepressant in non-psychotic postnatal depression and in depression following the menopause, and that oestrogen may augment the effect of antidepressants concurrently administered. Both hormone replacement therapy (HRT) and the combined oral contraceptive pill have been shown to improve the premenstrual syndrome (PMS). However for all of these conditions, antidepressants are also effective and for PMS there is robust evidence for the efficiency of the selective serotonin re-uptake inhibitor (SSRI) group of antidepressants. HRT with oestrogens reduces the risk of developing Alzheimer's disease.

However, attempts to prevent or treat puerperal psychosis with oestrogen have not been successful.

Clinically, administration of progesterone during HRT is associated with lowered mood and an increase in PMS-like symptoms even in hysterectomized patients. Concerns about the effect on mood in vulnerable individuals have been expressed in relation to progesterone-only contraception.

In summary, the popular view of PMS and postnatal depression as a progesterone-deficiency disorder is questionable scientifically. Its treatment by progesterone is not based on any robust evidence of clinical efficacy, indeed there is some evidence that it is 'depressogenic'.

Whilst the evidence for oestrogen therapy is more encouraging, its efficiency remains to be proven by more randomized controlled trials.

On balance, treatment with oestrogens should not be the first line treatment for a postnatal depressive illness but may be useful if antidepressants are not tolerated or are ineffective.

🔑 Key Points

- Although few psychotropic drugs are known to be teratogenic or to have adverse effects on the developing fetus or neonate, no psychotropic drug is of proven safety
- It is therefore very important that psychotropic medication should not be prescribed lightly during pregnancy or lactation and that such drugs should be prescribed only where there are positive indications for their use
- Close collaboration between obstetrician and psychiatrist is recommended before treatment of a mental illness with psychotropic medication
- Breastfeeding should not be routinely suspended in mothers who require psychotropic medication
- There is an adequate range of psychotropic drugs available to treat safely the pregnant or lactating woman who is mentally ill

CASE HISTORY

Mrs B

42-year-old professional, married for 16 years and in comfortable circumstances. No family history of psychiatric disorder, nor a previous personal history. However, she had always been anxious with marked obsessional (perfectionist) personality traits and in the past had not coped well with changes.

She had a long history of infertility investigations and had conceived her two children with IVF.

Following the birth of her first child, she found it difficult to adjust to her new lifestyle and suffered from self-doubt and mild anxiety and depression which spontaneously resolved following her return to work at six months postpartum.

Four years later following the birth of her second child, she became severely depressed. By six weeks postpartum she had marked psychomotor slowing and impaired concentration and efficiency. She had early morning wakening and her mood and coping abilities were worst in the morning (diurnal variation of mood). She was very anxious and had panic attacks triggered by intrusive morbid thoughts of some terrible harm coming to her infant. She had overvalued ideas of guilt and incompetence and actively concealed her state from her health visitor and GP. A good friend insisted that she seek help.

Within two weeks of starting a tricyclic antidepressant, dothiepin 150 mg (she was breastfeeding) she began to recover and was quite well by three months postpartum. She reduced her antidepressants gradually and stopped taking them six months later and has remained well.

Neonatology

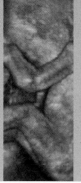

OVERVIEW

More than half a million babies are born every year in the UK, 4 million in the USA and 132 million worldwide. In the developed world less than 1 per cent of these babies will die, and at least half the deaths are amongst very premature babies with a birth weight of less than 1.5 kg. The picture is very different in the developing world, where the death rate is between 20 and 80 per 1000. The 29 countries in sub-Saharan Africa suffer the highest perinatal mortality rates in the world, around 80 per 1000 live births. In the developing world babies are dying from infections (including malaria and neonatal tetanus), malnutrition, lethal congenital malformations and hypoxic ischaemic encephalopathy.

THE CHALLENGE OF NEONATOLOGY

Neonatology is a relatively new sub-specialty that has achieved some spectacular successes, most notably improving the outcome for very premature babies threefold over the last thirty years. Considerable challenges remain; for example there has been very little advance in the treatment of seizures and noso-comial infection is still a problem. Antenatal diagnosis of a whole range of disorders from cystic adenomatoid malformation of the lung through to dilatation of the renal pelvis has resulted in large numbers of asymptomatic infants presenting to the neonatologist. For many of these conditions there is insufficient information about the natural history of the disorder if left untreated, and this information

could help management decisions. Early discharge ('drive-through' delivery) and choice in the place of delivery has fragmented the delivery of 'well baby' care. This means that all those who come into contact with newborns need to be informed about issues such as prophylaxis against vitamin K deficiency bleeding, promotion of breastfeeding, the management of jaundice and the implementation of child health screening policies.

ORGANIZATION AND DELIVERY OF NEONATAL CARE

About 10 per cent of all babies in the UK are admitted to neonatal units, with a wide range between hospitals from 4 to 35 per cent. Most of these admissions are for 'special care'; for example jaundice requiring phototherapy or blood glucose monitoring. Maternity units which provide 'transitional care', usually on postnatal wards staffed with midwives with experience and expertise in the care of the well small baby, have reduced admissions to their special care nurseries to 5 per cent. About 2 per cent of babies need full intensive care, mainly because they are born very prematurely and need artificial ventilation for respiratory distress syndrome (RDS). This roughly equates to a need for 1.1 intensive care cots per 1000 live births. The number of babies treated with intensive care techniques has grown rapidly, doubling in the 1980s. The increasing demand has led to a growth in the number of centres offering neonatal intensive care in the UK, with at least half of this work currently being carried out in units with fewer than four intensive care beds. Fluctuations in demand lead to transports over long distances. Table 22.1 gives a sample from the current UK definitions of special care, high-dependency care, and intensive care. The British Association of Perinatal Medicine has published these definitions in full, together with comprehensive standards for staffing, service size and management of neonatal intensive care services. These represent best practice in the UK and can be used to audit local services.

Table 22.1 – Categories of babies requiring neonatal care

Level 1 intensive care (maximal intensive care)

Care given in an intensive care nursery that provides continuous skilled supervision by qualified and specially trained nursing and medical staff.
Examples of level 1 intensive care include babies who are:
1. receiving assisted ventilation (including continuous positive airways pressure) and in the first 24 hr following withdrawal.
2. <27weeks' gestation and/or less than 1000 g for the first 48 hr post-delivery.

Level 2 intensive care (high-dependency intensive care)

Care given in an intensive care nursery which provides continuous skilled supervision by qualified and specially trained nursing staff who may care for more babies than in Level 1 care. Medical supervision is not so immediate as in Level 1 care.
Examples of level 2 intensive care includes babies who are:
1. requiring parenteral nutrition.
2. requiring oxygen 40–60% or have arterial lines or chest drains.

Special care

Care given in a special care nursery, transitional care ward, or postnatal ward which provides care and treatment exceeding normal routine care. A mother who is supervised by qualified nursing staff may undertake some aspects of special care.
Examples of special care includes babies who are:
1. being given IV glucose and electrolyte solutions.
2. being tube fed.
3. undergoing phototherapy.
4. receiving special monitoring (for example frequent glucose or bilirubin estimations).
5. needing constant supervision (for example babies whose mothers are drug addicts).

Resuscitation

The vast majority of babies achieve a remarkably smooth transition from intrauterine to extrauterine life, breathing within a minute of birth. Fetal lungs are filled with fluid and during labour, production of this fluid ceases and reabsorption begins, influenced by catecholamines. More lung fluid is squeezed out of the thorax during delivery. Finally, the infant takes his first gasp, establishing an air–liquid interface that moves rapidly down through the lungs. The last vestiges of lung fluid are absorbed by the lymphatics and the pulmonary capillaries. At the same time as the lungs are filled with air, the blood supply to them increases dramatically. Pulmonary blood flow is low in fetal life because a high resistance is actively maintained in the pulmonary capillaries. Immediately after birth the pulmonary vascular resistance starts to fall. The fall is driven by the release of vasoactive substances including prostaglandins and nitric oxide, and by the presence of oxygenated blood in the pulmonary capillaries themselves.

Infants who fail to breathe after birth may do so as a result of a deprivation of oxygen and blood supply to the brain before birth (hypoxia-ischaemia or asphyxia), or because they have a central nervous system or muscle disease or because they are systemically ill with infection. The possible placental and other mechanisms that cause hypoxia-ischaemia are discussed on page 122. The asphyxiated infant may have taken his last gasp (terminal apnoea) at birth or be in the phase of primary apnoea. An infant in terminal apnoea is unlikely to recover without intubation and positive pressure ventilation. Infants who have never breathed have failed to establish any air-liquid interface and bag and mask resuscitation is ineffective. Our understanding of the newborn's response to asphyxia is based on the classic primate experiments of Dawes. The changes in respiration and heart rate following asphyxia are illustrated in Fig. 22.1.

All professionals who attend deliveries must be able to recognize when a baby is not establishing normal respiration and circulation, and be trained to initiate resuscitation. Certain situations are clearly high risk, and a person with intubation skills should be present at the delivery. Examples of such situations are given below.

The Apgar score

The Apgar score is a tool that assists in the recognition of an infant who is failing to make a successful transition to extrauterine life. The Apgar score was

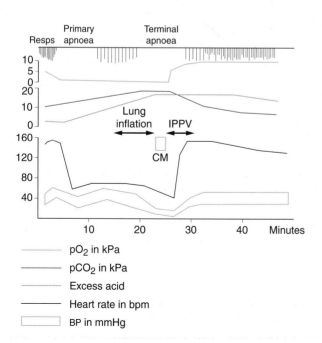

Figure 22.1 The response to asphyxia (from the Northern Region handbook, with permission). IPPV: intermittent positive pressure ventilation. CM: cardiac massage.

🔑 Key Points

Deliveries where a trained neonatal resuscitator should be present

- Preterm deliveries
- Vaginal breech deliveries
- Thick meconium staining of the amniotic fluid
- Significant fetal distress
- Significant antepartum haemorrhage
- Serious fetal abnormality (e.g. hydrops, diaphragmatic hernia)
- Rotational forceps or vacuum deliveries
- Caesarean section — unless elective and under regional anaesthesia
- Multiple deliveries

designed to do this, and in this respect it performs admirably. The reason for a low Apgar score may not be asphyxia, but the baby certainly has a problem and the sooner it is recognized and treated the better. The original Apgar score (Table 22.2) includes an item (grimace) which reports the infant's response to a suction catheter applied to the nostrils. However, frequent application of a suction catheter in this way can cause bradycardia, and although regular recording of the Apgar score is to be encouraged this item carries less weight than the heart rate, colour or breathing pattern. The Apgar score is usually awarded at one and five minutes. If the Apgar score is still low at five minutes further observations should be made at intervals. The Apgar score cannot replace a detailed narrative describing the baby's condition, the resuscitative efforts and the response to

resuscitation. Recording the Apgar score is helpful because it has become an internationally recognized shorthand way of summarizing a baby's condition at birth and his response to resuscitation.

Additional points in management

Basic resuscitation

Infants fall into one of three categories within a minute of birth:

1. Pink, breathing, and active with a heart rate of >100 beats per minute.

Leave this baby alone, preferably with his mother. If the baby has been given to you at the resuscitaire, dry him, wrap him in a warm towel and give him back to the mother. Do not suck him out; this risks producing a vagal bradycardia and cools him.

2. Not breathing regularly, but with a heart rate of >100 and centrally cyanosed.

Dry the baby and place under a radiant heat source wrapped in a warm dry towel. Drying often provides enough stimulation to induce breathing, but gentle rubbing can also be used. Offer supplementary oxygen. If there is no response, begin active resuscitation and call for help.

3. Not breathing or has a heart rate of <100 or is pale.

This baby is in need of prompt resuscitation and will not recover without it. Dry him quickly, place on the resuscitation surface in a warm dry towel and call for help. Initiate basic resuscitation with mask ventilation. If the heart rate remains less than 60 bpm commence chest compressions. If there isn't a rapid response proceed to intubation as soon as a person with the necessary skill arrives. Stay to help; a full-blown resuscitation is a job for at least two people.

Table 22.2 – The Apgar score

	Score	0	1	2
A	Appearance: central trunk colour	Pale	Blue	Pink (extremities often blue)
P	Pulse rate*	Absent	<100	>100
G	Grimace	Nil	Grimace	Cry or cough
A	Activity (muscle tone)	Limp	Some flexion	Well flexed
R	Respiratory effort	Absent	Gasping or irregular	Strong cry

* best to record the actual rate

Lung inflation through a face mask

Position the baby face upward on a resuscitation surface; a head down slope is not necessary. The head should be supported in a neutral position to keep the tongue from obstructing the back of the pharynx. Gently suction the mouth and nostrils to remove debris. Choose a face mask which covers the baby's mouth and nose but does not press on the eyes or overhang the chin (Fig. 22.2a). Hold the mask over the baby's face with one hand, using some of the fingers of the same hand to support the jaw (Fig. 22.2b). Begin to ventilate the lungs with air or oxygen using the source provided.

Use of drugs during resuscitation

Drugs are very rarely required during neonatal resuscitation and deciding to use them is a job for an experienced operator. Most babies respond to adequate oxygenation. Very occasionally a mother has received pethidine shortly before delivery, and the baby has depressed respiration as a result. This is much less common in clinical practice than in theory. Naloxone is a specific opiate antagonist that can reverse the effects of pethidine. Naloxone administration should not be used as a substitute for ineffective resuscitation, and is specifically contraindicated in babies born to drug-abusing mothers.

Ethical issues surrounding resuscitation

This is an area that generates a great deal of anxiety. A junior doctor suddenly faced with a very preterm or abnormal baby is not in the right place at the right time, nor are they sufficiently experienced to make a value judgement about resuscitation of a very preterm or malformed baby. Ideally this situation should be avoided by prior warning, so that a discussion can be held between the most senior paediatrician available, the obstetrician and the parents, also involving the staff which will be present at the delivery. The most senior paediatrician available should attend the delivery of a very preterm infant. Increasingly prior discussion can be achieved because of better antenatal diagnosis and warning of impending preterm delivery. If the parents, after

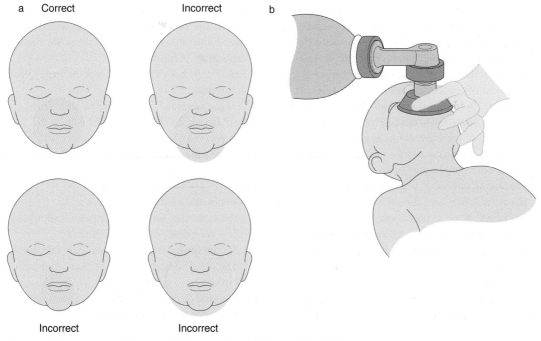

a   Correct   Incorrect   b

Incorrect   Incorrect

Figure 22.2 Correct use of the face mask. (Resuscitation of Newborn Babies, 1998 RCPCH and RCOG BMJ Publications, with permission.)

being informed of the chance of intact survival, do not wish active resuscitation of their baby who will be born at 23 or 24 weeks' gestation, most neonatologists would support their decision and offer 'comfort care' only. Experience teaches that it is wise to warn the parents beforehand that sometimes there is a surprise and the baby is bigger and more mature than expected, in which case it may be appropriate to offer intensive care on a 'wait and see' approach. If there is not time to consult with the parents, or there is any conflict or doubt, then full resuscitation should be offered. Most tiny babies who die do so very quickly, within 24 hours, and the period of intensive care allows time for the parents to take in the situation and to grieve afterwards because they are certain that 'everything has been done'. This course of action avoids the possibility of anger developing because of doubt remaining in the parent's minds.

CARE OF THE NORMAL TERM NEWBORN

Examination of the well term newborn

A thorough physical examination of every neonate is accepted as good practice and forms a core item of the child health surveillance programme in the UK. The aims of the neonatal examination are:

- diagnosis of congenital malformations (present in about 10–15 per 1000 babies; see Table 22.3)
- diagnosis of common minor problems, with advice about management or appropriate reassurance if no intervention is indicated (e.g. Mongolian Blue spots, jaundice, naevi)
- continuing screening, begun antenatally, to identify those babies who should be offered specific intervention, e.g. hepatitis vaccination
- health education advice, e.g. regarding breast feeding, cot death prevention, immunization, safe transport in cars
- general parental reassurance

For some babies early diagnosis may make an enormous difference to their subsequent health: for example in congenital cataract and urethral valves. For others, parental reassurance that their infant is

Table 22.3 – Prevalence of serious congenital malformations per 1000 live births in England and Wales (source: Office for National Statistics)

Congenital heart disease	6-8
Developmental dysplasia of the hip	1.5
Talipes	1.5
Down's syndrome	1.5
Cleft lip and/or palate	1.2
Urogenital (hypospadias, undescended testes)	1.2
Spina bifida/anencephaly	0.5

normal and general advice is all that is required. Every newborn infant deserves at least one full examination. At present this is usually carried out by a doctor, although in some areas midwives are being trained to perform this task. For recording purposes it is useful to have a checklist printed or stamped in the baby's notes to serve as an aide-mémoire. Items are merely ticked if normal but any abnormalities are marked distinctively and a full description written out. The examination should be dated and signed. A suggested order for the examination is as follows.

- Introduce yourself to the mother; ask her about any antenatally diagnosed problems which may need follow-up, any family problems (deafness, dislocation of hips).
- Remove the baby's clothes except the nappy; look at the skin.
- Feel the anterior fontanelle for tension (leave until later if the baby is crying!); palpate the sutures (craniosynostosis is a disorder with premature fusion of the sutures), check the scalp for swellings (a cephalhaematoma is the most common).
- Measure the head circumference.
- Look at the face for colour (cyanosis/pallor/jaundice – see below) or any peculiarities.
- Listen to the heart and estimate heart rate; normally 110–150 beats per minute but can drop to 80 in sleep.
- Count the respiratory rate; normally less than 60 breaths per minute. The lungs can also be auscultated but this is seldom informative.
- Palpate the abdomen; feel for masses including large bladder or kidneys.

- Examine the eyes; check that it is possible to obtain a red reflex using an ophthalmoscope to exclude cataract. Fundal examination is not routine.
- Examine the ears, nose and mouth (cleft palate).
- Examine the neck, including the clavicles.
- Examine the arms, hands, legs and feet.
- Remove the nappy.
- Feel for the femoral pulses.
- Examine the genitalia and anus.
- Turn the baby to the prone position and examine his back and spine; assess tone.
- Return the infant to the supine position and evaluate the central nervous system.
- Examine the hips.
- Make sure you have not omitted anything.

Common minor problems

Erythema toxicum

Erythema toxicum (Fig. 22.3) is a common rash which appears on the second or third day, and takes the form of a white pinpoint 'head' on an oval erythematous base. If the spots are biopsied, massive numbers of eosinophils are found.

Transient neonatal pustular melanosis

Transient neonatal pustular melanosis is commoner in black babies. The eruption starts with small pustule-like spots present at birth and which rapidly progress to a hyperpigmented macule resembling a freckle that fades in a few weeks.

Milia

Milia (Fig. 22.4) are tiny yellowish-white spots, especially common on the nose and elsewhere on the face, which disappear spontaneously over a month or two.

Mongolian blue spots

Mongolian blue spots (Fig. 22.5) are blue–black macular lesions usually situated over the base of the spine commoner in Afro-Carribean or Asian infants. They fade slowly over the first few years.

Port wine stains

Port wine stains are due to a malformation of the capillaries within the dermis. Port wine stains in the region of the trigeminal nerve are sometimes associated with intracranial vascular abnormalities (Sturge-Weber syndrome). Laser therapy can now produce an excellent cosmetic improvement for large facial lesions.

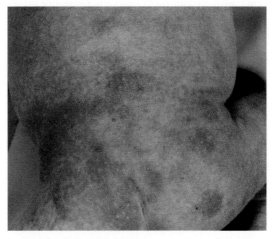

Figure 22.3 Erythema toxicum.

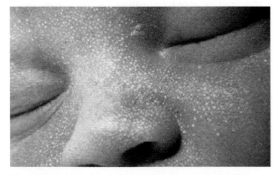

Figure 22.4 Milia (from *A Colour Atlas of the Newborn*, Milner RDG & Herber SM. Wolfe Medical Publications 1994, with permission).

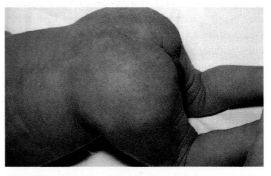

Figure 22.5 Mongolian blue spot (from *A Colour Atlas of the Newborn*, Milner RDG & Herber SM. Wolfe Medical Publications 1994, with permission).

Strawberry naevi

Strawberry naevi are not usually present at birth but appear within the first month. These increase until 6–9 months and then regress, so no treatment is offered unless the naevi interfere with vision or the airway.

Skin tags/extra digits

These should be surgically removed; the old practice of tying a silk thread around them produces a cosmetically inferior result. As these are often familial, examination of the parents will often provide proof of this.

Sacral pits

Sacrococcygeal pits which are in the natal cleft do not communicate with the dura, but any midline lesion which is higher than this should arouse suspicion. Imaging of the spinal cord below the lesion must be done, with ultrasound or magnetic resonance imaging (MRI).

Screening for developmental dysplasia of the hip

Early diagnosis of developmental dysplasia of the hip (DDH) in the neonatal period and expert management can be expected to produce a normal hip, while treatment initiated after the six months of life undoubtedly gives much worse results, even after prolonged and aggressive surgical treatment. Although it is not possible to detect all cases using the current screening methods, this should not be used as an excuse for a poor quality screening programme, as many cases are detectable. The cornerstone of the screening strategy for DDH remains a careful history and clinical examination, using the Ortolani–Barlow manoeuvres. These tests are difficult to describe in words and are best taught by demonstration. Sadly, despite initial confidence in the ability of the Ortolani and Barlow tests to detect DDH, the number of cases diagnosed late (0.2 per 1000) has not reduced. Some dislocated hips are not detectable with clinical examination in the newborn period and others may dislocate later, perhaps due to a shallow acetabulum that progresses to dislocation when weight bearing begins. There may have been a genuine increase in the incidence of the condition.

Ultrasonography can now be added to clinical

<table>
<tr><td>🔧 Key Points</td></tr>
</table>

Screening strategy for using ultrasound in the detection of DDH

- Breech presentation (whether delivered by caesarean section or vaginally)
- Family history of dysplastic hip
- Any deformity suggesting intrauterine compression, or oligohydramnios
- Clicky hip on clinical examination, or one with restricted abduction
- If sufficient manpower available consider first-born females

examination as a further tool for detecting DDH. Ultrasound can detect clinically stable but anatomically abnormal hips, and show normality in clinically suspect hips. DDH is commoner following breech presentation, in females, if there is oligohydramnios, and in those with a positive family history. Many hospitals now offer hip ultrasound examinations to selected high-risk groups; few hospitals have the manpower for universal screening.

Biochemical screening

Screening for phenylketonuria (1 in 13,000 infants) using dried blood spots collected onto filter paper (the Guthrie test) was introduced in 1969. Milk feeds need to be established first, and midwives collect blood by heel prick on the fifth to ninth day of life, posting the cards to the laboratory. The same system was expanded to include a screen for congenital hypothyroidism (1 in 3000) from 1981. Audit of the combined programme shows that it has been extremely successful. Virtually all infants with congenital hypothyroidism now start treatment by 28 days of age and have a better IQ as a result.

The dried blood spot can be used to screen for cystic fibrosis (measuring imunoreactive trypsin) and haemoglobinopathies such as sickle cell haemoglobin or thalassaemia. Tests are also available for a whole host of other rare conditions including maple syrup urine disease, homocystinuria, tyrosinaemia, biotinidase deficiency, galactosaemia, medium chain acyl-CoA dehydrogenase deficiency, Duchenne muscular dystrophy, fragile X syndrome and congenital adrenal hyperplasia but none have been implemented. Widespread screening for neonatal neuroblastoma using vanillyl mandelic acid (VMA) levels in urine did not prove cost-effective in Canada and seems unlikely to be introduced world-wide, apart from in Japan where the incidence is peculiarly high.

Prevention of vitamin K deficiency bleeding (haemorrhagic disease of the newborn)

Vitamin K deficiency bleeding (VKDB) occurs in three forms:

- Very early VKDB. This is limited to babies whose mothers have taken drugs which interfere with the manufacture of vitamin K-dependent clotting factors, such as antituberculous or anticonvulsant drugs. These mothers should be given extra vitamin K (5 mg daily) in the last month of pregnancy.
- Classical VKDB presents on days 2–7 of life, with bleeding from the umbilical stump, bruising or melaena. The mortality of classical VKDB is low, and the disorder can be prevented by a single dose of vitamin K given to the baby by any route.
- Late VKDB occurs virtually exclusively in babies who are breastfed, unless they have liver disease. Small warning bleeds from the gums are a common feature, but the worst problems are associated with the high (50 per cent) chance of intracranial haemorrhage, which can cause permanent neurological handicap.

Late onset VKDB can be prevented by a single intramuscular dose of vitamin K given at birth, but a single oral dose is ineffective. Intramuscular vitamin K has become less popular since the suggestion that it may be linked to later childhood leukaemia. Although confirmation is lacking, a definite refutation of this hypothesis is unlikely because of the enormous numbers of babies who would need to be involved in a trial. The UK Department of Health has recently endorsed two alternative regimens, either a single dose of intramuscular vitamin K or repeated oral doses. What is clear is that all infants must be offered vitamin K prophylaxis; there is no longer any place for selective regimens. If parents refuse vitamin K for their baby after counselling, the reasons for the refusal should be clearly documented.

Confirmation of the diagnosis of VKDB is obtained from coagulation tests, which show a normal platelet count and prolonged thrombin and prothrombin times. Treatment is with IV vitamin K and fresh frozen plasma.

Jaundice

At least two-thirds of all babies develop jaundice in the first week of life, and jaundice is the most common reason requiring readmission to hospital at this time. This reflects the immaturity of the liver's excretory pathway for bilirubin at a time of heightened production. In healthy term infants bilirubin rises over the first few days, and jaundice is not apparent on the first day of life. Any visible jaundice in the first 24 hours must be urgently investigated, and assumed to be due to haemolysis (rhesus incompatibility, ABO incompatibility, G6PD deficiency) until proved otherwise. Neonatal 'physiological' jaundice is contributed to by a high neonatal haematocrit, short red cell survival, breastfeeding and an initial absence of gut bacteria. Although neonatal jaundice is usually benign, it is a dangerous fallacy to assume that healthy term newborns are immune from kernicterus (yellow staining of the basal ganglia by bilirubin). In the current era of short postpartum hospital stay kernicterus has re-emerged in this group. Survivors are severely handicapped by athetoid cerebral palsy, classically with accompanying sensorineural deafness, paralysis of upgaze and dental enamel dysplasia. The level of unconjugated bilirubin at which kernicterus can occur in well term infants is not known with certainty, but appears to lie somewhere between 425 and 600 μmol/L. Only 1 in 770 normal term infants reach a level above 425 μmol/L. The risk of kernicterus is probably greater for an infant of 37 weeks' compared to one of 41 weeks' gestation (see case history).

The key to successful kernicterus prevention lies in detecting the very few healthy (usually breastfed) babies who are likely to develop a serum unconjugated bilirubin of more than 425 μmol/L. It is possible to predict the peak serum bilirubin from an early level measured before neonatal discharge. Infants 'track' for serum bilirubin, so that an infant who is on the 50th centile at 48 hours (136 μmol/L) will not develop a dangerous level unless a new complication develops. An infant with a similar level at 24 hours, however, is tracking along the 95th centile and needs a repeat estimation. Such an infant may not be suitable for early discharge unless the parents are willing

CASE HISTORY

Baby Kieran was born at 35 weeks' gestation, by normal vertex vaginal delivery weighing 2.7 kg. His mother had gone into labour following preterm rupture of membranes. Baby Kieran was in excellent condition at birth, with Apgar scores of 9[1] and 9[5] and a cord pH of 7.34. He required no resuscitation and went to the postnatal ward with his mother. The midwives noted jaundice for the first time when the child was about 28 hours old. The bilirubin was checked about 24 hours later and revealed a result of 279 µmol/L. On the following day the same doctor examined him who thought that the jaundice was unchanged and allowed him to go home. Midwives visited baby Kieran at home who reassured his young, first-time mother that his jaundice was not serious. He became lethargic. On the eighth day his concerned parents took him to the local casualty department, where he was noted to be very jaundiced, cool and feeding poorly. Blood was taken in the A&E department at midnight which revealed a serum bilirubin of 570 µmol/L. Baby Kieran was admitted to the ward where the following morning he was noted to be irritable, tense on handling and to be extending his neck (opisthotonic). He is handicapped with sensorineural hearing loss and athetoid cerebral palsy. He was recently awarded substantial damages after a successful claim of medical negligence.

to return to the hospital. In the meanwhile, all those who come into contact with babies in the first week of life need education about assessment of jaundice. All too often the early signs of bilirubin encephalopathy (lethargy, irritability, poor suck, shrill cry) are ignored. Assessing the level of jaundice from clinical examination can be difficult, especially in racially pigmented babies. Various transcutaneous bilirubinometers are under evaluation and may assist in reducing the traffic of blood samples (and babies) to and from maternity hospitals. One simple cheap device, the Gosset icterometer, consists of a plastic strip with coloured bars, and this can improve the clinical assessment of jaundice in the home (Fig. 22.6). The dermal zones of Kramer use the fact that jaundice stains the skin from the head to the feet in babies, and when the hands and feet are involved a level of more than 300 µmol/L can be anticipated. Babies who are thought to have a bilirubin level of more that 340 µmol/L should have a serum bilirubin estimation carried out. If this level is confirmed phototherapy should be offered, and at present this requires readmission to hospital in most areas of the UK. Phototherapy, used correctly, is a remarkably effective treatment and is capable of converting a fifth of the circulating unconjugated bilirubin to harmless photoisomers within a few hours.

Management of common malformations

Gastroschisis

This abdominal wall defect has increased in frequency in recent years and is usually diagnosed antenatally. Although the abnormality is a dramatic one, often with much of the gut outside the body (Fig. 22.7a), the defect is not usually associated with other malformations and is amenable to surgery. The immediate management involves preventing heat loss by wrapping the exposed gut in clingfilm, and general intensive care support. Surgery is carried out as an emergency. Usually the operation is a one-stage procedure but occasionally there is not enough room in the abdominal cavity. During a staged closure the exposed bowel is protected with a silo which is gradually reduced in size over a week or two. The prognosis is good with 90 per cent of individuals leading normal lives after neonatal surgical repair. Unfortunately a small proportion of children have long-term problems, including short gut syndrome, liver damage from prolonged total parenteral nutrition, and later adhesions.

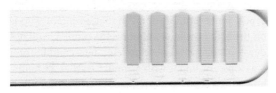

Figure 22.6 The Gosset icterometer.

Exomphalos (omphalocele)

This condition is distinct from gastroschisis because the bowel herniates into the umbilical cord rather than through an abdominal wall defect (Fig. 22.7b). The two conditions can be distinguished antenatally and were recognized as definitely distinct in 1967.

Exomphalos results from a failure of closure of one of the embryological folds that form the anterior abdominal wall. Infants with this condition frequently have other major malformations including heart disease. The liver is often included in the defect and its lobulation is frequently abnormal. This may be associated with Beckwith–Weidemann syndrome, which is characterized by exomphalos, macroglossia, visceromegaly, gigantism and hyperinsulinaemic hypoglycaemia. These children have a high incidence of malignancies outside the neonatal period, and the genetic defect has been localised to chromosome 11.

Spina bifida

Spina bifida has become a very rare neonatal condition. The incidence was falling before the discovery that maternal folate ingestion could go some way to preventing the problem, and many parents now choose to terminate the pregnancy if an open lesion is diagnosed on a routine fetal anomaly scan. In 1993 the Office of National Statistics recorded over 500 terminations of pregnancy for CNS defects but only 81 spina bifida live births in England and Wales, compared to over 1000 spina bifida births in 1974. Babies born with spina bifida often have a small skin covered lesion (a meningocoele) which was not diagnosable with antenatal ultrasound. These are easily removed surgically, and the prognosis depends on whether or not the sac contained any nerve roots (making the lesion a myelomeningocoele) and whether the spinal cord becomes tethered. The main neurological problems in the survivors are incontinence of the bladder and bowel with gait abnormalities due to involvement of the lower sacral nerves.

Hydrocephalus

Hydrocephalus often accompanies spina bifida, because most children with this condition have the Arnold–Chiari malformation. Indeed, the low-lying cerebellar tonsils are the anatomical features behind the 'lemon' and 'banana' signs that are detected antenatally. Dilated ventricles in the brain occurring without an associated spina bifida malformation are also quite common although the number of live births in the UK has declined from 313 in 1974 to 71 in 1993, largely as a result of antenatal diagnosis and termination of pregnancy. Congenital hydrocephalus not associated with spina bifida may be a single genetic abnormality or may be associated with other congenital CNS malformations such as the Dandy-Walker malformation. Congenital aqueduct stenosis is the most common of these. There is a rare genetic sex-linked form of aqueduct stenosis confined to males, associated with flexion and adduction defects of the thumbs.

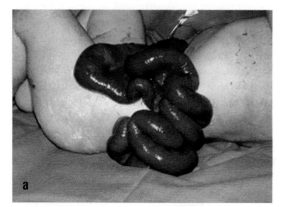

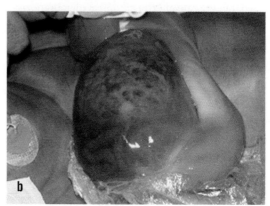

Figure 22.7 (a) gastroschisis, (b) exomphalos.

Cardiac defects

Although antenatal cardiac diagnosis is possible in expert hands, most major cardiac lesions are still unsuspected antenatally. Congenital heart disease affects about 8 per 1000 live births, and 30–40 per cent of these children will be symptomatic in early infancy. Important physical signs of heart disease include central cyanosis, poor peripheral perfusion, respiratory distress and heart murmurs although serious cardiac malformation can be present without a murmur. Echocardiography has revolutionized the early diagnosis of congenital heart disease and cardiac catheterization is now rarely necessary. Any suspicion of the cyanotic conditions of transposition of the great vessels, pulmonary atresia or tetralogy of Fallot should be followed by administration of prostin E2 to maintain ductal patency and transfer to a regional cardiac centre without delay. The prognosis for many congenital cyanotic heart lesions is now excellent although complex heart disease with pulmonary atresia remains an exception.

Diaphragmatic hernia

This defect remains a challenge, and the survival has not improved from the 50–60 per cent achieved since the mid-1970s. The reason for the considerable mortality in this condition is the associated pulmonary hypoplasia. Modern management consists of paralysis and artificial ventilation from birth, decompression of the bowel, and delayed surgery. Surfactant, nitric oxide, and oscillatory ventilation have all been tried, but the role of extra corporeal membrane oxygenation (ECMO) remains unproven. Antenatally diaphragmatic hernia is an indication for delivery in a centre with facilities for neonatal intensive care. Long-term problems include poor pulmonary function, scoliosis, gastro-oesopheageal reflux and neurological impairment.

Congenital cystic adenomatoid malformation of the lung (CCAM)

This condition is increasingly diagnosed antenatally, and as in many other conditions antenatal diagnosis has altered our perception of the natural history. The malformation consists of a mass of cysts lined by proliferating bronchial or cuboidal epithelium with intervening portions of normal lung. The defect is almost always restricted to one lung, usually only one lobe is affected. CCAM is a cause of hydrops and these infants are often stillborn. Other babies present with symptoms of acute respiratory distress and some are asymptomatic. The management of asymptomatic infants with a confirmed diagnosis of CCAM (using computerized tomography scanning) is controversial, but increasingly early operation is recommended because of the risk of infection in the abnormal lobe.

Cleft lip and palate

This common disorder causes great distress to parents, and the parent support groups have encouraged the recent drive towards very early lip closure. Whilst this can be done before the baby goes home for the first time it is the long-term results of this condition which are important. A recent survey revealed that many children suffer from mid-facial hypoplasia and dental problems in later childhood. Optimal management requires referral to a large centre which deals with many cases each year and includes a team incorporating dentists and speech therapists.

Infant feeding

Breastfeeding

Breast milk is the ideal food for babies for the first 4–6 months of life. Human milk contains the carbohydrate lactose, and the proteins casein, a-lactalbumin, immunoglobulin and lactoferrin. Human milk is whey predominant (60:40 whey/casein ratio) and is easily digested. Lactoferrin combines with other anti-infective agents such as lysozyme, and the overall effect is to ensure that breast-fed babies are well protected from gastrointestinal and other infections. The fat in human milk is predominantly unsaturated and there are long chain polyunsaturated fatty acids (LCPUFAs) which may provide important precursors for the infant's nervous system. Cow's milk contains much more protein than human milk (3.5 g/dL versus 1 g/dL), the protein is casein predominant and the whey protein differs from human milk (β-lactoglobulin not α-lactalbumin). Casein is the constituent of milk which forms a curd precipitate with acid.

There is a delay of 48 hours before copious milk secretion begins in women. This is unusual; in all animals except guinea pigs lactogenesis takes place within hours of parturition. Lactogenesis is initiated by the slowly falling progesterone levels in the presence of a high prolactin concentration. In an attempt to reverse the trend away from breastfeeding, the World Health Organization has proposed ten steps as a core item of its Baby Friendly Hospital Initiative. This programme has been very successful; for example neonatal infection was reduced from 23 to 3.4 per cent in one Romanian hospital.

Formula feeding

Modern formula milks are adjusted (humanized) so that the protein content and the whey/casein ratio is nearer that of human milk. Manufacturers do this by adding demineralized whey (from cheese production) and lactose but differences in the fatty acid and amino acid composition remain, and formula milk cannot contain any of the anti-infective agents. There is no evidence to support the claim that formulae with a higher casein content are more satisfying for the hungry and demanding baby. Additives are required to emulsify and thicken the milk. Water is required to reconstitute milk powder. Some products sold as 'natural mineral water' contain unacceptably high levels of sodium and nitrate for babies and are unsuitable for rehydrating dried formula milk.

Unmodified 'doorstep' cow's, sheep's and goat's milk are completely unsuitable foods for babies less than a year old. The electrolyte composition is vastly different from human milk and they are highly allergenic. Soy formulae have no lactose, the carbohydrate being derived from corn syrup and sucrose. Soy protein is nutritionally inferior to human milk protein and infants grow less well on soy milk. The only reason to use soy formula is if the infant has a cow's milk allergy or requires a lactose-free formula.

Hypoglycaemia

Healthy term babies of appropriate weight, particularly those who are breast-fed on demand, have lower

🔧 Key Points

The WHO Ten Steps to successful breastfeeding
- Have a written breastfeeding policy that is routinely communicated to all healthcare staff
- Train all healthcare staff in the skills necessary to implement this policy
- Inform all pregnant women about the benefits and management of breastfeeding
- Help mothers initiate breastfeeding within half an hour of birth
- Show mothers how to breastfeed and how to maintain lactation even if they are separated from their infants
- Give newborn infants no food or drink other than breast milk unless medically indicated
- Practise rooming-in (allow mothers and infants to stay together) 24 hours a day
- Encourage breastfeeding on demand
- Give no artificial teats or pacifiers (also called dummies or soothers) to breastfeeding infants
- Foster the establishment of breastfeeding support groups and refer mothers to them on discharge from the hospital or clinic

blood glucose concentrations than formula-fed babies in the first 2–3 days of life. They also have raised ketone body concentrations and the neonatal brain can use ketone bodies as an alternative fuel. Healthy term babies who are breastfeeding on demand do not need to have their blood glucose concentrations measured. There is no agreement on a lower limit of normal in this situation; bedside testing with reagent strips is notoriously inaccurate, and there is no evidence that a lower limit exists below which asymptomatic 'hypoglycaemia' is damaging. Recognition of these facts makes the use of supplementary feeding less likely and encourages breastfeeding.

However, there are babies who are at high risk of developing symptomatic hypoglycaemia. Occasionally an apparently healthy term baby has a rare condition such as idiopathic hyperinsulinaemic hypoglycaemia of infancy (formerly called neisidioblastosis) or medium chain acyl coenzyme A dehydrogenase (MCAD) deficiency which will manifest as symptomatic hypoglycaemia in the first days of life. In these situations prolonged symptomatic hypoglycaemia can occur which is undoubtedly damaging to the brain (see case history). A difficult balance needs to be struck between screening for, and preventing,

CASE HISTORY

Hypoglycaemia

Baby Jack was born at 35 weeks' gestation, the second twin. He was in good condition at birth and did not require resuscitation. He went to the postnatal ward with his mother and brother. Because he was preterm, and of low weight, glucose screening was instituted. The blood glucose measured using a Yellow Springs glucometer (this hospital did not use glucose testing stix in view of their inaccuracy) was 1.1 at four hours and remained between 0.7 and 1.5 over the first night in spite of formula feeds of increasing volume. Baby Jack was asymptomatic until the morning, when he had a seizure. At this point he was admitted to the nursery and a glucose infusion commenced. Cranial ultrasonography revealed a large intracerebral haemorrhage. Subsequent investigation led to a diagnosis of transient hyperinsulinaemia of prematurity that resolved. Baby Jack has an evolving spastic hemiplegia.

Infants at risk of developing symptomatic hypoglycaemia

- Intrauterine growth restriction
- Infants of diabetic mothers
- Preterm infants
- Infants who have suffered fetal distress in labour
- Infants who are large-for-dates – possibility of undiagnosed maternal gestational diabetes

symptomatic hypoglycaemia in at-risk infants and recognizing symptomatic hypoglycaemia in infants who are ill whilst avoiding overinvestigation and overtreatment for the normal term baby whose mother is trying to establish breastfeeding. Unnecessary supplementary feeds are the principle reason why mothers abandon breastfeeding.

Symptoms of hypoglycaemia in the newborn are vague and include apathy/floppiness, apnoea and excessive jitteriness. These non-specific symptoms can also be due to sepsis. If a term baby of normal weight is sleepy (perhaps from the pethidine given to the mother) they will need help to feed directly from the breast or to be given expressed colostrum if they cannot suck, not a glucose level. However if the symptoms worsen the baby must be examined fully by a paediatrician and investigations considered to exclude sepsis and/or hypoglycaemia. Checking a glucose level in this situation is not an excuse for omitting a proper examination. Early jaundice, fever, tachypnoea and poor capillary refill are indications for investigation and treatment.

Symptomatic hypoglycaemia should be prevented in at-risk babies by screening and supplementary feeding. Small for gestational age babies can require as much as 12 mg/kg per min to maintain glucose levels. Symptomatic hypoglycaemia in term babies is rare, and investigation and treatment is an emergency. Blood samples for true glucose, insulin and ketone body levels should be collected at the same time as commencing an IV infusion of 10 per cent dextrose. Boluses of dextrose should be avoided.

CARE OF THE ILL TERM NEWBORN

A brief description of a few of the more common and serious illnesses that afflict term newborns follows.

Birth trauma

Birth trauma is thankfully rare in modern neonatal practice, but occasional cases are still encountered.

Erb's palsy is caused by damage to the brachial plexus. It is more common in large babies, particularly in those where delivery is complicated by shoulder dystocia. A brachial plexus lesion is revealed by lack of movement in the arm; initially the arm is flaccid. After 48 hours an upper palsy can be distinguished from a complete palsy. In an upper root palsy (C5, C6, sometimes C7) the arm is internally rotated and pronated, there is no active abduction or elbow flexion (Fig. 22.8, the waiter's tip position). In a complete palsy of upper and lower roots the arm is flail; there may be a ptosis and a Horner's syndrome due to damage to the stellate ganglion adjacent to C8 and T1. Phrenic nerve palsy should be considered in these cases. Whilst the prognosis of brachial plexus

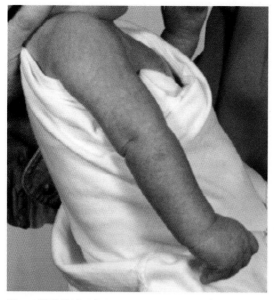

Figure 22.8 Erb's palsy.

lesions is generally good, with most series reporting an initial recovery rate of 75–95 per cent, a recent study of the long-term effects revealed a surprisingly high incidence of later problems in childhood. The results of surgical nerve repair have improved markedly since the early days and babies who have no recovery in biceps function by three months should be referred to a specialist.

Subgaleal (subaponeurotic) haemorrhage

The subaponeurotic space is potentially very large, lying as it does outside the skull and below the scalp (Fig. 22.9). Babies who bleed into this space can become shocked, and there is a mortality of 20 per cent. The condition is fortunately rare after normal vertex vaginal delivery but is reported in as many as 6 per 1000 babies delivered by the ventouse. The current recommendation of the UK Royal College of Obstetricians is that the ventouse is to be preferred for instrumental delivery, and this will mean that early recognition of subgaleal haemorrhage becomes more important. The clue to the diagnosis is a boggy swelling of the scalp that crosses suture lines. The baby's head circumference will have increased at least 1 cm from the birth measurement. When appropriately recognized and treated with blood transfusion the long-term prognosis is good.

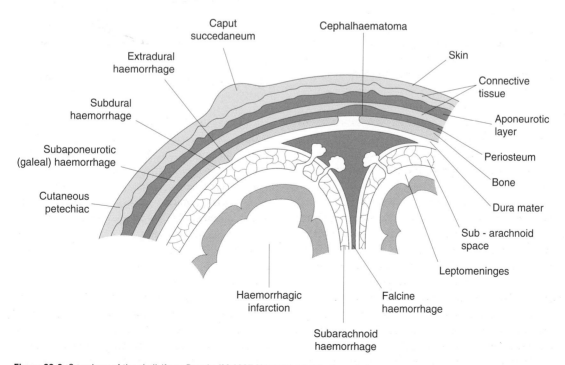

Figure 22.9 Coverings of the skull (from Rennie JM 1997 Neonatal cranial ultrasound, Cambridge University Press, with permission).

Transient tachypnoea of the newborn

Transient tachypnoea of the newborn (TTN) is the commonest respiratory disease of term infants, occurring in 4 per 1000. The disease is due to delayed clearance of lung liquid and is much more common after Caesarean Section delivery, particularly without labour. At term the incidence falls between 37 and 40 weeks (Fig. 22.10), and this finding has implications for the timing of elective Caesarean Section at term. Fortunately the disease is usually mild, but sometimes requires intubation and ventilation with the associated risk of complications this involves.

Meconium aspiration syndrome

Meconium aspiration syndrome (MAS) is a disease of post-term pregnancies, with an incidence of about 1:1000 total births in Europe and 2–6 per 1000 in the USA. Meconium can be aspirated before or after birth. Fetuses do not normally draw amniotic fluid into the airway but gasp when asphyxiated and the co-existence of asphyxia is the main determining factor in

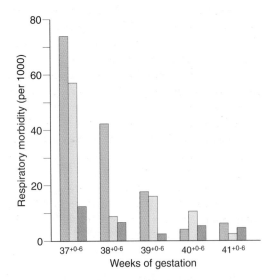

Figure 22.10 Respiratory morbidity (TTN plus RDS) at term in infants admitted to the NICU, Rosie Maternity Hospital, Cambridge by each week of gestation and mode of delivery. (From Morrison, Rennie and Milton 1995 Neonatal respiratory morbidity and mode of delivery at term: influence of timing of elective caesarean section. British Journal of Obstetrics and Gynaecology 102:101–106, with permission.)

MAS. Asphyxia exerts its own detrimental effect on lung function and is associated with the development of persistent pulmonary hypertension that complicates the treatment of MAS still further. These problems, together with a pre-existing aspiration of meconium into the airway which is not amenable to even the most aggressive suctioning at delivery, combines to make MAS a very serious neonatal illness.

The fact that some cases cannot be prevented by tracheal toilet should not discourage attempts at preventing meconium entering the airway at birth. Suctioning on the perineum has been shown to be effective in preventing MAS. Meconium in the airway creates a ball-valve effect in which air can be sucked past the obstruction but not exhaled past it, and the substance acts as a chemical irritant to the airways. Any reduction in the load is useful.

Persistent pulmonary hypertension

The term persistent pulmonary hypertension (PPHN) is preferable to that of persistent fetal circulation because the placenta is no longer in the circuit. In this disorder the baby is cyanosed because there is a failure of the usual rapid postnatal fall in pulmonary vascular resistance. There is no parenchymal lung disease, but the pulmonary capillaries are structurally abnormal, possessing excess smooth muscle that persists into smaller branches than usual. PPHN can occur as a primary disorder or as a complication of asphyxia, infection (such as group B streptococcus) and pulmonary hypoplasia. The diagnosis should be suspected in a baby who remains hypoxic in 100 per cent oxygen and whose chest X-ray is normal. Echocardiography confirms the right to left shunt at atrial and/or ductal level and excludes a differential diagnosis of congenital heart disease. Nitric oxide has recently been confirmed as effective treatment for PPHN and is now the therapy of choice if warmth, artificial ventilation, oxygen and/or alkali therapy do not succeed in correcting the acidosis.

Group B streptococcal septicaemia (see Chapter 15)

Early onset group B streptococcal septicaemia (GBS) disease is preventable. There can be no doubt about the effectiveness of selective intrapartum prophylaxis, which has been confirmed by meta-analysis showing a thirty-fold reduction in GBS disease. More than a decade has passed since the first clinical trial that demonstrated the effectiveness of prophylaxis, but still prevention strategies have not been implemented widely or consistently, and the incidence of neonatal GBS disease has not declined. Two alternative strategies exist. In the first, intrapartum antibiotic prophylaxis is offered to women identified as GBS carriers through prenatal screening cultures collected at 35–37 weeks' gestation, and to women who develop premature onset of labour or rupture of membranes before the screening is done. In the second, intrapartum antibiotic prophylaxis is provided to women who have one or more risk conditions at the time of labour or membrane rupture. Screening is not done. Clinical trials have not been done to compare the efficacy of the two strategies, and both are in use in different parts of the world.

Hypoxic ischaemic encephalopathy (HIE)

Seizures are the hallmark of this condition, and HIE is the commonest cause of early onset seizures in a term baby. There are many other causes of neonatal seizure, for example meningitis, stroke, and hypoglycaemia. A diagnosis of HIE should be considered when there is a combination of:
- fetal distress;
- birth depression (low Apgar score requiring resuscitation);
- metabolic acidosis on cord pH or an early neonatal sample;
- seizures;
- renal impairment (blood in the urine and a low urine output);
- alteration of central nervous system state – the baby is not normally conscious between seizures, but is irritable or lethargic with abnormal primitive reflexes.

The diagnosis should be confirmed by checking a serum calcium and glucose, performing a lumbar puncture to exclude meningitis and carrying out a cranial ultrasound scan. This may be normal or show a loss of the gyral pattern with obliterated ventricles suggesting cerebral oedema. Early electroencephalogram (EEG) often confirms electrical seizure activity and the background pattern can help in prognosis; a normal background even in the presence of frequent

seizures is reassuring whereas a very depressed or deteriorating background is an indication of a poor prognosis. An MRI scan, if available, is another investigation which confirms the diagnosis and helps in prognostication. The parents of many of these children pursue medical negligence claims on their behalf, sometimes many years later, and this means that the neonatal notes need to be kept in meticulous detail and preserved for up to 80 years.

CARE OF THE INFANT OF AN INSULIN-DEPENDENT DIABETIC MOTHER

This is described in Chapter 16.

CARE OF THE INFANT WITH INTRAUTERINE GROWTH RESTRICTION

Infants with intrauterine growth restriction (IUGR) may be symmetrically small, suggesting intrauterine infection or chromosomal abnormality. They may also be light, but with normal length and head size, suggesting onset of growth restriction later in pregnancy. Infants who are small for dates tolerate the stress of labour badly and are prone to HIE. Their low glycogen stores make them vulnerable to hypoglycaemia if adequate provision of glucose is not made after birth. Early feeding is indicated in this group, with pre-feed estimation of blood glucose for at least 48 hours, with the aim to keep the level higher than 2.6 mmol/L. Babies who cannot tolerate enteral feeds, or whose glucose does not reach a satisfactory level, or who become symptomatic must have IV dextrose. IUGR babies who were found to have reversed end-diastolic flow in the umbilical artery antenatally are at increased risk of necrotizing enterocolitis. These babies must be fed IV initially, with a cautious introduction of milk.

MANAGEMENT OF THE PRETERM INFANT

The prognosis for preterm infants has improved dramatically over the last thirty years, with survival rates for infants delivered beyond 30 weeks approaching

95 per cent. Neurological handicap, including cerebral palsy, sensorineural deafness, visual handicap and developmental delay, remains a problem in 10 per cent of survivors below 30 weeks (Fig. 22.11). School failure, poor attention span and behavioural difficulties afflict a further proportion of these children. The future priorities in neonatal intensive care must include achieving more intact survival.

Management of many of the complications of prematurity is beyond the scope of this chapter, and the reader is directed to standard textbooks. A few of the major conditions are discussed below.

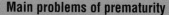

Main problems of prematurity

- Respiratory distress syndrome
- Chronic lung disease
- Intraventricular haemorrhage, parenchymal cerebral haemorrhage
- Periventricular leukomalacia
- Infection
- Necrotizing enterocolitis
- Patent ductus arteriosus
- Jaundice

Respiratory distress syndrome, chronic lung disease

The incidence of respiratory distress syndrome (RDS) is strongly related to gestational age, occurring in virtually 100 per cent of infants delivered at 26 weeks' gestation, 40–50 per cent at 30–31 weeks and about 5 per cent at 35 weeks. RDS is a condition of increasing respiratory distress, commencing at, or shortly after, birth and increasing in severity until progressive resolution occurs among the survivors, usually between the second to fourth day. It is due, at least in part, to insufficiency of pulmonary surfactant. RDS is manifest by respiratory distress (cyanosis, tachypnoea, grunting and recession) and respiratory failure is diagnosed by blood gas analy-

sis. An X-ray film showing ground glass appearance and air bronchograms (Fig. 22.12), will confirm the diagnosis although these radiological features are not pathognomic of RDS. Antenatal steroids and postnatal surfactant have combined effects and have helped to reduce the mortality and morbidity from this condition. Artificial ventilation remains the mainstay of management, although the modern trend is for gentle ventilation, aiming to reduce barotrauma and minimize the risk of chronic lung disease (CLD). CLD still afflicts as many as 50 per cent of babies weighing less than a kilo at birth, and these infants spend many months in oxygen sometimes only to succumb later to winter viral infections or cor pulmonale.

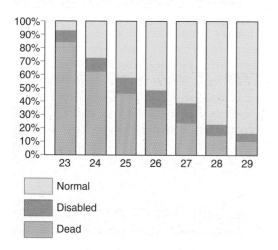

Figure. 22.11 Outcome for preterm infants by week of gestation.

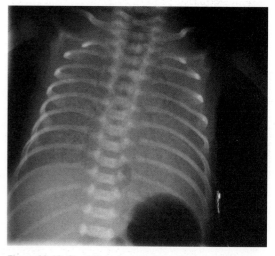

Figure 22.12 Chest X-ray in respiratory distress syndrome.

Preterm brain injury

The neonatal brain is vulnerable to injury, and both intracranial parenchymal haemorrhage and periventricular leukomalacia are associated with handicap in childhood. Intracranial haemorrhage is common in preterm infants, and occurs in the germinal matrix region. The germinal matrix is situated in the floor of the lateral ventricle. Bleeding into the germinal matrix often extends into the lateral ventricle of the brain, this is called germinal matrix-intraventricular haemorrhage (GMH-IVH). GMH-IVH can resolve but is sometimes complicated by persisting enlargement of the lateral ventricles or even progressive hydrocephalus. In these cases the risk of handicap is over 50 per cent. GMH-IVH can be diagnosed with ultrasound during life (Fig. 22.13). Uncomplicated

GMH-IVH that is bleeding not followed by ventricular dilatation or accompanied by a parenchymal lesion carries a good prognosis. Only about 4 per cent of ex-preterm infants with no GMH-IVH or an uncomplicated GMH-IVH will develop major neuro-developmental sequelae. Ventricular enlargement is often a sign of periventricular myelin loss and brain shrinkage, rather than raised intracranial pressure hydrocephalus. Brain growth is an important differentiating feature. The presence of progressive hydrocephalus requiring treatment increases the risk of serious sequelae in preterm infants to about 75 per cent.

Bleeding into the substance of the brain is usually followed by breakdown of tissue into a porencephalic cyst (Fig. 22.14). The outlook for infants with such a cyst can be surprisingly good but many have a hemiplegia. Periventricular leukomalacia (PVL) is the

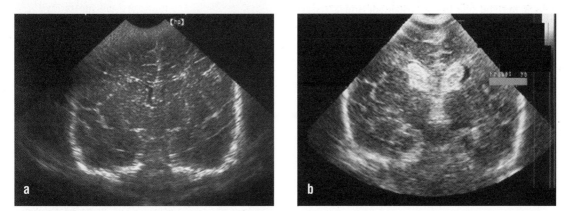

Figure 22.13 Cranial ultrasound scans made in the coronal plane (a) normal scan (b) intraventricular haemorrhage distending the ventricular cavity.

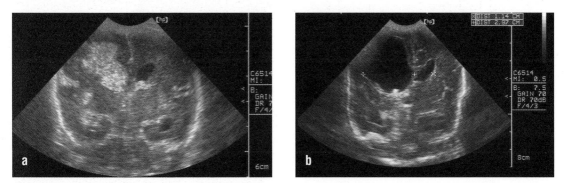

Figure 22.14 Evolution of a right-sided parenchymal lesion (a) into a porencephalic cyst (b) seen on coronal cranial ultrasound scans. The time interval between the scans was two months.

term used to describe multiple small cysts that are visualized within the periventricular white matter (Fig. 22.15). MRI scanning later in childhood shows a paucity of myelin in such cases, and the lesion is a very reliable predictor of later cerebral palsy. Cerebral palsy is almost universal in cases with bilateral occipital PVL. Factors that predispose to PVL include prolonged rupture of membranes, chorioamnionitis and neonatal hypocarbia.

Necrotizing enterocolitis

This serious gastrointestinal disease affects 2–5 per cent of preterm infants. The characteristic clinical presentation is of a preterm infant less than seven days old in whom enteral formula feeding has been commenced. Feeding is accompanied by abdominal distension, increased volume of gastric aspirate, which may be bile or bloodstained, and a tender abdomen. Abdominal X-ray may reveal the characteristic signs of intramural gas, a sentinel loop or even gas in the portal tract. Treatment involves omission of enteral feeds and surgery for perforation or for failure to respond to medical management. Mortality is about 10–20 per cent and is highest in very preterm infants who develop necrotizing enterocolitis in the first week of life. Long-term complications include stoma requirement, short bowel syndrome and nocturnal diarrhoea.

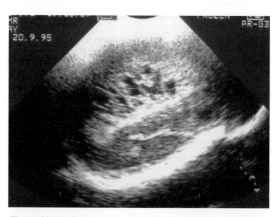

Figure 22.15 Cystic periventricular leukomalacia seen in parasaggital tangential section.

References for further reading

Rennie JM, Roberton NRC. *A Manual of Neonatal Intensive Care. 4th Edition*. London: Arnold, 2000.

Rennie JM, Roberton NRC. *Textbook of Neonatology. 3rd Edition*. Edinburgh: Churchill Livingstone, 1999.

Roberton NRC. *A Manual of Normal Neonatal Care. 2nd Edition*. London: Arnold, 1996.

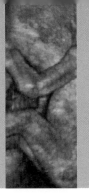

Appendices

Appendix 1: Medicolegal issues

The increase in patient expectations and greater transparency of medical decision-making leading to the 'demystification' of medicine has made it much more common for patients to take legal action against doctors, healthcare professionals and medical institutions. Added to this, the level of financial settlement in many cases make it attractive for patients to attempt legal action, or for lawyers to fight a case on a 'no win, no fee' basis. Whilst it is entirely right for patients and their relatives to seek redress in the courts for negligent actions of healthcare professionals, the trend throughout the 1990s has been for an inexorable increase in litigation. Obstetrics and gynaecology are at the forefront of specialties prone to this increase.

It is practically impossible to practice obstetrics for any length of time without becoming involved in a legal action. It used to be said that, when something goes wrong, patients simply want an apology, not financial compensation. Whether or not this is less true nowadays the threat of possible litigation must not stop an honest and open discussion with the patient or relatives. It is not an admission of liability in this context to say 'I am sorry', particularly if an unfortunate combination of circumstances has taken place which has placed the patient at risk without necessarily a negligent action having occurred.

The following are major areas that contribute to, or influence the outcome of, medicolegal cases.

Notekeeping
- Each sheet of patient notes must have the patient's name and hospital number recorded.
- Each entry must have date and time recorded.
- Signatures must be legible, and accompanied by the name printed, grade and a bleep/pager number given.
- Do not write sarcastic or derogatory comments in the notes.
- Avoid abbreviations apart from those that are universally recognized.
- Use permanent, dark coloured ink.

Inappropriate delegation
Never ask a more junior member of the team to perform a procedure or counsel a patient unless this falls within the normal remit for their grade, or you know that they are competent in the procedure.

Skills awareness and appropriate seniority
- Do not perform a procedure that you have only infrequently performed, or believe yourself to be inexperienced to perform.
- If your results for a particular procedure give you, staff or patients cause for concern, seek advice from an appropriate colleague or management when these procedures arise.
- You may be extremely competent at a particular procedure, but if either the condition or procedure are associated with significant mortality or morbidity and you are in a training grade, seek supervision from a senior colleague.

Consent
- Consent must be full and informed. This means that the patient must be informed of the likely outcome of the procedure in terms of success rate, and the resulting functional ability.
- Both the common, and the rare but potentially catastrophic, complications of a procedure should be discussed.
- The doctor who is likely to perform a procedure should obtain consent for this personally, and not delegate to other staff except in emergency situations.
- A patient not able to speak the same language as the doctor must be counselled with an interpreter

(preferably not a family member acting as the interpreter) present. The consent form should include the name of the interpreter.

- For patients under 16, normally the parent or guardian would sign the consent form. Failing this, the institution's legal adviser should be consulted.
- In an emergency situation, you may not be able to obtain full, informed consent. As long as you are acting in a reasonable way in the patient's best interest, you are unlikely to suffer recourse.

Communication

- A basic rule is to be as open and frank as possible with patients.
- The line of communication is between patient and doctor. Patients often do not like sensitive or confidential issues to be discussed with relatives, so beware of this.
- If there has been a clinical or other problem complicating a patient's care, the most senior member of the medical team should speak directly to the patient, if only for their reassurance.
- Effective communication must exist between different doctors, nurses and other healthcare professionals.

Guidelines and protocols

You may, occasionally, have to stray from the accepted institution or procedural protocol. If you do this, you must be sure that you have a good reason for it, and/or a senior colleague is aware of your proposed management.

Finally, the Bolam test

For a patient to bring a successful legal action against a doctor for negligence, the following conditions must be fulfilled.

- The doctor owes a duty of care to the patient.
- That duty of care is breached.
- The injury caused is as a result of the breach of that duty of care.

Appendix 2: Ethics in obstetric practice

The specialty of obstetrics is a hot-bed of ethical dilemmas. New developments in assisted conception, genetic diagnosis and fetal therapy present ethical problems of mind-boggling complexity. Physicians are required to have a sound knowledge of ethical principles in order that their decisions are defensible to their peers, their patients and in a Court of Law. Obstetrics is unique in that the physician is often dealing with two patients, both inextricably linked and whose interests usually, but do not always, coincide.

A fundamental understanding of bioethical principles is required to work out pragmatic solutions to these difficult problems. Bioethics is a secular, disciplined study of morality in healthcare, which is not based on theology or religion or professional consensus, personal conscience or law.

Fundamental to the doctor-patient relationship is the principle of beneficence. It is the core ethical principle of the Hippocratic writings – 'Declare the past, diagnose the present, foretell the future; practice these acts. As to disease, make a habit of two things – to help or at least do no harm.'

Beneficence requires the physician to assess objectively the various diagnostic and therapeutic options and to implement those that protect and promote the health-related interests of the patient by securing for the patient the greatest balance of clinical benefits over harm. For centuries, beneficence was the guiding principle for a doctor in clinical decision-making. In simple terms, beneficence was the essence of clinical judgement. At the beginning of the last century, it became apparent that beneficence was not enough. Too often beneficence-based decisions led to paternalism or to the physician over-riding the patient's wishes or intentions.

Beneficence has to be balanced by the principle of respect for autonomy, which accepts that patients have their own perspective on their health-related and other interests and should have the freedom to choose alternatives based on their values and beliefs. The essence of modern bioethics, therefore, is a balance between the beneficence-based obligations and autonomy-based obligations of the physician. In the majority of clinical situations, these coincide, but when there is conflict, patient autonomy should prevail unless, in the opinion of the physician, the patient requests a course of action that offends his professional conscience and under these circumstances he must refuse to carry out her request. Occasionally the private conscience of the physician, which is based on their up-bringing, personal experience or religious traditions, will justify their withdrawal from certain issues, such as termination of pregnancy. Private conscience does not justify the physician being judgmental or denying the transfer of their patient to a colleague whose private conscience is not affected by the issue.

Peculiar to bioethics applied to the pregnant woman, is the status of the fetus. The fetus is not a person and has no rights in law. Thus, it could be postulated that the fetus does not have moral status, i.e. having the property of a human being to whom obligations are owed. This concept is increasingly being challenged, especially as after 24 weeks' gestation the fetus is independently viable, albeit sometimes with technical support. Modern bioethicists argue that we should grant the independently viable fetus moral status, i.e. that the physician and pregnant woman have beneficence-based obligations to the fetal patient. In other words, the physician should regard the viable fetus as their patient. This may, on rare occasions, cause conflicts when the autonomy-based decision of the mother, as regards her viable fetus, is at odds with the professional judgement of the physician. Some examples and solutions are outlined below.

Case 1

On a routine ultrasound scan at 20 weeks' gestation, a fetus is diagnosed as having a lumbo-sacral spina bifida. The Obstetrician looking after the woman has strong religious beliefs that termination of pregnancy is wrong. What is the ethical solution?

Spina bifida is associated with a high risk of infant death or serious handicap. Legally the woman has the right to ask for termination of pregnancy under Section E of the United Kingdom Abortion Act: 'there is a substantial risk that if the child were born it would suffer from such physical or mental abnormalities as to be seriously handicapped'. Furthermore, as the fetus is less than 24 weeks' gestation it is considered pre-viable and it does not have the moral status of being a patient unless the woman confers that status, something she is free to withhold. A decision to carry out termination of pregnancy is justified in respect of her autonomy-based decision. The Obstetrician can avoid performing this procedure as a matter of personal conscience, but in terms of professional conscience, is obliged to refer the patient to another Obstetrician, who has no objections to performing termination of pregnancy.

Case 2

On an ultrasound scan at 34 weeks' gestation, a fetus is found to have the 'double bubble' sign of duodenal atresia. A rapid karyotype from a fetal blood sample taken by cordocentesis reveals that the fetus has Trisomy 21. The parents ask for termination of pregnancy. What is the ethical solution?

A fetus at 34 weeks has no rights in law. Nevertheless, it is viable and, therefore, has acquired the moral status of being a fetal patient. Duodenal atresia is a condition that is usually cured by surgery. Down's syndrome is a condition associated with a low IQ, but the child usually has a normal, but dependent life. Under Section E of the UK Abortion Act, there is no definition of 'serious abnormality'. To some Obstetricians, the case described here would fit the description of serious abnormality and they would recommend that termination of pregnancy would be justified under the Abortion Act and in terms of maternal autonomy. However, on ethical grounds, such a decision would be difficult to justify because Down's syndrome does not necessarily result in a life not worth living. Beneficence-based obligations to the second patient, i.e. the fetus, would not justify causing its death. It would, therefore, be reasonable on ethical grounds to deny maternal autonomy in this case and turn down her request for termination of pregnancy.

Case 3

A woman at 38 weeks' gestation has severe poorly controlled pre-eclampsia. The fetus is well-grown, but has a fetal heart tracing suggesting fetal acidaemia. The cervix is unfavourable suggesting a long labour is likely. The Obstetrician recommends Caesarean Section but the woman and her partner refuse to accept this advice. Thus, there is conflict between the beneficence-based judgement of the Obstetrician and the autonomous decision of the woman. Theoretically, in this case, it would be possible to obtain a Court Order to carry out Caesarean Section against the woman's wishes. The basis for this would be that the life of the fetus (the second patient) is at risk and Caesarean Section is the optimal means of saving its life. Caesarean Section would also be of benefit to the mother, in that it would reduce her chances of having an eclamptic seizure, renal failure and other consequences of severe pre-clampsia. However, it is generally agreed that obtaining a Court Order to perform

Caesarean Section would be an unwise step to take. The solution should be to attempt to persuade the prospective parents of the wisdom of performing Caesarean Section for the safety of herself and her unborn child. This persuasion should not be strident or threatening, but carefully reasoned and respectful. If this fails, then all attempts should be made to control the pre-eclampsia and recommend to the woman the second best option which would be induction of labour.

It may be asked why maternal autonomy was overridden in Case 2 above and not in Case 3. In Case 2, the woman demanded an action that ethically would be difficult to justify. A decision not to perform a termination of pregnancy can thus be successfully defended. In Case 3, the Obstetrician would have to carry out an operation on a woman against her express wishes with the possible accusation that an assault is being carried out on her body. This would be an unwise course of action and one that would be difficult to defend.

These three cases only touch on the complexity of the ethical considerations that affect day-to-day obstetric decision-making. It is a constant challenge to all healthcare workers in obstetrics, but it is also one of the reasons why obstetrics is such an interesting and exciting specialty.

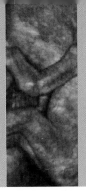

Index

Abbreviations used. The reader is referred to page ix for any abbreviations used but not explained in the index. Substances (e.g. hormones and biochemical compounds) have not been indexed under their abbreviated form (e.g. PTH) but under their full form (e.g. Parathyroid hormone).